35
12
× 150
25
2
400

HANDBOOK OF VETERINARY ANESTHESIA

ROMAN T. SKARDA,
Dr. med. vet., Ph.D.
Diplomate A.C.V.A.

Associate Professor
Department of Veterinary Clinical Sciences
The Ohio State University
College of Veterinary Medicine
Columbus, Ohio

RICHARD M. BEDNARSKI, D.V.M., M.S.
Diplomate A.C.V.A

Associate Professor
Department of Veterinary Clinical Sciences
The Ohio State University
College of Veterinary Medicine
Columbus, Ohio

Illustrations by Tim Vojt

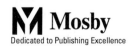

Mosby
Dedicated to Publishing Excellence

Executive Editor: Linda L. Duncan
Developmental Editor: Melba Steube
Project Manager: Gayle May Morris
Production Editor: Mary Cusick Drone
Manuscript Editor: Anne Stephens
Manufacturing Supervisor: Karen Lewis
Design Manager: Susan Lane
Cover: Tim Vojt

SECOND EDITION

Printed in the United States of America
Composition by Clarinda
Printing/binding by RR Donnelly and Sons

Mosby–Year Book, Inc.
11830 Westline Industrial Drive
St. Louis, Missouri 63146

Library of Congress Cataloging in Publication Data
Muir, William, 1946-
     Handbook of Veterinary anesthesia/William W. Muir III, John A.E.
     Hubbell, Roman Skarda; illustrations by Tim Vojt.—2nd ed.
         p.   cm.
     Includes bibliographical references and index.
     ISBN 0-8016-7656-8
     1. Veterinary anesthesia—Handbooks, manuals, etc.   I. Hubbell,
     John A. E.   II. Skarda, Roman.   III. Title.
     SF914.M85 1994
     636.089'796—dc20   94-24404
                                                               CIP

94   95   96   97   98   /   9   8   7   6   5   4   3   2   1

HANDBOOK OF

VETERINARY ANESTHESIA

SECOND EDITION

WILLIAM W. MUIR, III
D.V.M., Ph.D.
Diplomate A.C.V.A.; A.C.V.E.C.C.

Professor
Department of Veterinary Clinical Sciences
The Ohio State University
College of Veterinary Medicine
Columbus, Ohio

JOHN A.E. HUBBELL
D.V.M., M.S.
Diplomate A.C.V.A.

Associate Professor
Department of Veterinary Clinical Sciences
The Ohio State University
College of Veterinary Medicine
Columbus, Ohio

M Mosby

St. Louis   Baltimore   Boston   Carlsbad   Chicago   Naples   New York
Philadelphia   Portland   London   Madrid   Mexico City   Singapore
Sydney   Tokyo   Toronto   Wiesbaden

Contributors

DIANE MASON, D.V.M., M.S.
Diplomate, A.C.V.A.
Department of Clinical Sciences
Kansas State University
College of Veterinary Medicine
Manhattan, Kansas

JULIE SMITH, D.V.M.
Department of Veterinary Clinical Sciences
Louisiana State University
College of Veterinary Medicine
Baton Rouge, Louisiana

NANCY ANDERSON, D.V.M.
Department of Veterinary Clinical Sciences
The Ohio State University
College of Veterinary Medicine
Columbus, Ohio

RAYMOND WACK, D.V.M., M.S.
Department of Veterinary Clinical Sciences
The Ohio State University
College of Veterinary Medicine
Columbus, Ohio

Preface to the Second Edition

The first edition of this handbook was designed to provide a ready reference on clinical veterinary anesthesia for students, practicing veterinarians, animal health technicians, and researchers who use animals in their experiments. Since its publication 5 years ago, new anesthetic drugs, equipment, and monitoring devices have appeared. This edition incorporates information on these advances and provides an update on the drugs and techniques previously described.

In addition to adding new information, we have attempted to increase the readability and utility of the text. Our goals were to clarify, but not oversimplify and to provide interested students and others with an information base on which to build a more complete and comprehensive understanding of the practice of clinical veterinary anesthesia. As Thomas Mann said, "Order and simplification are the first steps toward mastery of a subject—the actual enemy is the unknown."

Edition two is the result of the labors of the Section of Anesthesiology of the Department of Veterinary Clinical Sciences of The Ohio State University. Advice from Dr. Ann Wagner, Earl Harrison, Jennifer Ford, Diane Hurley, Stephen Drab, and Beverly Ventura is greatly appreciated. Significant contributors to this edition include Roman Skarda, Rich Bednarski, Diane Mason, Julie Smith, Nancy Anderson, and Ray Wack. Our thanks to Frances Crowell for typing the manuscript.

William W. Muir, III
John A.E. Hubbell

Preface to the First Edition

The purpose of this preface is to serve as a dedication, prologue, and means of expressing gratitude. Briefly, this handbook of veterinary anesthesiology is dedicated to the veterinary student and practicing veterinarian. It was designed to be used by veterinary students, residents, and veterinary practitioners requiring an immediate source of information relating to the practice of veterinary anesthesia, cardiopulmonary emergencies, and euthanasia. Recent versions have been completely rethought, rewritten, and expanded.

The present edition is the result of the labors of the Section of Anesthesiology of the Department of Veterinary Clinical Sciences at The Ohio State University.

The material contained within this handbook is based upon the collective clinical experiences, research, and teaching activities of each of the contributors. Technical advice and suggestions were offered by Mary Ferguson, Sarah Flaherty, Earl Harrison, William Sheehan, Tom Sherman, Peter Hellyer, and Mark Leonard. Ideas and contributions to earlier versions of this final document were provided by Elaine Robinson, Cheryl Buchanan, and Karen Rosenberry Spenser. The final version is principally due to the concentrated and combined efforts of myself, Richard Bednarski, John Hubbell, Roman Skarda, Clifford Swanson, and Diane Mason. Our individual interests and dedication to teaching have made this work enjoyable. We have attempted to summarize and simplify what has become a very large and oftentimes confusing topic. It is not our intent to have this handbook replace more comprehensive textbooks of veterinary anesthesia, but to supplement them.

William W. Muir, III
John A.E. Hubbell

"To look back is to relax one's vigil."

BETTE DAVIS

"It's what you learn
after you know it all
that counts."

ANONYMOUS

Contents

HANDBOOK OF VETERINARY ANESTHESIA

CHAPTER ONE

Introduction to Anesthesia

"There are no safe anesthetic agents; there are no safe anesthetic procedures; there are only safe anesthetists."

ROBERT SMITH

OVERVIEW

The art and practice of anesthesia are based on a general understanding of (1) the terms that describe the effects of anesthesia on animals, (2) the pharmacology of anesthetic drugs and their antagonists, (3) the correct methods of anesthetic drug administration, and (4) the ways to respond to anesthetic-related complications or emergencies. This chapter outlines commonly used terms, the general uses for anesthetics, and routes of administration of anesthetic drugs and drug combinations used to produce chemical restraint and anesthesia in animals.

GENERAL CONSIDERATIONS

I. Anesthesia and/or chemical restraint is a reversible process; the purpose of anesthesia is to produce a convenient, safe, effective, yet inexpensive means of chemical restraint so that clinical procedures may be expedited with a minimum of stress, pain, discomfort, and toxic side effects to the patient or to the anesthetist

II. Criteria for selection of drugs and techniques
   A. Species, breed, age, and relative size of the patient
   B. Physical status and specific disease processes of the patient and concurrent medication
   C. Demeanor of the patient and the presence of pain

D. Personal knowledge and experience
E. Available assistants and their training
F. Familiarity with available equipment
G. Length and type of operation or procedure to be performed

III. Patient responses can vary because dosages and techniques are developed for the "average, normal" animal; thus it is essential that the practitioner know how to modify anesthetic techniques

IV. Definitions

A. Medical terms in practice of anesthesia

Akinesia: Loss of motor response (movement) caused by paralysis of motor nerves

Analgesia: Loss of sensitivity to pain

Anesthesia: Total loss of sensation in a body part or in the whole body, generally induced by a drug that depresses the activity of nervous tissue either locally (peripherally) or generally (centrally)

Local anesthesia: Analgesia limited to a local area

Regional anesthesia: Analgesia limited to a local area, generally an extremity

General anesthesia: Loss of consciousness in addition to loss of sensation; ideally includes hypnosis, hyporeflexia, analgesia, and muscle relaxation; can be produced with a single drug or by a combination of drugs

Surgical anesthesia: Loss of consciousness and sensation accompanied by sufficient muscle relaxation and analgesia to allow surgery to be performed without pain or movement by the patient

Balanced anesthesia: Surgical anesthesia produced by a combination of two or more drugs or anesthetic techniques, each contributing its own pharmacological effects; includes tranquilizers, narcotics, nitrous oxide, and muscle relaxants

Dissociative anesthesia: A central nervous system (CNS) state characterized by catalepsy, good peripheral analgesia, and altered consciousness; produced by drugs like ketamine

Catalepsy: State in which there is malleable rigidity of the limbs and the patient is generally unresponsive to aural, visual, or minor painful stimuli

Hypnosis: Artificially-induced sleep or a trance resembling sleep from which the patient can be aroused by stimuli

Narcosis: Drug-induced stupor or sedation in which the patient is oblivious to pain, with or without hypnosis

Neuroleptanalgesia: Hypnosis and analgesia produced by the combination of a neuroleptic drug and an analgesic drug

Sedation: Mild degree of CNS depression in which the patient is awake but calm; a term often used interchangeably with tranquilization; with sufficient stimuli the patient may be aroused; produces a dose-dependent depression of the cerebral cortex

Tranquilization, ataraxia, neurolepsis: State of tranquility and calmness in which the patient is relaxed, awake, and unconcerned with its surroundings and potentially indifferent to minor pain; sufficient stimulation will arouse the patient; tranquilizers act by depressing the hypothalamus and the reticular activating system

V. Clinical jargon

Bag: "The animal was bagged." The rebreathing bag on the anesthetic machine was squeezed to inflate the animal's lungs during anesthesia

Block: "The leg was blocked." Local anesthesia was produced at a specific site, locally or regionally

Bolus: "A bolus of thiobarbiturate was administered." A specified quantity of drug was rapidly administered intravenously

Breathed: The animal was breathed six times a minute." The lungs were either manually or mechanically inflated

Crashed: "The animal was crash induced." Anesthesia was rapidly introduced using intravenous (IV) techniques, although inhalation anesthetics (mask induced) can also be rapidly induced

Deep: "The animal is in a deep stage of anesthesia." The anesthetic drugs produced maximal CNS depression. The greater the degree of CNS depression, the deeper the anesthesia. This term is used in direct contrast to the term *light,* which implies minimal CNS depression. Animals that are "light" demonstrate active corneal and palpebral reflexes, may develop nystagmus, and occasionally lift their heads or move a limb

Down: The animal was "knocked down" or "put down." The animal was given a drug or combination of drugs that produced recumbency. The term *put down* is also used to denote euthanasia

Dropped: The animal was dropped." The animal received drugs that produce recumbency

Extubated: "The animal was extubated." The endotracheal tube was removed from the airway. The term is the opposite of "intubated"

Hit or stick a vein: "I hit the vein on the first attempt." A successful venipuncture was performed

Induced: "The animal was induced." The animal was given a drug or drugs that produced anesthesia

Intubated: "The animal was intubated." An endotracheal tube was placed through the nose or mouth into the trachea

Mask induced: "The animal was mask induced." A face mask was used to produce anesthesia. Because face masks are used to supply gaseous or volatile anesthetics, the term also implies that an inhalation anesthetic was used

Pre or post: "A preanesthetic was administered." Anything administered or done before anesthesia is considered to be in the preanesthetic period. Occurrences following the discontinuation of anesthetic drugs are considered postanesthetic

Pushed: "The thiobarbiturate was pushed." An IV drug or fluids was administered either rapidly or in amounts greater than usually given

Ran a strip: "I ran a strip on that animal." An electrocardiogram was obtained

Reversed: "The animal was reversed." A drug's effects were antagonized by administering a specific antagonist. For example, the opioid antagonist naloxone can be administered to reverse the effects of morphine

Spiked: "The animal spiked a fever," or "The fluids were spiked with potassium." Depending on the clinical situation, *spiked* may mean a sudden rapid increase or that some substance (K^+) or drug was added to a solution

Stabilized: "The animal is stable" or "The animal has been stabilized." Cardiopulmonary variables or the "depth" of anesthesia has been returned to or is within acceptable limits

Topped-off: "The animal was topped off with a thiobarbiturate." An additional drug was administered to produce the desired effect. The term implies that the original calculated dosage was insufficient to produce the desired effect

Tubed: "The animal was tubed." An endotracheal tube was placed in the trachea through either the mouth or nasal cavities (see also intubated)

USE OF ANESTHETICS

   I. Restraint
   - A. Radiography
   - B. Cleaning, grooming, dental prophylaxis
   - C. Biopsy, bandaging, splinting, cast application
   - D. Capture of exotic and wild animals
   - E. Transportation
   - F. Manipulation
     1. Catheterization
     2. Closed reduction of luxations or fractures
     3. Wound care
     4. Obstetrics
  II. Anesthesia (see Definitions: Anesthesia)
 III. Control of convulsions
 IV. Euthanasia

TYPES OF ANESTHESIA (ACCORDING TO ROUTE OF ADMINISTRATION)

Acupuncture
Controlled hypo-
    thermia
Electroanesthesia
Field block*
Infiltration*
Inhalation*

Intramuscular*
Intraosseous
Intraperitoneal
Intratesticular
Intrathoracic
Intravenous*

Oral*
Rectal
Regional nerve
    block
Subcutaneous
Topical*

EFFECT OF ROUTE AND METHOD OF ADMINISTRATION OF ANESTHETIC DRUG

I. Given intravenously (Fig. 1-1): onset of action is immediate; peak effect is rapidly obtained; duration of action is short, and effects are generally more intense than with other routes

II. Given intramuscularly or subcutaneously: onset of action may take 10 to 15 minutes; peak effect may not be obtained for many minutes to hours and depends on the blood supply to the tissues at the site of injection, drug absorption, and the rate of metabolism of the drug; duration of action is more prolonged than by the IV route

III. Rapidity of injection: rapid injections generally cause more intense effects because of decreased bolus drug effects; especially true when cardiac output is low

IV. Concentrations of solutions
   A. Drugs should be administered on a unit/kg basis (e.g., mg/kg); most drugs list concentration as unit/ml (e.g., mg/ml) or percent (%); percent solutions can be converted to unit/ml (a 1% solution contains 10 mg/ml); therefore a 0.5% solution contains 5 mg/ml, and a 3% solution contains 30 mg/ml
   B. Increasing drug concentration increases the intensity and duration of the immediate drug effect
   C. Increasing concentrations may increase vascular irritation

---

*Route commonly used in veterinary medicine.

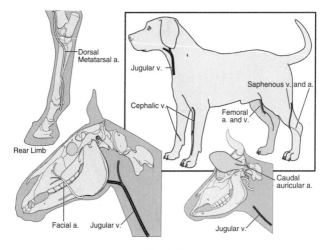

Fig. 1-1

The jugular, cephalic, femoral, and saphenous veins are used in the dog (illustrated) and the cat for intravenous administration of fluids and drugs. The jugular vein is the most frequently used vein in horses, cattle, sheep, and goats. Various arteries are catheterized to directly monitor arterial blood pressure or anaerobically obtain blood samples for pH and blood gas analysis.

V. Onset of action of inhalation drugs requires absorption of gas from alveoli into the blood, then diffusion of anesthetic into the CNS

VI. Duration of drug action is primarily determined by the pharmacokinetic profile of the drug (metabolism and elimination); but it is also influenced by the effect of the drug on the CNS, hemodynamics, and metabolism

CHAPTER TWO

Patient Evaluation and Preparation

"For every mistake that is made for not knowing,
a hundred are made for not looking."

ANONYMOUS

OVERVIEW

Anesthesia is more than just the delivery of anesthetic drugs to the patient. Safe anesthesia includes selecting the appropriate drugs for each procedure, assessing the physical status of the patient, noting the administration of concurrent medication, and familiarity with the anesthetic drugs being used. This chapter outlines preoperative evaluation as it relates to subsequent anesthetic management.

GENERAL CONSIDERATIONS

I. The preanesthetic evaluation (history and physical examination) dictates the choice and dose of anesthetics to be used

II. The history and physical examination are the basis of patient evaluation; the need for further workup is indicated by abnormalities found during physical examination *or* historical information that suggests altered bodily functions

III. Laboratory tests are no substitute for a thorough physical examination

IV. An open airway must be maintained in every patient

V. A patent intravenous route must be maintained for all high-risk patients

VI. Unexpected events must be anticipated

PATIENT EVALUATION

I. Patient identification
   A. Case number or identification
   B. Signalment
      1. Species
      2. Breed
      3. Age
      4. Sex
   C. Body weight
II. Client complaint and anamnesis (history)
   A. Duration and severity of illness
   B. Concurrent symptoms or disease
      1. Diarrhea
      2. Vomiting
      3. Hemorrhage
      4. Epilepsy
      5. Heart failure
      6. Renal failure
   C. Level of activity (exercise tolerance)
   D. Recent feeding
   E. Previous and current administration of drugs (see Chapter 12)
      1. Organophosphates
      2. Insecticides
      3. Antibiotics
         a. Sulfonamides
         b. Chloramphenicol
         c. Streptomycin, neomycin, polymyxin B
      4. Digitalis glycosides
      5. β-blockers
      6. Calcium channel blockers
      7. Diuretics
      8. Catecholamine-depleting drugs
   F. Previous anesthetic history and reactions

CURRENT PHYSICAL EXAMINATION

I. General body condition
   A. Obesity
   B. Cachexia
   C. Pregnancy
   D. Hydration
   E. Temperature
   F. Calm or excited
   G. Nervous or apprehensive (stress)
II. Cardiovascular
   A. Heart rate (Table 2-1)
   B. Arterial blood pressure and pulse pressure
   C. Capillary refill time (<1.5 sec)
   D. Auscultation (cardiac murmurs)
III. Pulmonary
   A. Respiratory rate and depth
      1. Usually 15 to 25 for small animals, 8 to 20 for large animals
      2. Tidal volume approximately 14 ml/kg
   B. Mucous membranes
      1. Pallor (anemia)
      2. Cyanosis (>5 g/dl of unoxygenated hemoglobin)
   C. Auscultation (breath sounds)
   D. Upper airway obstruction
   E. Percussion

TABLE 2-1

NORMAL HEART RATE AND MEAN ARTERIAL BLOOD PRESSURE RANGES

ANIMAL	HEART RATE	ARTERIAL BLOOD PRESSURE
Dog	70-80	70-90
Cat	145-200	80-100
Cow	60-80	90-120
Horse	30-45	70-90
Colt	50-80	60-80
Sheep, goat	60-90	80-110
Pig	60-90	80-110

IV. Hepatic
   A. Jaundice
   B. Failure of blood to clot
V. Renal
   A. Oliguria/anuria
   B. Polyuria/polydipsia
VI. Gastrointestinal
   A. Diarrhea
   B. Vomiting
   C. Parasites
   D. Distention
VII. Nervous system and special senses
   A. Seizures
   B. Fainting
   C. Coma
   D. Glaucoma
VIII. Metabolic and endocrine
   A. Temperature
   B. Hyperthyroidism/hypothyroidism
   C. Hyperadrenocorticism/hypoadrenocorticism
   D. Diabetes
IX. Integument
   A. Hydration
   B. Neoplasia (pulmonary metastasis)
   C. Subcutaneous emphysema (fractured ribs)
   D. Parasites (fleas, mites); (anemia)
   E. Hair loss
   F. Burns (fluid and electrolyte loss)
   G. Trauma
X. Musculoskeletal
   A. Muscle mass (% fat)
   B. Weakness
   C. Electrolyte imbalance (hypokalemia)
   D. Ambulatory or nonambulatory
   E. Fractures

PRESURGICAL LABORATORY WORKUP (Tables 2-2 and 2-3)

I. Minimum laboratory evaluation
  A. Plasma protein
  B. Packed cell volume
  C. Hemoglobin
II. Other laboratory tests (Tables 2-4 and 2-5)
  A. Complete blood count
  B. Blood gases
  C. Hemostasis
  D. Albumin
III. Blood chemistry profile
  A. Electrolytes
  B. Blood urea nitrogen
  C. Creatinine
  D. Aspartate aminotransferase, alanine aminotransferase
  E. Bile salts
IV. Urinalysis (normal findings given in parentheses)
  A. Specific gravity (1.01 to 1.03)
  B. Physiochemical evaluation
    1. pH (7.0 to 7.5, meat diet; 7.0 to 8.0, vegetable diet)
    2. Protein (negative)
    3. Acetone (negative)
    4. Bilirubin (negative)
    5. Blood (negative)
  C. Microscopic evaluation of urine sediment
    1. Casts (negative or rare)
    2. Red blood cells (RBC) (negative)
    3. White blood cells (WBC) (negative)
    4. Epithelial cells (negative)
    5. Bacteria (negative)
    6. Crystals
      a. Oxalate (normal finding)
      b. Triple phosphates (normal finding)
      c. Urates (normal finding)
      d. Calcium carbonate (normally found in horse only)

TABLE 2-2
NORMAL HEMATOLOGIC VALUES

	DOG	CAT	COW	HORSE	SHEEP	PIG
Plasma protein (g/dl)	6-7.5	6-7.5	6-7.5	6-7.5	6.3-7.1	6-7.5
PCV (%)	35-54	27-46	23-43	25-45	30-50	30-48
Hb (g/dl)	12.5-19	8.5-16	8-13	10-16	10-16	10-15
Total leukocytes ($\times 10^9$/L)	6.5-19	4.5-16.5	4-12	5-15	4-12	6.5-20
Neutrophil — segmented($\times 10^9$/L)	3-11.5	3-13	1.4-6	2.3-8.5	1-6	3-15
Neutrophil — band ($\times 10^9$/L)	0-0.3	0-0.3	0-0.1	0-0.1	0-0.1	0-0.5
Lymphocytes ($\times 10^9$/L)	1.2-5.2	1.2-9	1.4-7	1-5	2-8	2-12
Monocytes ($\times 10^9$/L)	0.2-1.3	0-0.7	0-0.8	0-0.7	0-0.6	0-0.6
Eosinophil ($\times 10^9$/L)	0-1.2	0-1.2	0-2	0-0.8	0-1	0-0.6
Basophil ($\times 10^9$/L)	rare	rare	0-0.2	0-0.3	0-0.1	0-0.1

PCV, Packed cell volume, *Hb*, hemoglobin.

TABLE 2-3
SERUM CHEMISTRY

	UNITS	DOG	CAT	HORSE	COW	SHEEP	PIG
CO_2 combining	mEq/L	16-30	15-25	25-35	21-32	—	—
Calcium	mg/dl	9.8-12.8	9.1-12.3	11.6-13.4	8.9-11.6	8.1-9.5	—
Phosphorus	mg/dl	2.5-7.3	2.8-8.7	1.5-5.1	4.5-8.2	3.5-6.7	5.3-9.6
Glucose	mg/dl	66-120	70-175	78-140	45-90	50-80	60-100
Creatine	mg/dl	0.7-1.3	0.7-1.8	0.9-1.4	0.8-1.5	—	1.0-2.7
Bilirubin (T)	mg/dl	0-0.2	0-0.2	0-1.1	0-0.3	—	—
Bilirubin (D)	mg/dl	0-0.2	0-0.1	0-0.8	0-0.2	—	—
Albumin	g/dl	2.6-3.6	2.5-3.9	2.2-3.4	2.8-4.1	2.4-3	—
Protein	g/dl	5.3-7.5	6.2-8.2	5.7-7.9	6.3-8.9	6.3-7.1	—
BSP		5% R	5% R	2-3.7 $t_{1/2}$	2.5-4 $t_{1/2}$	—	3% R
BUN	mg/dl	6-30	15-33	19-33	6-32	5-20	8-24
Cholesterol	mg/dl	106-330	50-275	50-105	60-240	—	—
ALP	IU/L	20-130	0-83	90-325	0-200	—	—
Amylase	IU/L	350-1950	700-1800	—	—	—	—
CK	IU/L	14-460	100-850	150-450	90-350	—	—

TABLE 2-3—cont'd
SERUM CHEMISTRY

	UNITS	DOG	CAT	HORSE	COW	SHEEP	PIG
LDH	IU/L	?	?	?	?	—	—
SDH	IU/L	—	—	4-20	6-30	—	—
AST	IU/L	10-50	15-36	220-600	55-100	—	—
ALT	IU/L	15-110	15-75	—	—	—	—
Na	mEq/L	145-155	150-170	137-143	137-148	140-145	139-152
K	mEq/L	4.0-5.4	3.7-6.0	3.2-4.5	3.5-5.1	4.9-5.7	4.4-6.7
Cl	mEq/L	104-117	111-128	98-105	84-102		100-105
Ca^{2+}	mg/dl	9.8-12.8	9.1-12.3	11.6-13.4	8.9-11.6		9.5-12.7
Mg	mg/dl	1.8-2.4	—	2.2-2.8	2.2-3.4	—	—
pH	Units	7.27-7.43	7.25-7.33	7.34-7.42	7.32-7.45	—	—
Po_2	mmHg	25-46	31-49	26-46	24-39	—	—
Pco_2	mmHg	28-49	35-49	39-53	34-53	—	—
HCO_3	mEq/L	18-25	18-22	23-31	23-31	—	—
Base excess	mEq/L	-6 to 0.5	-6 to -3	-1 to 5	-1 to 4.2	—	—
Cortisol 0 hr	µg/dl	1-4.8	—	1-4.4	1-2.7	—	—
Cortisol 2 hr IM ACTH	µg/dl	5-26	—	5.1-14.6 (8 hr)	2.7-6	—	—
T_3 (RIA)	ng/dl	50-200	60-200	—	—	—	—
T_4 (RIA)	µg/dl	1-4	1.5-5	—	—	—	—

ACTH, Adrenocorticotropic hormone; *ALP,* alkaline phosphatase; *ALT,* alanine aminotransferase; *AST,* aspartate aminotransferase; *BSP,* bromosulphalein; *BUN,* blood urea nitrogen; *CK,* creatinine kinase; *LDH,* lactate dehydrogenase; *R,* retention; *SDH,* sorbitol dehydrogenase; $T_{1/2},$ half-life; $T_3,$ triiodothyronine; $T_4,$ thyroxine.

TABLE 2-4
ARTERIAL BLOOD GASES

	NORMAL VALUES (21% O_2)	VALUES ROUTINELY OBSERVED DURING ANESTHESIA
pH	7.4 ± 0.2	7.25 - 7.45
$Paco_2$ mm Hg	40 ± 3	30 - 60*
Pao_2 mm Hg	94 ± 3	250 to 500 (100% O_2) up to 250 (50% O_2)
Base excess	0 ± 1	-4 to -10

*The development of respiratory acidosis during anesthesia is common; its degree of severity depends in part on the drugs used, the depth of anesthesia, the duration of anesthesia, and patient status.

FURTHER PRESURGICAL TESTS

 I. Electrocardiography
   A. Traumatized patients
   B. Irregular rhythm on physical exam
 II. Radiology
   A. Thorax
   B. Abdomen
 III. Ultrasonography

PHYSICAL STATUS

 I. Identify status
   A. Class I: normal patient with no organic disease
   B. Class II: patient with mild systemic disease
   C. Class III: patient with severe systemic disease that limits activity but is not incapacitating
   D. Class IV: patient with incapacitating systemic disease that is a constant threat to life
   E. Class V: moribund patient not expected to live 24 hours with or without an operation
 II. Designate emergency operation by an "E" after appropriate classification

PATIENT PREPARATION

 I. Withhold food
   A. Withholding food and its duration is species dependent (see species-specific recommendations)

TABLE 2-5
HEMOSTASIS AND TEMPERATURE

	UNITS	DOG	CAT	HORSE	COW	SHEEP	PIG
Platelets	1000/µl	150-400	150-400	100-400	200-800	250-800	200-700
PT	seconds	10-12	6.5-9	15-19	23-28	13-17	—
APTT	seconds	18-24	14-20	55-110	55-80	35-50	—
Normal body temperature							
Farenheit		101.5-102.5 (small breed) 99.5-101.5 (large breed)	100-102.5	99.5-101.5 (foal) 99-100.5 (adult)	101.5-130.5 (calf up to 1 yr) 100-102.5 (ox)	102-104	102-104 (piglet) 100-102 (adult)
Centigrade		38.5-39.2 (small breed) 37.5-38.6 (large breed)	37.8-39.2	37.5-38.6 (foal) 37.2-38 (adult)	38.6-39.8 (calf up to 1 yr) 37.8-39.2 (ox over 1 yr)	38.9-4	38.9-40 (piglet) 37.8-38.9 (adult)

PT, Prothrombin time; APTT, activated partial thromboplastin time.

    A. Do not withhold food for excessive periods in neonates, animals under 5 pounds, or birds

II. Correct or compensate for
    A. Dehydration (hypovolemia)
    B. Anemia, blood loss, or hypoproteinemia
    C. Acid-base and electrolyte abnormalities
    D. Cardiac dysfunction
    E. Respiratory distress
    F. Renal dysfunction
    G. Hemostatic defects
    H. Temperature

III. Specific preparation for intended procedure
    A. Thoracic
    B. Abdominal
    C. Orthopedic
    D. Ophthalmologic

IV. Other considerations
    A. Fluid and caloric needs during and following anesthesia
    B. Special medications (inotropes, antiarrhythmics)
    C. Duration of surgery
    D. Needs of the surgeon

PLAN FOR ANESTHETIC MANAGEMENT

I. Formulation of anesthetic care plan
    A. Planned surgical procedure
    B. Positioning
    C. Selection of drugs: emphasis on the control of pain during all phases of the preoperative, intraoperative, and postoperative periods
    D. Airway management
    E. Fluid management
    F. Body temperature management
    G. Monitoring
    H. Possible untoward effects and response to anticipated problems

II. Assembling of emergency drugs and equipment

CHAPTER THREE

Drugs Used for
Preanesthetic Medication

"Dying is nothing, but pain is a very serious matter."
HENRY JACOB BIGELOW, 1871

OVERVIEW

Preanesthetic medications are an important factor in safe anesthetic management. When used appropriately, they minimize stress and the cardiopulmonary depression and deleterious effects associated with many intravenous and inhalation anesthetics.

Routine preanesthetic medications are classified in four categories. *Anticholinergics,* although controversial, limit excessive salivary secretions and prevent bradycardia. *Phenothiazine and butyrophenone tranquilizers* produce a calming effect and decrease the amount of general anesthetic required to produce anesthesia. α_2-*Agonists and tranquilizer or opioid drug combinations* produce sedation, analgesia, and sleep without producing general anesthesia. *Opioids* produce an analgesic effect and are potentially calming.

GENERAL CONSIDERATIONS

Purposes of preanesthetic drugs
  I. Aid in animal restraint by modifying behavior (produce a calming effect or sedation)
  II. Reduce stress
  III. Eliminate or minimize pain
  IV. Produce muscle relaxation
  V. Decrease the amount of potentially more dangerous drugs

used to produce sedation, muscle relaxation, analgesia, or general anesthesia

VI. Produce safe and uncomplicated induction, maintenance, and recovery from anesthesia

VII. Minimize the adverse and potentially toxic effects of concurrently administered drugs, and drugs used to produce general anesthesia

VIII. Minimize autonomic reflex activity, whether of sympathetic or parasympathetic origin

DRUG CATEGORIES

I. Anticholinergics (e.g., atropine, glycopyrrolate, scopolamine)

A. Competitively antagonize the action of acetylcholine on structures innervated by postganglionic, parasympathetic (cholinergic) nerve fibers and on smooth muscles that are influenced by acetylcholine but lack innervation; referred to as parasympatholytics, anticholinergics, or antispasmodics

B. Are primarily used to prevent salivary secretions and to inhibit the bradycardic effects of vagal stimulation

C. Atropine and scopolamine may produce drowsiness and potentiate the effects of central nervous system (CNS) depressant drugs; large doses may stimulate cerebral areas, leading to restlessness, disorientation, and delirium, an effect more common in ruminants

D. Glycopyrrolate, a quaternary ammonium drug, does not cross the blood-brain or placental barriers

E. Reduce glandular secretions of the respiratory tract, gastrointestinal tract, oral and nasal cavities

1. The accumulation of excessive secretions in the oral cavity of small animals (e.g., cats) may predispose to upper airway obstruction and laryngospasm

2. Increased secretory activity may occur after parasympatholytic drug effects subside; this is called a postparasympatholytic rebound phenomenon

3. Gastric pH is increased (i.e., less acidic); gastrointestinal motility and contractions of the bladder and ure-

ter are reduced; intestinal motility may be decreased for several hours in horses, an effect that could cause colic

F. Produce bronchodilation (increased physiological dead space) and mydriasis

G. Inhibit bradycardia caused by reflex increases in vagal tone (e.g., laryngeal or ocular stimulation and vagovagal reflexes)

   1. Parasympatholytics may induce a sinus tachycardia or occasionally precipitate ventricular arrhythmias; anticholinergic drugs cause sinus bradycardia to progress through various stages of first- and second-degree atrioventricular block before the establishment of sinus tachycardia

   2. Atropine sulfate may stimulate vagal nuclei in the medulla and thus induce an initial sinus bradycardia; glycopyrrolate does not cross the blood-brain or placental barrier and therefore is devoid of CNS or fetal effects

   3. Vagal reflexes produced by traction on visceral organs or during ocular surgery are not always successfully treated with parasympatholytic drugs

   4. General anesthetics, opioids, α_2-agonists, digitalis glycosides, hyperkalemia, acidosis, and injection of calcium salts augment vagal effects and may precipitate bradycardia

      a. Halothane, methoxyflurane, enflurane, isoflurane, and barbiturates may enhance parasympathetic effects by suppressing sympathetic tone

      b. Large doses of a phenothiazine tranquilizer may produce a CNS induced cholinergic effect and sinus bradycardia; they are adrenolytic

H. Administer intramuscularly (IM) or subcutaneously (SC) (intravenously [IV] for emergencies)

   1. Atropine sulfate (0.01 to 0.02 mg/lb) or glycopyrrolate (0.005 mg/lb) increases heart rate and dries secretions in small animals. The duration of action of atropine sulfate is 60 to 90 minutes; for glycopyrrolate it is 2 to 4 hours

   2. Since the value of routinely using parasympatholytics

in large animal species is questionable, therapy should be directed to specific needs; the following dosages have not been adequately evaluated

    a. Horses: atropine, 0.02 to 0.04 mg/lb; glycopyrrolate, 0.0015 to 0.003 mg/lb

    b. Ruminants: not recommended; atropine temporarily decreases secretions, which become more viscid; proper positioning of the head and neck is of the utmost importance to prevent pooling of the solution in the pharynx and subsequent aspiration

    c. Pigs: atropine (0.02 mg/lb); glycopyrrolate (0.0015 mg/lb)

I. Produce untoward reactions

    1. Atropine may cause an initial bradycardia after intravenous administration

    2. Cardiac arrhythmias, particularly sinus tachycardia and first- and second-degree atrioventricular block, are observed after intravenous administration of atropine or glycopyrrolate; ventricular arrhythmias may occur after intravenous atropine administration

    3. Sinus tachycardia increases myocardial oxygen consumption and can precipitate heart failure in patients with preexisting cardiovascular disease

    4. Atropine may cause depression in dogs and cats; restlessness, delirium, and disorientation in ruminants

    5. Colic in horses is due to ileus

II. Tranquilizers, neuroleptics, and sedatives (e.g., phenothiazines, butyrophenones, benzodiazepines, and α_2-agonists) (Table 3-1)

    A. Phenothiazines (e.g., acepromazine, promazine), butyrophenones (e.g., droperidol, azaperone)

        1. Mode of action

            a. Calming and neurologic effects appear to be mediated by depression of the reticular activating system and antidopaminergic actions in the CNS; drug actions in the brain stem can cause a loss of vasomotor regulation

            b. Suppression of the sympathetic nervous system (depresses mobilization of catecholamines centrally and peripherally)

    c. Phenothiazine tranquilizers lower seizure threshold in animals with epilepsy; butyrophenones do not

    d. Phenothiazines and butyrophenones produce a marked antiemetic effect by inhibiting dopamine interaction in the chemoreceptor trigger zone in the medulla

2. Physical properties

    a. Water soluble

    b. Can be mixed with other water-soluble drugs

3. Produce mental calming, decrease motor activity, and increase threshold for responding to external stimuli

    a. Not noted for analgesic activity, but improve the analgesic effect of drugs with analgesic activity

    b. Excessive doses of phenothiazines and butyrophenones cause apparent involuntary (extrapyramidal) musculoskeletal effects and hallucinatory activity in some animals, particularly horses

    c. The calming effect can be temporarily reversed with an adequate stimulus; most evident in excitable or apprehensive animals

4. Calms vicious or nervous animals

5. Cardiopulmonary effects

    a. α-Adrenergic blockade (epinephrine may cause a paradoxic drop in blood pressure [BP])

        (1) Hypotension occurs more frequently in excited or apprehensive patients. Reflex tachycardia may occur in response to hypotension

        (2) Severe reactions include hypotensive crisis and (rarely) bradycardia resulting in death

        (3) Phenylephrine (α-agonist) and fluids can be used to increase blood pressure following intravenous fluid administration

    b. Reflex tachycardia due to hypotension; centrally induced bradycardia

    c. Antiarrhythmic effects: epinephrine-induced cardiac irregularities can be prevented by reducing central sympathetic, ganglionic, and peripheral (adrenal) activity

    d. Direct depression of the myocardium and vascular smooth muscle

TABLE 3-1

INTRAVENOUS DOSAGES OF COMMONLY USED TRANQUILIZERS, SEDATIVES, AND NARCOTICS (mg/lb)

AGENT	DOG	CAT	HORSE	COW	GOAT	PIG
Major tranquilizers						
Acepromazine	0.05-0.2	0.05-0.3	0.01-0.04	0.02-0.04	0.02-0.04	0.1-0.3
Promazine	0.3-0.5	0.5-1.5	0.1-0.5	0.1-0.5	0.1-0.5	0.5-1.5
Minor tranquilizers						
Diazepam	0.1-0.2	0.1-0.2	0.01-0.004	0.01-0.04	0.01-0.04	0.1-0.2
Midazolam	0.1-0.2	0.1-0.2	0.01-0.02	—	—	—
Sedatives						
Xylazine	0.2-0.5	0.2-0.5	0.2-0.5	0.01-0.05	0.01-0.03	Not effective
Detomidine	—	—	5-10 µg/lb	1-5 µg/lb	—	—
Chloral hydrate	—	—	10-15	20-30	15-25	20-30
Azaperone	—	—	0.1-0.2	—	—	0.5-1

TABLE 3-1—cont'd

INTRAVENOUS DOSAGES OF COMMONLY USED TRANQUILIZERS, SEDATIVES, AND NARCOTICS (MG/LB)

AGENT	DOG	CAT	HORSE	COW	GOAT	PIG
Opioid agonists and partial agonists*						
Morphine	0.2-0.5	0.05-0.01	0.02-0.05	—	—	0.2-0.4
Meperidine	0.2-0.5	0.1-0.2	0.2-0.5	—	—	0.2-0.5
Oxymorphone	0.05-0.1	—	0.01-0.05	—	—	—
Methadone	0.1-0.3	—	0.03-0.06	—	—	—
Fentanyl	0.001-0.003	—	0.03-0.06	—	—	—
Pentazocine	0.1-0.2	0.05-0.01	0.2-0.4	—	—	0.1-0.2
Butorphanol	0.05-0.1	—	0.005-0.1	—	—	0.1-0.2
Neuroleptanalgesics						
Fentanyl-droperidol (0.4 mg fentanyl + 20 mg droperidol/ml)	1 ml/30-60 lb	1 ml/20 lb				1 ml/50 lb
Acepromazine-oxymorphone	0.1-0.2 mg/lb (Acepromazine)† 0.4 mg/lb (Oxymorphone)†					

Intramuscular dose is 2 to 3 times the intravenous dose. Lower drug dosages should be used in sick patients.

*Antagonists are used whenever drug reversal is desired. Analgesia may be reversed also.

1. Flumazinil: 0.1 mg/lb benzodiazepines
2. Yohimbine: 1-2 mg/lb α₂-agonists
   Atipamazole: 0.05-0.2 mg/lb α₂-agonists
3. Naloxone: 15 μg/5 lb opioids

†Dogs and cats only.

    e. Ganglionic blocking activity

    f. Reduces respiratory rate first, but may decrease tidal volume when administered in large doses; decreases respiratory center sensitivity to increases in CO_2

6. Potentiates the ventilatory and cardiovascular depressant effects of α_2-agonists, opioids, and drugs used to produce general anesthesia

7. Useful as antiemetics

8. Most have antihistaminic properties; phenothiazines and butyrophenones should be avoided when skin testing for allergies

9. Most phenothiazine tranquilizers cross the placental barrier relatively slowly

10. Many phenothiazine tranquilizers, including acepromazine and promazine, can cause erection and temporary or permanent prolapse of the penis in stallions

11. Azaperone (a butyrophenone tranquilizer) produces calming and prevents fighting and cannibalism in pigs; also used as preanesthetic medication

12. Primary area of metabolism is the liver

13. Clinical effects are present for 4 to 8 hours, but may last up to 48 hours or longer in aged animals or animals with portocaval shunts

14. Commonly used phenothiazines include acepromazine and promazine; butyrophenone tranquilizers presently used in veterinary practice are droperidol and azaperone (Table 3-2)

15. Dose (see Table 3-1)

16. Side effects

    a. Akathisia: restless condition in which the patient needs to be in constant motion

    b. Acute dystonic reactions: hysteria, seizures, ataxia

    c. Tachycardia or (rarely) bradycardia

    d. Hypotension

    e. Hypothermia

    f. Inhibited platelet function

    g. Butyrophenone tranquilizers (e.g., droperidol, azaperone) cause excitement and extrapyramidal effects in horses at relatively low doses

B. Benzodiazepines (e.g., diazepam, midazolam), sometimes referred to as minor tranquilizers
   1. Mode of action
      a. Exert many of their pharmacologic effects by enhancing the activity of CNS inhibitory neurotransmitters (γ-aminobutyric acid, glycine) and opening chloride channels, thereby hyperpolarizing membranes; also produce their effects by combining with CNS benzodiazepine (BZ_1, BZ_2) receptors
      b. Depress the limbic system, thalamus, and hypothalamus (reducing sympathetic output), thereby inducing a mild calming effect
      c. Reduce polysynaptic reflex activity, resulting in muscle relaxation
      d. Cause minimal CNS depression, and produce anticonvulsant effects in most animals; may cause disorientation and agitation after rapid intravenous administration
      e. Stimulate appetite and pica in some animals
   2. Physical properties
      a. Diazepam is solubilized by mixing with 40% propylene glycol, ethyl alcohol, sodium benzoate, or benzoic acid; propylene glycol is a cardiovascular depressant and may produce hypotension, bradycardia, cardiac arrhythmias, and apnea if administered IV in large dosages too rapidly
      b. Midazolam is water soluble
   3. Produce minimal or no calming in normal animals; calming effects observed in sick, depressed, or debilitated animals
      a. Muscle relaxation
      b. Anticonvulsant
      c. Behavior modification
   4. Cardiopulmonary effects
      a. Minimal hypotensive effects are observed after intravenous administration
      b. Bradycardia and hypotension have occurred after rapid intravenous administration
      c. Respiratory rate and tidal volume are minimally affected

TABLE 3-2
COMMONLY USED ANALGESIC AND TRANQUILIZER COMBINATIONS FOR INTRAVENOUS USE*

ANIMAL	DRUGS	RECOMMENDED INTRAVENOUS DOSAGES	UNTOWARD EFFECTS
Dog	Acepromazine-meperidine	0.05-0.1 mg/lb 0.1-0.3 mg/lb	Hypotension
	Acepromazine-oxymorphone	0.05-0.1 mg/lb 0.05-0.1 mg/lb	Hypotension
	Acepromazine-butorphanol	0.05 mg/lb 0.1-0.2 mg/lb	Bradycardia Hypotension
	Diazepam-fentanyl	0.1-0.2 mg/lb 0.005 mg/lb	Bradycardia
	Droperidol-fentanyl (Innovar-Vet)	1 ml/30-60 lb	Bradycardia/apnea
Cat	Acepromazine-oxymorphone	0.1 mg/lb IM 0.04 mg/lb	Excitement
	Acepromazine-butorphanol	0.05 mg/lb 0.1-0.2 mg/lb	Bradycardia Hypotension
Horse	Xylazine-morphine‡	0.3 mg/lb 0.1-0.3 mg/lb	Bradycardia Hypotension

TABLE 3-2—cont'd

COMMONLY USED ANALGESIC AND TRANQUILIZER COMBINATIONS FOR INTRAVENOUS USE*

ANIMAL	DRUGS	RECOMMENDED INTRAVENOUS DOSAGES	UNTOWARD EFFECTS
	Xylazine-meperidine	0.3 mg/lb 0.5 mg/lb	Hypotension
	Xylazine-butorphanol	0.3 mg/lb 0.01 mg/lb	Ataxia
	Xylazine-acepromazine	0.3 mg/lb 0.025 mg/lb	Hypotension
	Meperidine-acepromazine	0.25 mg/lb 0.025 mg/lb	Hypotension
Pig	Droperidol-fentanyl (Innovar-Vet)	1 ml/40 lb (under 200 lb) 1 ml/80 lb (over 200 lb)	Respiratory depression
	Azaperone	0.5-2.0 mg/lb	
Ruminants			
Cow	Xylazine	0.02-0.05 mg/lb	Respiratory depression, bradycardia
Sheep	Xylazine	0.05-0.1 mg/lb	
Goat†	Xylazine	0.005-0.05 mg/lb	

*Lower doses should be used in sick patients.
†Variable response
‡Detomidine (1 to 5 µg/lb IV) can be substituted for xylazine in horses.

5. Produce excellent muscle relaxation in animals and reduce muscle spasms and spasticity; effects are additive or synergistic with other drugs used to produce general anesthesia (e.g., barbiturates)
6. Increase seizure threshold
7. Effects on gastrointestinal activity undetermined
8. Use in pregnancy not investigated
9. Diazepam is eliminated in the urine and feces after metabolism by the liver; duration of action is 1 to 4 hours
10. Diazepam increases appetite in domestic cats and ruminants, probably in all species
11. Dose (see Table 3-1)
12. Side effects
   a. Ataxia, particularly evident in large animal species
   b. Paradoxical increase in anxiety and fear response in some animals
   c. Pronounced CNS depression in neonates possible
   d. Diazepam painful if administered IM
13. Antagonists: benzodiazepine effects can be antagonized by benzodiazepine antagonists (e.g., flumazinil: 0.005 to 0.01 mg/lb IV)

C. Xylazine, detomidine, medetomidine
   1. Mode of action
      a. Produce CNS depression by stimulating presynaptic α_2-adrenoceptors in the CNS and peripherally; this decreases norepinephrine release centrally and peripherally; the net result is a decrease in CNS sympathetic outflow and decreases in circulating catecholamines and other stress-related substances; the CNS effects of α_2-agonists can be antagonized by α_2-receptor antagonists (e.g, yohimbine, tolazoline, atipamazole)
      b. Comparative drug selectivity for α_2- vs. α_1-receptors

DRUG	α_2-SELECTIVITY
Clonidine	220:1
Xylazine	160:1
Detomidine	260:1
Medetomidine	1620:1
Dexmedetomidine	dextro (active)-isomer of medetomidine

   c. Polysynaptic reflexes are inhibited (centrally acting muscle relaxant), but the neuromuscular junction is not influenced; depress internuncial neuron transmission

   d. Induce a sleeplike state comparable to phenothiazines, only more pronounced

   e. Produce analgesia by stimulating CNS α_2-receptors

   f. Effects are additive when combined with other depressant and analgesic drugs used to produce chemical restraint or general anesthesia

   g. Demonstrate both parasympathetic (bradycardia) and α_1- and α_2-receptor stimulatory activity

2. General properties

   a. Produce calming effect/sedation, muscle relaxation, and analgesia

     (1) Xylazine: 20 to 40 minutes

     (2) Detomidine: 90 to 120 minutes

     (3) Medetomidine: 45 to 90 minutes

   b. Can be administered epidurally or subarachnoidally to produce regional or segmental analgesia

3. Cardiopulmonary effects

   a. Slow heart rate due to decreased CNS sympathetic outflow and increased parasympathetic activity; may initiate sinus bradycardia or first- or second-degree atrioventricular blockade; complete or third-degree atrioventricular block occurs rarely

   b. Increase cardiac sensitivity to catecholamine-induced arrhythmias during halothane anesthesia; this effect is caused by α_1- and possibly α_2-adrenoceptor stimulation; this effect is transient, coincides with the increase in arterial BP, and is not observed after detomidine or medetomidine administration

   c. Cardiac output may decrease by 30% to 50% and coincides with decreases in heart rate and increases in peripheral vascular resistance

   d. Initially increase BP (α_1- and α_2-adrenoceptor stimulatory effect), then reduce BP to below control values because of decreases in CNS sympathetic outflow

      e. Decrease norepinephrine release from sympathetic nerve terminals

      f. Cause bradycardia

      g. Initially increase peripheral vascular resistance

      h. Depress respiratory centers centrally

      i. Decrease respiratory center sensitivity and increase threshold to increases in P_{CO_2}; decrease tidal volume and respiratory rate with an overall decrease in minute volume when administered in large dosages IV

      j. May induce stridor and dyspnea in horses and brachycephalic dogs with upper airway obstruction

4. Gastrointestinal system

      a. Suppress salivation, gastric secretions, and gastrointestinal motility; may stimulate pica and appetite at low doses

      b. Cause vomiting in dogs and cats

      c. Depress swallowing reflex

      d. Suppress insulin release by stimulating presynaptic α_2-receptors in the pancreas, resulting in an increase in plasma glucose concentration and glucosuria

      e. Excellent for treating colic

5. Absorption, fate, and excretion

      a. Rapidly absorbed after intramuscular or subcutaneous administration

      b. Relatively rapidly metabolized by the liver and excreted in the urine

      c. Active metabolites possible; over 20 identified

6. Other

      a. Produce profound sleep in dogs, cats, foals, and small ruminants; this is partially reversible with doxapram hydrochloride (0.05 to 0.2 mg/lb IV)

      b. Xylazine crosses the placenta, but an abortifacient effect has not been noted in pregnant mares; neither were there observable effects upon gestation or parturition; xylazine may induce premature delivery in cattle

      c. Highly excited or nervous animals may react adversely by becoming extremely ataxic, reacting violently or viciously when approached or touched, or showing inadequate response to the drug

d. Effect is oxytocin-like in ruminants; this activity has not been reported in mares or small animals

e. Clinical value in pigs is questionable because of their relatively rapid metabolism

7. Side effects

   a. Severe respiratory depression (respiratory acidosis)

   b. Bradyarrhythmias

   c. Hypotension

   d. Ataxia in large animals

   e. Sweating in horses

   f. Diuresis

   g. Occasional severe inflammatory response if administered SQ in horses or cattle

8. α_2-Antagonists

   a. Yohimbine (0.25 mg/lb IV)

   b. Tolazoline (1 to 2 mg/lb IV)

   c. Atipamazole (0.05 to 0.2 mg/lb)

III. Opioids

A. Mode of action

1. Act by reversible combination with one or more specific (opiate and nonopiate) receptors in the brain and spinal cord to produce a variety of effects, including analgesia, sedation, euphoria, dysphoria, and excitement

2. Referred to as opioid agonists, agonist-antagonists, and antagonists

   a. Consist of a wide variety of naturally occurring (opiate) derivatives and synthetically manufactured drugs

   b. Classified according to analgesic activity or addiction potential

   c. Commonly used opioids include morphine, meperidine, oxymorphone, and fentanyl; pentazocine, butorphanol, and buprenorphine are drugs with opioid agonist-antagonist effects

   d. Analgesic potency

     (1) Morphine: 1

       (2) Meperidine: 0.5

       (3) Oxymorphone: 5-10

       (4) Fentanyl: 100

       (5) Pentazocine: 0.1

       (6) Butorphanol: 2-5

       (7) Buprenorphine: 3-5

       (8) Etorphine: 1

   3. Senses not interfered with by opioid agonists or agonist-antagonists

     a. Touch

     b. Vibration

     c. Vision

     d. Hearing

B. Are used before, during, or after surgery for analgesia

   1. Fentanyl, alfentanil, and oxymorphone are generally used during surgery as a part of a balanced anesthetic technique

   2. Can be administered epidurally or subarachnoidally to produce regional or segmental analgesia

C. Produce analgesic action at doses lower than needed for sedation (dosage tailored to individual animal)

D. Effects in addition to sedative actions

   1. Behavioral changes (e.g., sedation, euphoria, or dysphoria)

   2. Reduction in response to external stimuli (animal may not recognize owner)

   3. Miosis in dogs and pigs, mydriasis in cats and horses

   4. Hypothermia caused by panting caused by resetting of the thermoregulatory center

   5. Sweating, particularly in horses

   6. Body temperatures in dogs by panting

E. Produce additive effects when used with other depressants (e.g., tranquilizers, barbiturates, inhalation anesthesia)

F. May be used in combination with tranquilizers and sedatives to produce neuroleptanalgesia (see Table 3-1)

G. Produce excellent sedation in dogs, but may cause excitement when given rapidly IV; cats and horses are particularly susceptible to the excitatory effect of opioids; this is typified by increased motor activity and pacing in horses

H. Purchase and use should be strictly controlled; increased security and accurate record keeping are required

I. Cardiopulmonary effects
   1. Bradycardia caused by stimulation of medullary vagal nuclei
   2. Possible hypotension caused by release of histamine
   3. Positive inotropic action when used in low dosages (morphine only) caused by release of epinephrine and norepinephrine from the adrenal and sympathetic nerve terminals
   4. Respiratory depression is dose-dependent (rate and tidal volume); raises the threshold of the respiratory center to increases in P_{CO_2}
   5. Reduced respiratory reserve capabilities
J. Gastrointestinal effects
   1. Salivation
   2. Nausea
   3. Vomiting in those species that can
   4. Nonpropulsive gastrointestinal hypermotility, increases in sphincter tone
   5. Defecation
K. Decrease urine production by increasing ADH release
L. Cross the placental barrier relatively slowly; useful for cesarean section because depressant effects can be antagonized
M. Extensively metabolized by the liver, and metabolites are eliminated in the urine; the opioid agonists vary in biologic half-life, most with durations of action ranging from 30 minutes to 3 hours in most species; morphine may produce effects lasting 6 to 8 hours in horses
N. May develop tolerance with continued use
O. Opioid agonist-antagonists
   1. Pentazocine, butorphanol, and buprenorphine antagonize the effects of other opioid agonists (e.g., morphine, meperidine, oxymorphone, fentanyl), but can produce mild CNS depression, euphoria, and analgesia when administered in therapeutic doses
   2. Butorphanol, an excellent cough suppressant
P. Opioid antagonists
   1. Classification
      a. Pure antagonist (e.g., naloxone)
      b. Partial antagonists (e.g., nalorphine, butorphanol, buprenorphine)

      c. Opioid antagonists may possess many of the same properties as opioids; naloxone possesses the least narcotic agonistic effects

   2. Mechanism of action

      a. Opioid antagonists compete with opioid drugs for their specific receptor sites

      b. Partial antagonists act in a fashion similar to opioid antagonists

         (1) Nalorphine can produce autonomic, endocrine, analgesic, and respiratory depressant effects

         (2) Nalorphine is about two thirds as potent as morphine as an analgesic

         (3) Nalorphine may add to existing respiratory depression

   3. Rapidly metabolized in the liver

   4. Dosage

      a. Naloxone: 1 to 15 μg/lb IV

      b. Nalorphine: 1 mg/5 lb IV

Q. Side effects

   1. Excitement, dysphoria

   2. Apnea

   3. Bradycardia

   4. Ataxia and incoordination

   5. Excessive vomiting

   6. Excessive sweating in horses

IV. Neuroleptanalgesia

A. A state of CNS depression and analgesia produced by the combination of a tranquilizer and analgesic drug; useful in dogs, cats, and pigs (see Definitions, Chapter 1)

B. The animal may or may not retain consciousness and is responsive to auditory stimuli; many animals defecate, some vomit

C. The only commercial combination is fentanyl (opioid) and droperidol (tranquilizer)

   1. Fentanyl

      a. Actions are similar to morphine, but 100 times more potent

      b. Respiratory and cardiovascular depressant

         (1) Decreases the minute volume response to CO_2

         (2) May produce a dramatic decrease in heart rate

2. Droperidol
   a. A butyrophenone tranquilizer
   b. Can be compared in its action to the phenothiazine tranquilizers; a potent antiemetic; do not administer to horses
   c. Prevents arrhythmias produced by exogenous epinephrine (exerts an adrenergic blocking action)
   d. Enhances the actions of barbiturates
3. This drug combination may cause dramatic behavior modification and aggressiveness in aged dogs
4. The veterinary product contains 0.4 mg/ml of fentanyl and 20 mg/ml of droperidol (Innovar-Vet)

D. Results of the drug combination
   1. Sedation-analgesia, ataxia, and/or recumbency
   2. Depression of ventilation (apnea may occur)
   3. Bradycardia
   4. Defecation and flatulence
   5. Analgesia for periods up to 40 minutes

E. Overdosages usually result in profound hypotension and respiratory depression; respiratory depression can generally be reversed by an opioid antagonist (e.g., nalorphine, levallorphan, naloxone)

F. Most animals are premedicated with a parasympatholytic (e.g., atropine or glycopyrrolate) to prevent bradycardia and excessive salivation

G. Neuroleptanalgesics are used in combination with barbiturates in dogs to eliminate the stimulatory effect of loud noises and produce better muscle relaxation
   1. Thiamylal (1 mg/lb) after Innovar-Vet (1 ml/30 lb IV)
   2. Sodium pentobarbital (3 mg/lb) after Innovar-Vet (1 ml/20 lb IV)

H. Other combinations of opioids and tranquilizers have been used to produce sedation and analgesia similar to that of Innovar-Vet
   1. Acepromazine (0.1 to 0.2 mg/lb) in combination with morphine (0.2 to 0.4 mg/lb IV or SC), meperidine (0.5 to 1 mg/lb IV), or oxymorphone (0.05 to 0.1 mg/lb IV) is used to produce neuroleptanalgesia in dogs; diazepam (0.1mg/lb IV) and oxymorphone (0.04 mg/lb IV), or acepromazine (0.1 mg/lb IM)

and butorphanol (0.1 to 0.2 mg/lb IM) are used in dogs and cats

2. The combination of xylazine (0.3 mg/lb IV) and morphine (0.1 to 0.3 mg/lb IV), or xylazine (0.3 mg/lb IV) and butorphanol (0.01 to 0.02 mg/lb IV) is commonly used for horses

I. Useful for short operative procedures and for cesarean section in small animals

J. Side effects
1. Respiratory depression
2. Bradycardia
3. Ataxia
4. Excitement
5. CNS and behavioral abnormalities in some breeds of dogs (e.g., Doberman Pinschers)

CHAPTER FOUR

Local Anesthetic Drugs and Techniques

"And don't give me any of those local anesthetics. Get me the imported stuff."

FROM THE CARTOON "HERMAN" UNIVERSAL PRESS SYNDICATE

OVERVIEW

Local anesthetics produce desensitization and analgesia of skin surfaces (topical anesthesia), local tissues (infiltration and field blocks), and regional structures (conduction anesthesia, intravenous regional anesthesia). Local anesthetic techniques are an alternative or adjunct to intravenous and inhalation anesthesia in high-risk patients. A number of anesthetic drugs are available; they vary in potency, toxicity, and cost. The most commonly used local anesthetic drugs are lidocaine hydrochloride and mepivacaine hydrochloride; they produce intermediate anesthetic duration (90 to 180 minutes), have a rapid onset of action, and provide anesthesia over a wide field. Vasoconstrictors (epinephrine) are occasionally incorporated with or added to a local drug to increase intensity and prolong anesthetic activity. Adding hyaluronidase increases tissue penetration in the region of infiltration, and hastens the onset of anesthesia.

GENERAL CONSIDERATIONS

I. Use sterile solutions and injection equipment
II. Do not inject into inflamed areas
III. Use undamaged needles
IV. Use as small a gauge of needle as practical

V. Aspirate for blood before injecting
VI. Use lowest effective concentration of local anesthetic drug
VII. Use smallest possible amount of local anesthetic (consider the use of a vasoconstrictor)

LOCAL ANESTHETICS

I. Mechanism of membrane and impulse conduction
   A. All clinically used local anesthetics are membrane-stabilizing agents
   B. They enter and occupy (by polar association) the membrane channels through which ions normally move
   C. The most immediate and apparent effect is to prevent the inflow of Na^+ and therefore block all subsequent ionic flow
   D. They prevent depolarization and therefore stop or retard conduction of impulses
II. Uptake
   A. The salt of the anesthetic base is an ionizable quaternary amine with little or no anesthetic properties of its own because it is not lipid soluble and is not absorbed in the nerve membrane
   B. After deposition in tissue that is slightly alkaline and has considerable buffering capacity, the anesthetic base is liberated as follows

$$RNH^+\ Cl^- \leftrightarrow Cl^- + RNH^+ \leftrightarrow RN + H^+$$
$$\text{Salt} \qquad \text{Cation} \quad \text{Base}$$

   C. The free anesthetic base is absorbed at the outer lipid nerve membrane, where anesthetic action takes place
III. Effect of tissue pH
   A. If sufficient local buffering capacity exists to remove the dissociated H^+, this reaction proceeds to the right to liberate active base and exert an anesthetic effect
   B. The pH is considerably below normal (more acid) in inflamed or infected tissues; in acid conditions, little free base dissociates from the anesthetic salt, resulting in poor local anesthesia

IV. Absorption
  A. Poor absorption through intact skin
  B. Absorption from
    1. Injured skin
    2. Mucous membranes
    3. Respiratory epithelium
    4. Intramuscular deposition
    5. Subcutaneous deposition
    6. Intravenous administration
V. Classification and function of nerve fibers
  A. Myelinated A-fibers
    1. α (Alpha): motor, proprioception
    2. β (Beta): motor, touch
    3. γ (Gamma): muscle spindles
    4. δ (Delta): pain, temperature
  B. Myelinated B-fibers (preganglionic sympathetic)
  C. Nonmyelinated C-fibers transmit
    1. Pain
    2. Temperature
VI. Priority of blockade
  A. B-fibers, C-fibers, $>A_\delta$-fibers $>A_\alpha$-fibers
  B. Sensation disappears in the following order: pain, cold, warmth, touch, joint, and deep pressure
VII. Blocking quality
  A. Potency: binding affinity to receptor protein (tetracaine $>$lidocaine $>$procaine)
  B. Latency is the time between injection and maximum effect
  C. Duration of action is related to the logarithm of the concentration (e.g., doubling the concentration increases the duration by only approximately 30%)
  D. Recovery time is the time it takes for normal sensation to return; it is dependent on outflow diffusion and gradual release of local anesthetic from the nerve membrane; it may be 2 to 200 times longer than induction time
VIII. Autoclaving of local anesthetic drugs: ampules of hydrochloride salts can be autoclaved at 120° C for 20 to 30 minutes

DRUGS USED FOR VASOCONSTRICTION

I. Epinephrine (adrenaline) or L-norepinephrine (levarterenol) 1:50,000 (1 mg/50 ml saline) or 1:200,000 (1 mg/200 ml saline)
II. Effects of vasoconstriction
    A. Maximal vasoconstriction is probably produced by the lower of these concentrations, but because of the instability of epinephrine, the higher concentration is used to increase shelf life
    B. Vasoconstrictors delay absorption, reducing the toxicity and increasing the margin of safety
    C. Vasoconstrictors increase intensity and prolong anesthetic activity
    D. Vasoconstrictors increase risk of cardiac arrhythmias and ventricular fibrillation

DRUGS USED TO HASTEN THE TIME OF ONSET OF ANESTHESIA

I. Hyaluronidase
    A. Increases the area of diffusion, resulting in a larger total area being desensitized
    B. Often produces rapid anesthesia
    C. Usually shortens anesthesia time because of increased absorption, unless a vasoconstrictor is used
    D. Does not substitute for precise, accurate technique; fascial planes are barriers
    E. Use five turbidity-reducing units per milliliter of local anesthetic solution
II. Combinations

$$\left.\begin{array}{l}\text{Hyaluronidase}\\\text{Epinephrine}\end{array}\right\} + \text{procaine} \rightarrow \left[\begin{array}{l}\text{Doubles the area anesthetized}\\\text{Increases duration of local}\\\text{anesthesia almost five times}\end{array}\right.$$

SPECIFIC LOCAL ANESTHETIC DRUGS

I. Ester-linked drugs (Table 4-1)
    A. Cocaine (alkaloid of the leaf of Erythroxylon coca)

B. Procaine hydrochloride (Novocain)
   1. Prototype of all other local anesthetics
   2. Standard drug for comparison of anesthetic effects
   3. Hydrolyzed in plasma by pseudocholinesterase
C. Chloroprocaine hydrochloride (Nesacaine)
   1. Minimal toxicity
   2. Good penetration
   3. Hydrolyzed by pseudocholinesterase
D. Tetracaine hydrochloride (Pontocaine)
   1. Ten to fifteen times more potent than procaine
   2. Relatively toxic
   3. Prolonged anesthetic effect
   4. Hydrolyzed by pseudocholinesterase

II. Amide-linked drugs
A. Lidocaine hydrochloride (Xylocaine, Lignocaine)
   1. Most stable drug in this group; not decomposed by boiling, acids, or alkali
   2. Superior penetration compared to procaine: effects evident in ⅓ the time; effects persist 1½ times longer; spreads over a wider field
   3. No tissue damage or irritation
   4. No allergy or hypersensitivity
   5. Sedative effects
   6. Antiarrhythmic
   7. Metabolized in the liver
B. Mepivacaine hydrochloride (Carbocaine)
   1. Similar to lidocaine
   2. No irritation or tissue damage
   3. Metabolized in the liver
C. Dibucaine hydrochloride (Nupercaine)
   1. Twenty times more potent than procaine
   2. Anesthetic effect is three to five times longer
D. Bupivacaine (Marcaine)
   1. Intermediate onset
   2. Decreased motor blocking potency
   3. Anesthetic effect is four to six hours
   4. Metabolized in the liver
E. LEA (Ropivacaine)
   1. Similar to bupivacaine
   2. Less cardiotoxic

TABLE 4-1
LOCAL ANESTHETICS

AGENT (GENERIC NAME)	TRADE NAME (REGISTERED BY)	CHEMICAL NAME	POTENCY RATIO (PROCAINE = 1)
Procaine	Novocain (Winthrop Stearns)	Para-aminobenzoic acid ester of diethylaminoethanol	1:1
Chloroprocaine	Nesacaine (Wallace & Tiernan)	Para-amino-2 chlorobenzoic acid ester of B-diethylaminoethanol	2.4:1
Lidocaine	Xylocaine (Astra Pharmaceutical Products)	Diethylaminoacet −2,6 xylidide	2:1
Mepivacaine	Carbocaine (Winthrop Laboratories)	1-methyl-2', 6'-pipecoloxylidide monohydrochloride	2.5:1
Tetracaine	Pontocaine (Winthrop Laboratories)	Parabutylamino benzoyl-dimethylaminoethanol-HCl	12:1
Hexylcaine	Cyclaine (Merck, Sharpe, and Dohme)	1-cyclo-hexamino 2-propylbenzoate	1-2:1
Dibucaine	Nupercaine (CIBA Pharmaceutical Products)	a-butyl-oxycin-choninic acid of diethylethylene-diamide	20:1
Bupivacaine	Marcaine (Breon Laboratories)	1-butyl-2', 6' pipecoloxylidide-HCl	8:1

TABLE 4-1—cont'd
LOCAL ANESTHETICS

TOXICITY RATIO (PROCAINE = 1)	DOSAGE (%)	STABILITY	COMMENTS
1:1	1-2 for infiltration and nerve block	Aqueous solutions are heat resistant, decomposed by bacteria	Hydrolyzed by liver and plasma esterase
0.5:1	1-2 for infiltration and nerve block	Multiple autoclaving accelerates hydrolysis and impairs potency	Immediate onset of action; 2 hr duration with epinephrine
0.5% 1:1 1% 1.4:1 2% 1.5:1	0.5-2 for infiltration and nerve block; topically 2-4	Aqueous solutions are thermostable; multiple autoclaving possible	Excellent penetrability; rate of onset twice as fast as procaine; 2 hr duration with epinephrine
Less toxic than lidocaine	1-2 for infiltration and nerve block	Resistant to acid and alkaline hydrolysis; multiple autoclaving possible	Absence of vasodilator effects makes addition of a vasoconstrictor unnecessary
10:1	0.1 for infiltration and nerve block; topically 0.2	Crystals and solutions should not be autoclaved	Slow onset of anesthesia (5-10 min); 2 hr duration; for eye installation
2-4:1	0.5-1 for infiltration; 2 for nerve block; 5 topically	Crystals and solutions are thermostable	Recommended for epidural and topical anesthesia
15:1	Topically 0.1	Thermostable, but precipitation by alkalies	Slowly detoxified
Greater margin of safety than lidocaine	0.25 for infiltration; 0.5 for nerve block; 0.75 for epidural block	Stable compound	Intermediate onset, lasting 4-6 hr

TOPICAL ANESTHETICS

I. Commonly used topicals
   A. Butacaine (Butya sulphate)
   B. Tetracaine (Pontocaine)
   C. Piperocaine (Metycaine)
   D. Proparacaine (Ophthaine)
   E. Cetacaine (Benzocaine)
II. Vascular effect: local anesthetic drugs are vasodilators, with the exception of cocaine (a vasoconstrictor) and lidocaine (minimal effect)
III. Toxicity dependent on
   A. Rate of absorption
   B. Rate of detoxification

METHODS OF LOCAL ANESTHETIC APPLICATION

I. Surface anesthesia
   A. Sprayed or brushed on mucous membranes (mouth, nose)
   B. Dropped into the eye
   C. Infused into the urethra
   D. Injected subsynovially (synovial membranes)
II. Infiltration anesthesia
   A. Diffuse infiltration of operative area
      1. Sensitive tissues: skin, nerve trunks, blood vessels, periosteum, synovial membranes, mucous membranes near orifices (mouth, nose, rectum, anus)
      2. Insensitive tissues: subcutaneous, fat, muscles, tendons, fascia, bone, cartilage, visceral peritoneum
   B. Techniques
      1. Bleb (very localized deposition of a small quantity)
      2. Layer by layer
   C. Uses
      1. Wound treatment
      2. Skin incision
         a. Surgical removal of superficial tumors
         b. Repositioning of fractured bones
III. Regional (perineural) anesthesia
   A. Linear block

B. Field block: contraindications
   1. Fissures of bones
   2. Fractures of bones
C. Epidural block
D. Paravertebral block
IV. Intraarticular anesthesia
V. Subsynovial anesthesia
VI. Intravenous regional anesthesia
VII. Refrigeration or hypothermic anesthesia

ANALGESIC ACTIVITY OF EPIDURALLY ADMINISTERED α_2-ADRENOCEPTOR AGONISTS

α_2-Adrenoceptor agonists such as clonidine, xylazine, detomidine, romifidine, medetomidine, and dexmedetomidine are used for their sedative, analgesic, anxiolytic, anesthetic sparing, and hemodynamic-stability properties; xylazine and detomidine injected epidurally in cattle and horses produce caudal (S3 to coccyx) localized analgesia with minimal impairment of motor function

I. Site of action
   A. The site of action of α_2-adrenoceptor agonists in epidural analgesia is unknown
   B. The antinociceptive effects of epidurally and intrathecally (subarachnoid) administered α_2-adrenoceptor agonists suggested are primarily the result of
      1. Stimulation of α_2-adrenoceptors in the spinal cord; receptor binding results in release of norepinephrine, hyperpolarization of dorsal horn neurons, and inhibition of substance P (pain) release, thereby producing behavioral analgesia in animals
      2. Inhibition of impulse conduction in primary afferent nerve fibers; C-fibers (pain, reflex responses, and postsympathetic transmission) are blocked to a greater extent than A-fibers (somatic motor function and proprioception differential nerve blockade)
   C. The antinociceptive effects of epidurally and intrathecally (subarachnoid) administered α_2-adrenoceptor ago-

nists are independent of opiate receptor mechanisms; the α_2-agonists may provide effective alternatives in pain states that are resistant to opioids

D. The addition of xylazine to an epidural solution containing lidocaine prolongs the duration of analgesia

II. Receptors

A. α_2-Adrenergic receptors are located on the dorsal horn of the spinal cord

B. The predominant α_2-adrenergic receptor in human cortex, and human and rat spinal cord is the α_2-A subtype

C. The density of α_2-adrenergic receptors in humans and rats is greater in the sacral cord than in the thoracolumbar cord

D. The density of α_2-adrenergic receptors in the spinal cord of domestic animals is unknown

III. Epidural xylazine

A. Xylazine is the most commonly used α_1-and α_2-agonist for epidural injection in cattle, horses, and pigs (Table 4-2)

1. Xylazine has a high affinity and selectivity for α_1- and α_2- receptors

2. Xylazine has local anesthetic properties that are independent of α-adrenergic stimulation

3. The exact proportion of α_1 versus α_2-adrenoceptor–mediated analgesia and local anesthesia within the spinal cord has not been determined for domestic animals

B. Clinical use of epidural xylazine

1. In cattle, xylazine (0.05 mg/kg expanded to a 5-ml volume with sterile saline) given in the epidural space at the first coccygeal intervertebral space produces anesthesia in the anal and perineal region for surgery and obstetric procedures (see Table 4-2)

2. Xylazine-induced caudal epidural anesthesia in cattle is associated with side effects

a. Marked sedation (head drop)

b. Mild ataxia

c. Bradycardia

d. Hypotension

e. Respiratory acidosis

      f. Hypoxemia

      g. Transient ruminal amotility

      h. Renal diuresis

    3. The side effects in cattle are dose dependent and partially reversed by administration of tolazoline (priscoline) (0.3 mg/kg intravenously [IV])

    4. In horses, xylazine (0.17 mg/kg) given in the epidural space at the first coccygeal intervertebral space produces anesthesia in the anal and perineal region for surgery and obstetric procedures, with minimal ataxia (Table 4-2)

    5. In pigs, xylazine (2 mg/kg) given in the epidural space at the lumbosacral interspace produces bilateral surgical anesthesia of the trunk caudal to the umbilicus and analgesia and paralysis of rear limbs, with minimal cardiovascular depression (see Table 4-2)

      a. Smaller doses of epidural xylazine (<1 mg/kg) do not produce surgical anesthesia

      b. Larger doses of epidural xylazine (>3 mg/kg) induce weakness of rear limbs for 36 hours or longer

IV. Onset and duration of analgesia

  A. Signs of analgesia develop within 20 to 30 minutes (compared to 5 to 10 minutes after epidural lidocaine)

  B. A mixture of xylazine and lidocaine can be used to shorten onset of analgesia to approximately 5 minutes and prolong analgesia to approximately 5 hours (see Table 4-2)

    1. Duration of analgesia is longer for the xylazine/lidocaine combination than for either drug used alone

    2. Approximate duration of analgesia after epidural drug administration is variable (see Table 4-2)

      a. 110 min after lidocaine

      b. 220 min after xylazine

      c. 330 min after xylazine-lidocaine combination

    3. Surgical and obstetric procedures can commence soon after injection without the need for additional anesthetic

V. Local anesthetic properties of xylazine

  A. Xylazine-induced epidural analgesia may be mediated by local spinal analgesic mechanisms because the sys-

TABLE 4-2

XYLAZINE-, XYLAZINE/LIDOCAINE-, AND DETOMIDINE-INDUCED ANALGESIA AFTER EPIDURAL ADMINISTRATION IN CATTLE, PONY, HORSE, PIG, AND LLAMA

SPECIES	AGONIST	CONCEN-TRATION OF DRUG (%)	DOSE (mg/kg)	VOLUME OF DILUENT (ml)
Cattle	Xylazine	2	0.05	5 ml of 0.9% NaCl
Pony	Xylazine	2	0.35	—
Horse	Xylazine	2	0.17	6 ml/450 kg with sterile water
	Xylazine	10	0.17	5 ml/450 kg with 2% lido-caine (0.22 mg/kg)
	Detomidine	1	0.06	10 ml/500 kg with sterile water
Pig	Xylazine	10	2	5 ml of 0.9% NaCl
	Xylazine	10	1 in large sows >180 kg 2 in small pigs <50 kg	10 ml of 2% lidocaine
	Detomidine	1	0.5	5 ml of 0.9% NaCl
Llama	Xylazine	10	0.17	2 ml/150 kg of sterile water
	Xylazine	10	0.17	1.7 ml/150 kg with 2% lido-caine (0.22 mg/kg)

TABLE 4-2—cont'd

XYLAZINE-, XYLAZINE/LIDOCAINE-, AND DETOMIDINE-INDUCED ANALGESIA AFTER EPIDURAL ADMINISTRATION IN CATTLE, PONY, HORSE, PIG, AND LLAMA

| SITE OF INJECTION | SPREAD OF ANALGESIA | ANALGESIA | | SIDE EFFECTS |
		ONSET (MIN)	DURATION (MIN)	
$C_0 1$-$C_0 2$	S3 to coccyx	10	>120	Sedation, ataxia, cardiopulmonary depression, ruminal hypomotility, diuresis
$C_0 1$-$C_0 2$	S3 to coccyx	20-30	240	Mild ataxia
S5-$C_0 1$	S3 to coccyx	30	200	—
S5-$C_0 1$	S3 to coccyx	5	300	Mild ataxia
$C_0 1$-$C_0 2$	T14 to coccyx	10-15	130-150	Sedation, ataxia, cardiopulmonary depression, diuresis
Lumbosacral	Umbilicus to coccyx	5	>120	Sedation, immobilization
Lumbosacral	Umbilicus to coccyx	5-10	300-480	
Lumbosacral	Umbilicus to coccyx	10	<30	Atipamazole (0.2 mg/kg IV) reverses sedation
$C_0 1$-$C_0 2$	S3 to coccyx	20	180	
$C_0 1$-$C_0 2$	S3 to coccyx	<5	330	Mild sedation occasional recumbency

temic administration of α_2-, or α_1- and α_2-adrenoceptor antagonists does not abolish the analgesic effect

1. Atipamezole (0.2 mg/kg) a potent α_2-adrenoceptor antagonist, when injected IV, does not abolish the analgesic effect of epidurally administered xylazine in pigs
2. Atipamezole (0.2 mg/kg) when injected IV, does not reverse xylazine-induced epidural immobilization in pigs
3. Tolazoline (0.3 mg/kg), an α_1- and α_2-adrenoceptor antagonist, when injected IV, does not reverse xylazine-induced epidural analgesia in cattle

VI. Epidural detomidine
   A. In horses, detomidine (0.06 mg/kg expanded to a 10-ml volume with sterile saline) given in the epidural space at the first coccygeal intervertebral space produces analgesia extending from the thoracic (T14) region to the coccyx (see Table 4-2)
      1. Detomidine-induced caudal epidural analgesia in horses is associated with side effects
         a. Marked sedation, head drop
         b. Bradycardia with second-degree, atrioventricular heart block
         c. Hypotension
         d. Hypercarbia
         e. Renal diuresis
      2. These side effects are dose dependent and can be partially antagonized by atipamezole (0.12 mg/kg IV), without affecting local analgesia

VII. Restraint: movements of head, shoulder, and forelimbs are not suppressed by epidural analgesia/anesthesia and should be controlled by physical or chemical restraint

VIII. Toxicity: no detrimental histologic effects on the spinal cord of ponies, horses, and pigs have been noted after epidural administration of xylazine

CHAPTER FIVE

Local Anesthesia in Cattle, Sheep, Goats, and Pigs

"The pain of the mind is worse than pain of the body."

PUBLILIUS SYRUS

OVERVIEW

The most commonly used local anesthetic techniques in ruminants are surface (topical) anesthesia, infiltration anesthesia, nerve block (conduction) anesthesia, epidural anesthesia, and intravenous (IV) regional anesthesia. The standing position is optimal for surgery in ruminants because it reduces the problems associated with bloat, salivation, recumbency-related regurgitation, and nerve or muscle damage.

The most commonly used local anesthetic techniques in appropriately tranquilized pigs are infiltration anesthesia, lumbosacral epidural anesthesia, and intratesticular injection.

CATTLE: LOCAL ANESTHESIA FOR STANDING LAPAROTOMY

I. Four techniques for inducing anesthesia of the paralumbar fossa in ruminants
   A. Infiltration anesthesia
   B. Proximal paravertebral anesthesia
   C. Distal paravertebral anesthesia
   D. Segmental dorsolumbar epidural anesthesia
II. Abdominal surgeries in which these anesthetic techniques may be used

53

ǀ

A. Rumenotomy
B. Cecotomy
C. Correction of gastrointestinal displacement
D. Intestinal obstruction
E. Volvulus
F. Cesarean section
G. Ovariectomy
H. Liver or kidney biopsy

III. Infiltration anesthesia
A. Line block
   1. Area blocked: skin, muscle layers, and parietal peritoneum along the line of incision
   2. Needle: 18-gauge, 1½- to 3-inch
   3. Anesthetic: 50 ml of 2% lidocaine
   4. Method: make multiple subcutaneous injections of 0.5 to 1 ml of anesthetic, 1 to 2 cm apart; then infiltrate the muscle layers and parietal peritoneum through the desensitized skin
   5. Advantages
      a. Easiest technique
      b. Use of routinely sized needles (2.5-cm, 20-gauge or smaller for skin block; 7.5- to 10-cm, 18-gauge for infiltrating the muscle layers and peritoneum)
   6. Disadvantages
      a. Large volume of anesthetic
      b. Lack of muscle relaxation
      c. Incomplete block of deeper layers of the abdominal wall
      d. Formation of hematomas along the incision line
      e. Increased cost due to larger amounts of anesthetic use and time required
   7. Complications
      a. Potential toxicity if significant amount of anesthetic (250 ml of 2% lidocaine hydrochloride solution) is injected into the peritoneal cavity in adult cattle (450 kg)
      b. Interference with healing
B. Inverted L block (Fig. 5-1)
   1. Area blocked: flank caudal and ventral to site of injection

2. Site: a line along the caudal border of the last rib and along a line ventral to the lumbar transverse processes from the last rib to the fourth lumbar vertebra (inverted L)
3. Needle: 18-gauge, 3-inch
4. Anesthetic: up to 100 ml of 2% lidocaine, evenly distributed
5. Method: Inject drug into the tissues bordering the dorsocaudal aspect of the last rib and ventrolateral aspect of the lumbar transverse processes, creating a wall of anesthetic enclosing the incision site

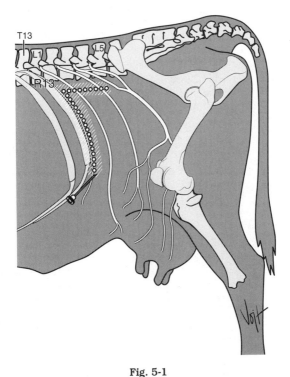

Fig. 5-1

Regional anesthesia of the cow's left flank using inverted L infiltration pattern.

   6. Advantages
      a. Similar to line block
      b. Absence of anesthetic agent from the incision line minimizes edema, hematoma, and possible interference with healing
   7. Disadvantages
      a. Large volume of anesthetic required
      b. Length of time required to infiltrate such a long line
      c. Incomplete block of the deep layers of the abdominal wall (particularly the peritoneum)
   8. Complications: similar to line block
IV. Specific nerve anesthesia
   A. Proximal paravertebral anesthesia (Farquharson technique)
      1. Area blocked: flank of side on which technique is performed
      2. Nerves blocked: dorsal and ventral branches of T13, L1, and L2 (and occasionally if L3 is blocked the animal may become ataxic)
      3. Site: 2.5 to 5 cm from midline (Fig. 5-2); T13 immediately in front of transverse process of L1; L1 immediately in front of transverse process of L2; L2 immediately in front of transverse process of L3
      4. Needle: 14-gauge, ½-inch needle, creating passage for a 16- or 18-gauge, 4½-inch needle, (up to 6 inches for bull)
      5. Anesthetic: 20 ml of 2% lidocaine at each site
      6. Method: Palpate the lumbar transverse processes, starting from L5 and moving forward. L1 may be difficult to feel; measure 5 cm (2 inches) from midline; palpate the lumbar dorsal processes; injection site is at a 90-degree angle to the spaces between the dorsal processes; pass the needle vertically down until hitting the cranial edge of the transverse process, and proceed down through the intertransverse ligament; inject 15 ml of 2% lidocaine below the ligament to block the ventral branch of the nerve (there should be minimal resistance to injection); withdraw the needle sufficiently to inject 5 ml of 2% lidocaine above liga-

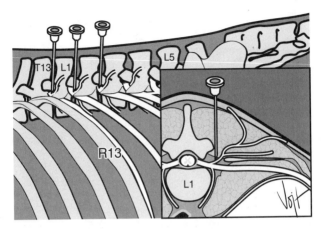

Fig. 5-2

Needle placement for proximal paravertebral nerve block in cattle. Left lateral aspect and cranial view of a transection of the first thoracolumbar vertebra at the location of the intervertebral foramen. R13 is the last rib, T13, L1, and L5 are the spinous proceses of the last thoracic and the first and fifth lumbar vertebrae.

    ment, level with dorsal surface of transverse process to block the dorsal branch (resistance to injection); if the first lumbar transverse process cannot be palpated, anesthetize the other nerves first, and then measure the distance between injection sites to find the site for blocking nerve T13

7. In sheep and goats, T13, L1, and L2 are desensitized similarly to the cattle method, but 2.5 to 3 cm off the midline and with less anesthetic (2 to 3 ml per site)

8. Advantages over local block
   a. Anesthesia of skin, musculature, and peritoneum
   b. No additional restraint required
   c. Large quantities of local anesthetic not required
   d. Shorter postsurgical convalescent period; incision site avoided

9. Disadvantages
   a. Procedure difficult in fat cattle and some beef cattle

      b. Arching of the spine due to paralysis of back muscles

      c. Anesthesia of abdominal viscera

      d. Bowing out toward the area of incision (after unilateral blockade) making the closure of the incision and navigation more difficult

  10. Complications

      a. Possible penetration of the aorta

      b. Possible penetration of the thoracic longitudinal vein (posterior) or vena cava

      c. Loss of the motor control of the pelvic limb due to caudal migration of drug (femoral nerve block)

B. Distal paravertebral anesthesia (Magda, Cakala, or Cornell technique)

  1. Area blocked: flank of side on which technique is performed

  2. Nerves blocked: dorsal and ventral rami of T13, L1, and L2

  3. Site: distal ends of lumbar transverse processes of L1, L2, and L4 (Fig. 5-3)

  4. Needle: 18-gauge, 3-inch

  5. Anesthetic: 10 to 20 ml of 2% lidocaine at each site

  6. Method: insert the needle ventral to the tips of the respective transverse process; inject anesthetic (up to 20 ml) in a fan-shaped infiltration pattern; withdraw the needle a short distance and reinsert it dorsal and caudal to the transverse process, and inject approximately 5 ml of the anesthetic

  7. Advantages of distal paravertebral nerve block over proximal paravertebral block

      a. Use of routinely sized needles

      b. Lack of risk of penetrating a major blood vessel

      c. Lack of scoliosis

      d. Minimal ataxia or weakness in the pelvic limb

  8. Disadvantages

      a. Large volume of anesthetic

      b. Variations in efficacy, particularly if the nerves follow a variable anatomic pathway

  9. Complications: none

C. Segmental dorsolumbar epidural block

  1. Area blocked: flank on both sides

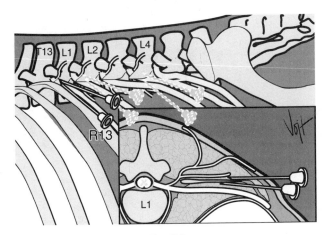

Fig. 5-3

Needle placement for distal paravertebral nerve blockades in cattle. Left lateral aspect and cranial view of a transection of the first lumbar vertebra at the location of the intervertebral foramen. R13 is the last rib, and T13, L1, L2, and L4 are the spinous processes of the last thoracic and first, second, and fourth lumbar vertebrae.

2. Nerves blocked: T13 and anterior lumbar nerves, depending on the total dose administered
3. Site: epidural space between L1 and L2 vertebrae
4. Needle: spinal, preferably 18-gauge, 4½-inch
5. Anesthetic: 8 ml of 2% lidocaine
6. Method: To reach the epidural space, insert the spinal needle 8 to 12 cm ventral and cranial at an angle of 10 to 15 degrees from vertical; piercing of the interarcuate ligament is felt as slight resistance during the insertion process; no blood or cerebrospinal fluid (CSF) can be aspirated, and also no resistance to the injection of anesthetic results after correct needle placement
7. Advantages over proximal or distal paravertebral anesthesia
   a. Only one injection
   b. Small quantity of anesthetic
   c. Uniform anesthesia and relaxation of the skin, musculature, and peritoneum (begins 10 to 20 min-

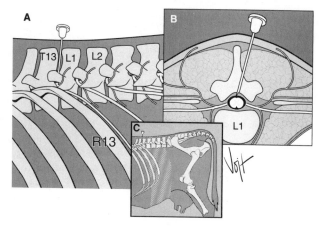

Fig. 5-4

Needle placement for segmental dorsolumbar epidural block. **A,** Left lateral aspect. **B,** Cranial view of a transection of the first lumbar vertebra at the location of the intervertebral foramen. **C,** *(inset)* Desensitized area of skin after segmental epidural anesthesia. R13 is the last rib; and T13, L1, and L2 are the spinous processes of the last thoracic and first and second lumbar vertebrae.

          utes after administration and continues for 45 to 120 minutes)
8. Disadvantages: difficult technique to perform
9. Complications
   a. Loss of motor control of the pelvic limbs due to overdose or subarachnoid injection
   b. Physiologic disturbance due to overdose or subarachnoid injection
   c. Potential for trauma to the spinal cord or venous sinuses

ANESTHESIA FOR OBSTETRIC PROCEDURES AND RELIEF OF RECTAL TENESMUS

I. Caudal epidural anesthesia and desensitization of the internal pudendal nerve are commonly used in ruminants for obstetric manipulations, caudal surgical procedures, and as an adjunct treatment for control of rectal tenesmus; these techniques are not effective in pigs

II. Cattle

    A. Low posterior or caudal epidural anesthesia (Fig. 5-5, *A*)

        1. Area blocked: anus, perineum, vulva, vagina

        2. Nerves blocked: coccygeal and posterior sacral nerves

        3. Site: first intercoccygeal space

        4. Needle: 18-gauge, 1½-inch (average dairy cow)

        5. Anesthetic: 5 to 6 ml of 2% lidocaine

        6. Method: Locate the sacrococcygeal joint by moving the tail up and down; this joint moves very little and is located just anterior to the anal folds; the first intercoccygeal joint is easily located by its movement; it is much wider and is posterior to the anal folds; insert the needle exactly at the midline of the sacrococcygeal space at a right angle to the skin surface; push the needle ventrally through the interarcuate ligament to the floor of the neural canal, which is at about 2 to 4 cm (¾ to 1½ inches); withdraw the needle slightly

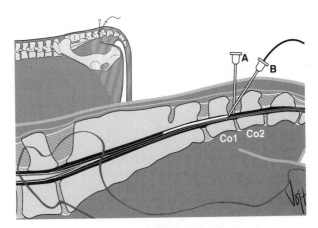

Fig. 5-5

Needle placement for **A,** caudal epidural anesthesia and **B,** continuous caudal epidural anesthesia in cattle. Co1 is the first coccygeal vertebra, and Co2 is the second coccygeal vertebra.

into epidural space and test by injecting 1 cc of air; no resistance should be felt

7. Advantages
   a. Minimal effect on cardiovascular and respiratory systems
   b. Little effect on organ systems
   c. Little problem with toxicity
   d. Good muscle relaxation
   e. Good postoperative analgesia
   f. Rapid recovery
   g. Relatively simple
   h. Inexpensive

8. Disadvantages
   a. Technically difficult if Co1-Co2 interspace is not identified
   b. Technically difficult if the sacrococcygeal interspace is ossified in older cow

9. Complications
   a. Rare
   b. Infection resulting in draining tracts or permanently paralyzed tail
   c. Possible ataxia and collapse due to overdose
   d. Hemorrhage due to puncture of a venous sinus

B. Continuous caudal epidural anesthesia (see Fig. 5-5, *B*)
   1. Indications: painful prolapse of the vagina and/or rectum that provokes severe continuous straining
   2. Nerves blocked: coccygeal and posterior sacral nerves
   3. Site: first intercoccygeal space
   4. Needle: 16- or 17-gauge, 2½-inch, thin-walled, Huber-point directional needle or Hustead needle
   5. Catheter: 30-cm, medical-grade vinyl tubing (0.036 cm outside diameter) or a commercially available epidural catheter with gradual markings
   6. Anesthetic: 3 to 5 ml of 2% lidocaine
   7. Method: Identify the first intercoccygeal joint as previously described; desensitize the skin and needle tract; with stylet in place and bevel directed craniad, advance the spinal needle for 5 to 8 cm approximately 45 degrees to vertical, until an abrupt reduction in resistance to needle passage is noted; remove the stylet

from the needle, and inject 3 ml of 2% lidocaine with minimal resistance; the test dose ensures proper placement of the needle in the vertebral canal; introduce the catheter aseptically introduced into the canal through the needle and advance it cranially approximately 3 cm beyond the tip of the needle (see Fig. 5-5, *B*); withdraw the needle, leaving the catheter in position; inject local anesthetic solution into the catheter at 3- to 5-hour intervals or as needed; place a catheter adapter on the free end of the catheter; secure the catheter at the entrance into the skin with adhesive tape sutured to the skin; place a protective sterile gauze over the free end of the catheter to allow the catheter to be used for many hours of infusion in the field

8. Advantages
    a. Similar to caudal epidural anesthesia
    b. Repeated administration of small fractional doses of local anesthesia
    c. No fibrosis of the extradural space from repeated standard epidural blocks
9. Disadvantages
    a. Similar to caudal epidural anesthesia
    b. Greater cost of equipment
    c. Acute tolerance to repeated injections
10. Complications
    a. Similar to caudal epidural anesthesia
    b. Kinking and curling of the catheter and occlusion of the tip with fibrin

C. Internal pudendal nerve block
    1. Indications
        a. Anesthesia and relaxation of the penis for examination
        b. Relief of tenesmus associated with vaginal and uterine prolapse
    2. Nerves blocked: internal pudendal (fibers of the ventral branches of S3 and S4), caudal rectal (fibers of the ventral branches of S3 and S4), and pelvic splanchnic nerves
    3. Site: identified by rectal palpation
    4. Needle: spinal, preferably 18-gauge, 3½-inch

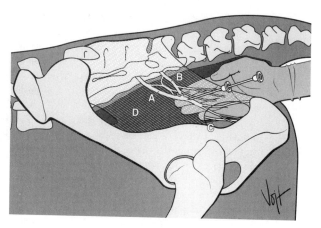

Fig. 5-6

Right hand and needle placement at the internal pudendal nerve on the medial side of the left pelvis. **A,** Internal pudendal nerve. **B,** Pelvic splanchnic nerves. **C,** Pudendal artery. **D,** Sacrosciatic ligament.

5. Anesthetic: up to 25 ml of 2% lidocaine per side
6. Method: use rectal palpation to locate the lesser sciatic foramen, a soft, circumscribed depression in the sacrosciatic ligament; find the nerve a finger's width dorsal to the pudendal artery present in the fossa; pass the needle through the disinfected skin in the ischiorectal fossa; deposit 15 ml of 2% lidocaine around the nerve; withdraw the needle 2 to 3 cm caudodorsally, and inject another 10 ml of the anesthetic in the area of the pelvic splanchnic nerve; repeat the procedure on the opposite side of the pelvis
7. Advantages
   a. No loss of tail tone
   b. No sciatic nerve involvement
   c. Ballooning of the vagina may aid in retention of the vagina after it is repositioned in a cow with prolapse
8. Disadvantages
   a. Technical difficulty and necessity of identifying the injection sites by rectal palpation

        b. Lack of cervical anesthesia

        c. Anesthesia of 3- to 6-hours' duration

     9. Complications: injury to the bull's penis, which must be protected from injury by replacing it into the prepuce

III. Sheep and goats: low posterior or caudal, epidural anesthesia

    A. Similar to that used in cattle

    B. No more than 0.5 to 1 ml of 2% lidocaine per 50 kg of bodyweight injected at the first coccygeal interspace or sacrococcygeal (S4-Co1) space (Fig. 5-7); excellent for tail docking in lambs and intravaginal obstetric procedures

ANTERIOR EPIDURAL ANESTHESIA

I. Anterior epidural anesthesia can be used for all procedures caudal to the diaphragm; the lumbosacral space is commonly

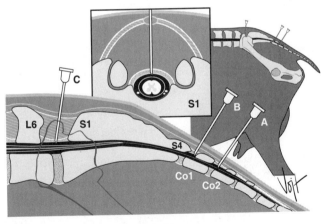

Fig. 5-7

Needle placement for caudal epidural anesthesia (**A** and **B**) and anterior epidural anesthesia (**C**) in the goat. **A,** Lateral aspect and cranial view of a transection to the first sacral vertebra. A needle is placed into **A,** the first intercoccygeal vertebral space; **B,** the sacrococcygeal space; and **C,** the lumbosacral space.

used in calves, sheep, and goats because the injection sites are usually palpable; this space is the only practical injection site for producing anterior anesthesia in pigs; the sacrococcygeal or first intercoccygeal space is the injection site of choice in adult cattle for producing anterior anesthesia because the technique is relatively simple and avoids trauma to the spinal cord and meninges; proper techniques should provide anesthesia of the following areas

  A. Perineal region

  B. Inguinal region

  C. Flank

  D. Abdominal wall caudal to the umbilicus

II. Increasing the dose of the anesthetic increases the area of blockade

III. Rapid epidural injections must be avoided to prevent consequences

  A. Discomfort to the patient

  B. Increased rate of vascular absorption, which can result in less drug for neural uptake; reduced neural uptake can result in the following

    1. Reduced duration of action

    2. Higher incidence of incomplete anesthesia

    3. Only a slight increase in segmental spread

IV. The technique is contraindicated in animals with certain known conditions

  A. Cardiovascular disease

  B. Bleeding disorders

  C. Shock or toxemic syndromes because of sympathetic block and consequent depression of blood pressure

V. The following complications may result from overdose or subarachnoid injection

  A. Transient loss of consciousness

  B. Flexor spasm

  C. Rapid muscular contractions

  D. Convulsions

  E. Respiratory paralysis

  F. Hypotension

  G. Hypothermia

VI. Small ruminants (sheep and goats)

  A. Landmarks and techniques for injection at the lumbosacral space are similar to those used in dogs (Fig. 5-7, C)

B. Dose: 1 ml of 2% lidocaine per 10 lb of body weight

C. Effect

1. Onset of posterior paralysis occurs in 2 to 15 minutes
2. Anesthesia generally reaches three fourths of the distance from pubis to umbilicus
3. Duration of action is 1 to 2 hours
4. Similar extent and duration of anesthesia can be achieved if only half the dose (0.5 ml/10 lb) is injected subarachnoidally (the space from which spinal fluid is aspirated into the syringe); true cerebral spinal fluid (CSF) anesthesia results with onset of posterior paralysis within 1 to 3 minutes
5. Gravity, not diffusion of drug in the CSF, determines the spread of anesthesia
6. Morphine (0.05 mg/lb) diluted with saline to a volume of 0.06 ml/lb can be injected epidurally following orthopedic procedures to produce 6-hour analgesia and sedation with minimal cardiopulmonary complications

VII. Pigs

A. Landmarks and techniques for injection at the lumbosacral space are similar to those used in dogs (Fig. 5-8)

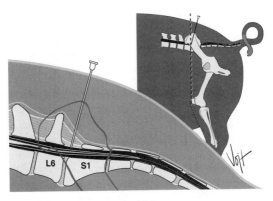

Fig. 5-8

Needle placement for epidural anesthesia in the pig. L6 is the sixth lumbar vertebra, and S1 is the first sacral vertebra.

B. Dose when using 2%:

STANDING CASTRATION	CESAREAN SECTION
4 ml/200 lb	10 ml/200 lb
6 ml/400 lb	15 ml/400 lb
8 ml/600 lb	20 ml/600 lb

C. Effect
  1. Onset of anesthetic action generally occurs within 5 minutes
  2. Maximum effect is within 15 to 20 minutes
  3. Duration of action is 120 minutes

LOCAL ANESTHESIA FOR DEHORNING

I. Cattle
  A. Area blocked: horn and base of the horn
  B. Nerves blocked: cornual branch of zygomaticotemporal (lacrimal) nerve, a portion of the ophthalmic division of the trigeminal nerve
  C. Site: temporal ridge, 2 cm from the base of horn (Fig. 5-9); needle penetration is from 1 cm (¼ inch) in small cattle to 2.5 cm (1 inch) in large bulls
  D. Needle: 18-gauge, 1- or 1½-inch
  E. Anesthetic: 5 to 10 ml of 2%
  F. Method: Palpate the lateral temporal ridge of the frontal bone. The nerve is relatively superficial, 7 to 10 mm deep (¼ to ½ inch) on the upper third of the ridge, lying between the thin frontalis muscle and the temporal muscle and can usually be palpated between these muscles; aspiration ensures that the needle point is not inadvertently intravascular; inject 2 to 3 cm in front of the horn
  G. Advantages
    1. Minimal systemic effects on the cardiopulmonary system
    2. Relatively simple procedure
  H. Disadvantages
    1. Cornual anesthesia does not result if the anesthetic is injected too deeply in the aponeurosis of the temporal muscle

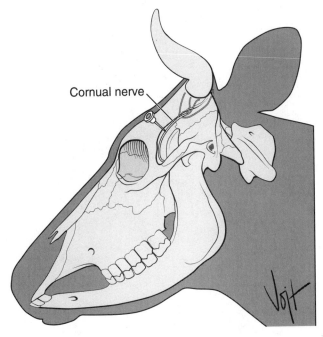

Fig. 5-9
Needle placement for desensitizing the cornual branch of the zygomatico-
temporal nerve in the cow.

      2. A second injection posterior to the horn may be required
         in adult cattle with well-developed horns

      3. Anesthesia of a fractured horn involving the frontal bone
         or sinuses may require a Peterson eye block

  I. Complications: none

II. Goats

    A. Area blocked: horn and base of the horn

    B. Nerves blocked: cornual branch of the zygomaticotempo-
       ral (lacrimal) nerve and cornual branch of the infratroch-
       lear nerve

    C. Site: halfway between lateral canthus of the eye and lat-
       eral base of the horn (lacrimal nerve) (Fig. 5-10, *A*) and

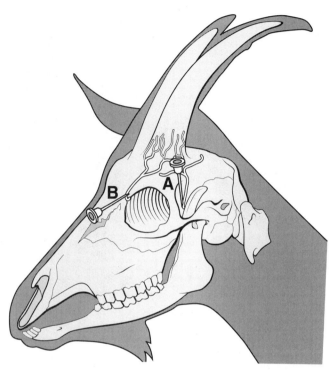

Fig. 5-10

Needle placement for desensitizing **A,** the cornual branch of the zygomati-cotemporal (lacrimal) nerve; and **B,** the cornual branch of the infratrochlear nerve in the goat.

halfway between medial canthus of the eye and medial base of the horn (cornual branch of infratrochlear nerve) (Fig. 5-10, *B*)

D. Needle: 22-gauge, 1-inch

E. Anesthetic: 2 to 3 ml of 2% lidocaine at each site in the adult goat; no more than 0.5 ml of 2% lidocaine for ring block at the horn base in young kids 7 to 14 days of age

F. Method: To reach the cornual branch of the zygomatico-temporal nerve, insert the needle as close as possible to the caudal ridge of the supraorbital process and 1 to 1.5 cm deep (see Fig. 5-10, *A*); to reach the cornual branch of the infratrochlear nerve, insert the needle dorsal and parallel to the dorsomedial margin of the orbit; inject the anesthetic in a line, since this nerve is frequently branched (see Fig. 5-10, *B*)

G. Advantages
   1. Alleviation of pain during dehorning
   2. Alleviation of pain during disbudding
H. Disadvantages
   1. Sedation of the animal is required if the frontal sinus will be entered during horn removal
   2. A total dose of 10 mg/kg (0.5 ml of 2% solution per kg or 1 ml of a 1% solution per kg) must not be exceeded to minimize adverse reactions
I. Complications: toxicity due to overdose of lidocaine and any of the following clinical signs
   1. Excitation
   2. Lateral recumbency
   3. Generalized tonic-clonic convulsions
   4. Opisthotonus
   5. Respiratory depression
   6. Cardiac arrest

LOCAL ANESTHESIA FOR THE EYE

I. At present, topical and regional anesthetic techniques are used in surgery of the eye and its associated structures; paralysis of the eyelids (without analgesia) is accomplished by selectively desensitizing the auriculopalpebral branch of the facial nerve (producing akinesia); anesthesia of the eye and orbit and immobilization of the globe are commonly achieved by the Peterson technique (Fig. 5-11)
   A. Area blocked: eye and orbit, orbicularis oculi muscle, *except* the eyelids
   B. Nerves blocked: oculomotor, trochlear, and abducens nerves, and the three branches of the trigeminal nerve (ophthalmic, maxillary, and mandibular)
   C. Sites: the points at which these nerves emerge from the foramen orbitorotundum

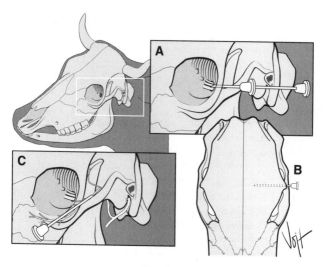

Fig. 5-11

Needle placement for Peterson eye block, with needle tip at the foramen orbitorotundum. **A,** Craniolateral aspect. **B,** Dorsal aspect. **C,** Needle placement for akinesia of the eyelids in the cow.

D. Needle: 14-gauge, 1-inch to serve as a cannula1; 18-gauge, 4½-inch

E. Anesthetic: 7 to 15 ml of 2% lidocaine at the foramen orbitorotundum; 5 to 10 ml of 2% lidocaine for desensitizing the auriculopalpebral nerve

F. Method

1. Fully extend cow's head in a standing position with frontal and nasal bones parallel to the ground
2. Surgically prepare area posterior and ventral to the eye
3. Inject several milliliters of anesthetic with a small-gauge needle into the skin and subcutaneously into the notch formed by the zygomatic and temporal process of the malar bone (where the supraorbital process of the frontal bone meets the zygomatic arch) (see Fig. 5-11)
4. Place a 14-gauge, ½- or 1-inch needle (to serve as a cannula) through the skin as far anterior and ventral as possible in the notch

5. Direct a straight, 18-gauge, 4½-inch needle with no syringe attached (to feel the bony landmarks) through the cannula in a horizontal and slightly posterior direction, until it strikes the coronoid process of the mandible
6. Reposition the point of the needle anteriorly until it passes medially around this bone
7. Advance needle slightly posteriorly and somewhat ventrally until it strikes a solid bony plate, which is at a depth of between 3 and 4½ inches
8. Inject 15 ml of 2% lidocaine anterior to the foramen rotundum
9. Blocking the auriculopalpebral branch of the facial nerve (see Fig. 5-11, *C*)
   a. Fill a 10-ml syringe with local anesthetic, attach it to the needle, and partially withdraw the cannula
   b. Withdraw the needle until it almost leaves the skin, and direct it posteriorly for 2 to 3 inches lateral to the zygomatic arch while injecting lidocaine
   c. If the upper lid is involved in the surgical procedure, make a line of infiltration with local anesthetic subcutaneously about 1 inch from the margin of the lid

G. Advantages
   1. Technique is useful for enucleation of the eyeball and removal of tumors from eye and eyelids
   2. Technique is quick, easy, safe, and effective if done properly
   3. Less edema and inflammation result than when eyelids and orbit are infiltrated
   4. Surgery of cornea (removal of tumors and dermoids) can be done easily without retraction or fixation forceps if the eyeball is proptosed
   5. Peterson eye block is safer than retrobulbar injections of local anesthetic, which often lead to orbital hemorrhage, direct pressure on the globe, penetration of the globe, damage to the optic nerve, or injection into the optic nerve meninges

H. Disadvantages
   1. The cow's head is difficult to keep horizontal when the animal is in a chute or stanchion with the head tied to one side; this makes the landmarks difficult to locate

2. If the needle point strikes the pterygoid crest, the anesthesia drug will be deposited at the wrong site; therefore no anesthesia results following injection of the local anesthetic
3. In 50% of cases, incomplete anesthesia of the upper eyelid results because of sensory innervation from other nerves
4. Blinking is prevented for several hours
5. Sterile saline solution should be applied to the eye frequently during surgery to keep the cornea moist
6. Antibiotic eye ointments should be applied to the cornea after orbital replacement of the globe
7. Sunlight, dust, and wind in the eye must be avoided to prevent keratoconjunctivitis
8. The lids may be sutured together until motor activity of the lids returns

I. Complications
   1. In procedures other than enucleation, keratitis may result from postoperative drying of the cornea because effective block prevents blinking for several hours
   2. Penetration of the turbinates and injection with local anesthetic into the nasopharynx and optic nerve meninges can cause severe central nervous system toxicity, including certain clinical signs
      a. Hyperexcitability
      b. Lateral recumbency
      c. Tonic-clonic convulsions
      d. Opisthotonos
      e. Respiratory arrest
      f. Cardiac arrest

LOCAL ANESTHESIA OF THE FOOT: THREE METHODS

I. Infiltrating the tissues around the limb with local anesthetic solution (ring block)
II. Desensitizing specific nerves (regional anesthesia)
III. Injecting local anesthetic solution into accessible superficial vein in extremity isolated from circulation by placing tourniquet on animal's leg (intravenous regional anesthesia)
   A. Area blocked: extremity distal to tourniquet

B. Veins used: *A*, common dorsal metacarpal vein; *B*, radial vein; *C*, plantar metacarpal vein in the thoracic limb (Fig. 5-12); cranial branch of the lateral saphenous vein, lateral plantar digital vein in the pelvic limb (see Fig. 5-12).

C. Needle: 18-gauge, 1½ inch

D. Anesthetic: 10 to 30 ml 2% lidocaine in adult cattle; 3 to 10 ml lidocaine in small ruminants and pigs

E. Method: place rubber tourniquet proximal to the metatarsal or metacarpal region for foot surgery, or at a more proximal position for surgery of the carpal or tarsal region; rapidly inject local anesthetic into the prominent vein, directing the needle either proximally or distally

F. Advantages
    1. No special skill or knowledge of anatomy of the limb is needed
    2. Only one injection is required, with little risk of introducing bacteria

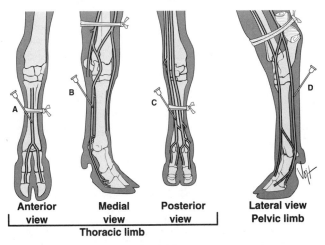

Anterior view	Medial view	Posterior view	Lateral view
			Pelvic limb

Thoracic limb

Fig. 5-12

Tourniquet and needle placement for intravenous regional anesthesia of the cow. In the thoracic limb, the needle tip is placed at **A,** the common dorsal metacarpal vein; **B,** the radial vein; or **C,** the plantar metacarpal vein. In the pelvic limb, the needle tip is placed at **D,** the cranial branch of the lateral saphenous vein.

   3. Onset of anesthesia distal to the tourniquet is rapid (5 to 10 minutes); anesthesia occurs last in the interdigital region
   4. Recovery is rapid after removal of tourniquet (5 to 10 minutes)
G. Disadvantages
   1. Inexplicable failure rate of 7%
   2. Occasional hematoma at the injection site
   3. Failure of anesthesia due to tourniquet slipping or extravascular injection
H. Complications: ischemic necrosis, severe lameness, and edema if tourniquet is left in place longer than 2 hours

TEAT AND UDDER ANESTHESIA OF CATTLE

 I. Techniques for surgical procedures on the forequarters and foreteats
   A. Paravertebral anesthesia of L1, L2, and L3 spinal nerves
   B. Segmental lumbar epidural anesthesia of L1, L2 and L3 spinal nerves
   C. Both techniques are difficult, and often result in cows lying down
 II. Techniques for surgical procedures of the caudal-most teats and escutcheon areas of the udder
   A. Desensitizing the perineal nerve in the standing cow
   B. High caudal epidural anesthesia in recumbent ruminants
   C. Lumbosacral epidural anesthesia in recumbent ruminants
III. Most surgical procedures on the teat (e.g., repair of a stenotic teat sphincter, repairs of teat fistulae and lacerations) are generally performed under local anesthesia
   A. Needle: 20- or 22-gauge, ½-inch or teat cannula
   B. Anesthetic: 6 to 10 ml of 2% lidocaine
   C. Methods
      1. Inverted V block: line infusion of the anesthetic using an inverted V pattern, which encloses the teat skin defect (Fig. 5-13, *A*)
      2. Ring block: local anesthetic infused into the skin and muscular tissue of base of the teat, after thorough cleaning of the external surface of the teat and quarter (Fig. 5-13, *B*)

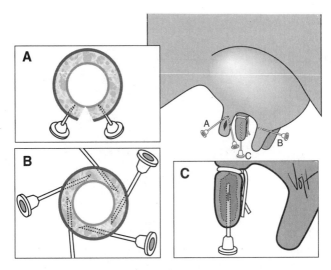

Fig. 5-13
Needle placement in the cow's teat. **A,** Inverted V block. **B,** Teat ring block. **C,** Tourniquet and cannula placement for teat cistern infusion.

    3. Teat infusion block
       a. Teat opening is cleaned
       b. Tourniquet is placed at the base of the teat
  D. Ten ml of 2% lidocaine is infused into teat cistern (Fig. 5-13 *C*)
       a. Mucous membrane of the teat cistern is anesthetized within 5 minutes; the muscular and skin layers remain sensitive; thereafter the remaining lidocaine is milked out and the tourniquet is removed

CHAPTER SIX

Local Anesthesia in Horses

**"A horse is dangerous at both ends and
uncomfortable in the middle."**

IAN FLEMING

OVERVIEW

Many diagnostic and surgical procedures can be performed safely
and humanely in the horse by coupling physical restraint and sedation with surface (topical) anesthesia, infiltration anesthesia,
nerve block (regional) anesthesia, or epidural anesthesia. Peripheral nerve blocks, intraarticular and intrabursal injections, and local infiltrations (ring block) are used to diagnose equine lameness
and to anesthetize surgical sites. Desensitization of the auriculopalpebral nerve is most frequently used to prevent voluntary
closure of the eyelids during examination and treatment of the eye.
Although regional anesthesia of the head can be induced by various techniques, the most frequently desensitized nerves of the head
are the supraorbital, infraorbital, and mandibular alveolar.

Caudal epidural anesthesia is used to facilitate surgery involving the tail, perineum, anus, rectum, vulva, vagina, and urethra
and for symptomatic relief of painful conditions during obstetric
manipulations.

Improper injection techniques contribute to inadequate anesthesia. Overdosing leads to more serious complications, including
ataxia of hindlimbs, hindlimb motor blockade, and recumbency.

REGIONAL ANESTHESIA OF THE HEAD

The most frequently desensitized nerves of the head
  I. Supraorbital (frontal)

II. Auriculopalpebral

III. Infraorbital

IV. Mandibular alveolar

ANESTHESIA OF UPPER EYELID AND FOREHEAD

I. Area blocked: upper eyelid except medial and lateral canthi

II. Nerve blocked: supraorbital (or frontal) nerve

III. Site: supraorbital foramen (Fig. 6-1, *A*)

IV. Needle: 22- to 25-gauge, 1-inch

V. Anesthetic: 5 ml of 2% lidocaine

VI. Method: palpate the supraorbital foramen about 5 to 7 cm above the medial canthus where it perforates the supraorbital process of the frontal bone; insert the needle into the foramen to a depth of 1.5 to 2 cm; inject 2 ml of lidocaine into the foramen: 1 ml as the needle is withdrawn and 2 ml subcutaneously over the foramen

VII. Use

A. Desensitization of the upper eyelid

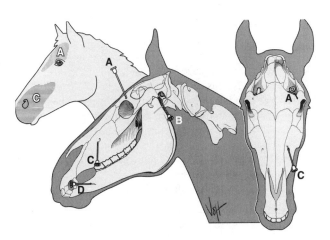

Fig. 6-1

Needle placement for nerve blocks on the head: **A,** supraorbital (or frontal); **B,** auriculopalpebral; **C,** infraorbital; **D,** mandibular alveolar nerves.

B. Blockade of the palpebral motor supply derived from the auriculopalpebral nerve

AKINESIA OF THE EYELIDS

I. Area blocked: paralysis of orbicularis oculi muscles; no desensitization

II. Nerve blocked: auriculopalpebral nerve (Fig. 6-1, *B*)

III. Site: caudal to posterior ramus of the mandible

IV. Needle: 22- to 25-gauge, 1-inch

V. Anesthetic: 5 ml of 2% lidocaine

VI. Method: insert the needle into the depression caudal to the mandible at the ventral edge of the temporal position of the zygomatic arch; inject local anesthetic subfascially as the needle is withdrawn

VII. Use: Examination of the eye; successful blockade of the motor nerve supply prevents the horse from closing the eyelids

ANESTHESIA OF THE UPPER LIP AND NOSE

I. Area blocked: upper lip and nostril, roof of nasal cavity, and related skin up to the infraorbital foramen

II. Nerve blocked: infraorbital nerve

III. Site: external opening of the infraorbital canal (Fig. 6-1, *C*)

IV. Needle: 22- to 25-gauge, 1-inch

V. Anesthetic: 5 ml of 2% lidocaine

VI. Method: find the bony lip of the infraorbital foramen, about halfway along and 2.5 cm dorsal to a line connecting the nasomaxillary notch and the anterior end of the facial crest; push the flat levator labii superioris muscle, which runs over the foramen, upward with the fingertips and place the needle tip at the foramen opening

VII. Use: simple lacerations in quiet or sedated horses

ANESTHESIA OF THE LOWER LIP

I. Area blocked: lower lip, all parts of mandible rostral up to and including the third premolar tooth (PM3)

II. Nerve blocked: mandibuloalveolar nerve

III. Site: within mandibular canal (Fig. 6-1, *D*)
IV. Needle: 20-gauge, 3-inch
  V. Anesthetic: 10 ml of 2% lidocaine
VI. Method: palpate the lateral border of the mental foramen as a ridge along the lateral aspect of the ramus in the middle of the interdental space; insert the needle into the mandibular canal as far as possible in a ventromedial direction; injection requires pressure, and fluid might partially drain back from the canal under the skin
VII. Use: simple lacerations in quiet or sedated horses

CAUDAL EPIDURAL ANESTHESIA

  I. Area blocked: tail, perineum, anus, rectum, vulva, vagina
 II. Nerves blocked: caudal nerves and last three pairs of sacral nerves
III. Site: epidural space in the first intercoccygeal space (Co1-Co2) (Fig. 6-2)
IV. Needles: spinal with stylet (spinal: 18-gauge, 2- to 3-inch; stylet: 2-gauge, 2-inch)

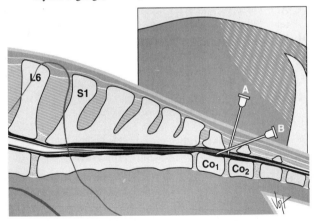

Fig. 6-2
Needle placement into **A** or **B**, caudal epidural space at the first intercoccygeal space (Co1-Co2). Stippled markings indicate desensitized subcutaneous area after caudal blockade.

V. Anesthetic: 6 to 10 ml of 2% lidocaine; other drugs can be considered (e.g., xylazine, xylazine-lidocaine combination) (see Chapter 4)

VI. Method

    A. Use proper restraint, depending on the horse's temperament; clip, surgically scrub, and disinfect the injection; make a skin wheal, and infiltrate the tissues down to the interarcuate ligament to minimize movement during insertion of the spinal needle

    B. Method A (see Fig. 6-2, *A*): insert the spinal needle into the epidural space in the center of the first intercoccygeal space at a right angle to the general contour of the croup, and press the needle ventrally in a median plane until it strikes the floor of the vertebral canal; withdraw the needle approximately 0.5 cm

    C. Method B (see Fig. 6-2, *B*): insert the spinal needle about 1 inch posterior to the first intercoccygeal space and slide its point ventrocranially at an angle of about 30 degrees to the horizontal plane and to its full length into the vertebral canal

    D. Test with a syringe of air for resistance to the injection; alternatively, fill the needle hub with isotonic saline solution and manipulate slightly until the solution is aspirated from the needle by subatmospheric epidural pressure (hanging drop technique); inject local anesthetic; needle can be left in place with stylet reinserted; maximum blockade may require 10 to 30 minutes, and it is not advisable to redose during this time if surgery is to be done with the horse standing

VII. Use

    A. Anesthesia of pelvic viscera without loss of hindleg motor control during obstetric manipulations

    B. Anesthesia of genitalia without loss of hindleg motor control during obstetric manipulations

    C. For standing surgical procedures of viscera and genitalia

        1. Caslick operation (for pneumovagina)

        2. Rectovaginal fistula repair

        3. Prolapsed rectum repair

        4. Urethrostomy

     5. Tail amputation

     6. Tenesmus prevention

VIII. Common causes for inadequate anesthesia or incomplete block

  A. Improper injection technique

     1. Use of solutions of diminished potency

     2. Inadequate dispersal of anesthetic

  B. Inappropriate angulation of the spinal needle

     1. Needle point strikes the dorsal aspect of the vertebral arch

     2. Deviation of the needle from the midline

  C. Horses that have fibrous connective tissue from previous epidural injections, which limits diffusion of anesthetic agent

  D. Anatomic peculiarities

     1. Presence of septa within the epidural space

     2. Presence of patent intervertebral foramina

IX. Complications

  A. Trauma to coccygeal nerve(s)

  B. Infection of the neural canal

  C. Extensive cranial migration of local anesthetic solution causing the following

     1. Ataxia

     2. Staggering

     3. Excitement

     4. Recumbency

REGIONAL ANESTHESIA OF THE LIMB

I. Perform peripheral nerve blocks on the most distal branches of the nerve trunks to gain as much information as possible in diagnosis of equine lameness; then conduct the examination proximally

II. The palmar (volar) digital nerves of the forelimb or the plantar digital nerves of the hindlimb branch dorsal to the fetlock at the level of the sesamoids, forming three digital nerves

  A. The anterior (or dorsal) digital nerve supplies sensory fibers to the anterior two thirds of the hoof

  B. The middle digital nerve (relatively unimportant)

C. The low palmar or plantar digital nerve, which is the most important clinically, supplies sensory fibers to the posterior third of the hoof, including portions, if not all, of the navicular area

PALMAR (VOLAR) OR PLANTAR DIGITAL NERVE BLOCK (Figs. 6-3, A and 6-4, A)

I. Area blocked: posterior third of the foot, including the navicular bursa

II. Nerves blocked: digital nerves

III. Site: palmar (volar)/plantar region of the pastern joint

IV. Needle: 20- to 25-gauge, 1-inch

V. Anesthetic: 2 ml of 2% lidocaine at each site

VI. Method: palpate the palmar (volar) or plantar nerve just palmar/plantar to the vein and artery, dorsal to the flexor tendon; insert the needle in the palmar/plantar region of the pastern joint, medially and/or laterally with the leg elevated or bearing weight

VII. Use: diagnosis of equine lameness

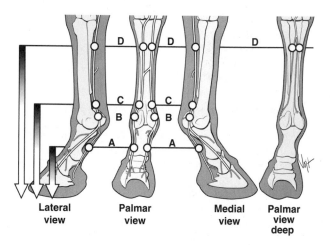

Lateral view **Palmar view** **Medial view** **Palmar view deep**

Fig. 6-3

Injection sites for nerve blocks on the left forelimb in the horse: **A,** palmar (digital); **B,** abaxial sesamoidean; **C,** low palmar; **D,** high palmar nerve.

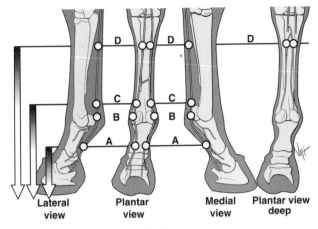

Fig. 6-4

Injection sites for nerve blocks on the left hindlimb in the horse: **A,** plantar digital; **B,** abaxial sesamoidean; **C,** low plantar; **D,** high plantar nerve.

ABAXIAL (BASILAR) SESAMOIDEAN NERVE BLOCK (Figs. 6-3, *B,* and 6-4, *B*)

  I. Area blocked: entire foot distal to the injection site, including the back of the pastern area and distal sesamoidean ligaments
 II. Nerves blocked: anterior and posterior digital nerves
III. Site: palmar region of the fetlock joint over abaxial surface of proximal sesamoids
 IV. Needle: 20- to 25-gauge, 1-inch
  V. Anesthetic: 3 ml of 2% lidocaine at each site
 VI. Method: palpate the digital nerve in the palmar region of the fetlock joint over the abaxial surface of proximal sesamoids, just palmar/plantar to the digital artery and vein; insert the needle subcutaneously at this site
VII. Use: diagnosis of equine lameness

PALMAR (VOLAR) OR PLANTAR NERVE BLOCK

  I. The palmar (volar) or plantar nerves can be desensitized at either a low site (low palmar/volar or low plantar nerve block) or a high site (high palmar/volar or higher plantar nerve block)

II. Midregion blocks (midmetacarpal or midmetatarsal) should be avoided because of the location of anastomotic branch, which transverses downward from medial to lateral

LOW PALMAR (VOLAR) OR PLANTAR NERVE BLOCK (Figs. 6-3, C and 6-4, C)

I. Area blocked: almost all structures distal to the fetlock and fetlock joint, except for a small area dorsal to the fetlock joint supplied by sensory fibers of the ulnar (Fig. 6-5) and musculocutaneous nerves (Fig. 6-7)

II. Nerves blocked: palmar or plantar nerves (medial/lateral: four-point block)

III. Site: medially and laterally at the level of the distal enlargements of metacarpals II and IV and metatarsals II and IV (splints)

IV. Needle: 20- to 25-gauge, 1-inch

V. Anesthetic: 2 to 3 ml of 2% lidocaine at each site

VI. Method

    A. Desensitize the palmar nerves (medial/lateral) by injecting the anesthetic between the flexor tendon and suspensory ligament

    B. Desensitize the palmar metacarpal and metatarsal nerves (medial/lateral) by injecting the anesthetic between the suspensory ligament and the splint bone

VII. Use: diagnosis of equine lameness

HIGH PALMAR (VOLAR) OR PLANTAR NERVE BLOCK (Figs. 6-3, D and 6-4, D)

I. Area blocked: palmar (volar) metacarpal or plantar metatarsal region and all of the digit distal to the fetlock

II. Nerves blocked: palmar or plantar nerves (medial/lateral)

III. Site: proximal quarter of the metacarpus or metatarsus proximal to the communicating branch of the medial and lateral palmar (volar) or plantar nerves

IV. Needle: 22-gauge, 1½-inch

V. Anesthetic: 2 to 3 ml of 2% lidocaine at each site

VI. Method: desensitize the medial and lateral palmar (volar) and plantar nerves by injecting anesthetic subfascially into the

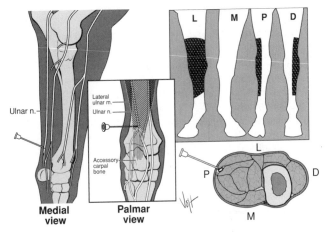

Fig. 6-5

Needle placement for ulnar nerve block: lateral, palmar, and cross-sectional views. Stippled markings indicate desensitized area (*L*, lateral; *P*, palmar; and *D*, dorsal views) after ulnar nerve block of the left forelimb.

groove between the suspensory ligament and the deep flexor tendon on both the medial and lateral sides

VII. Use

    A. Diagnosis of equine lameness

    B. The ulnar, median, and musculocutaneous nerves must be desensitized to produce complete anesthesia of the forelimb from the carpus distally

ULNAR NERVE BLOCK (see Fig. 6-5)

   I. Area blocked: lateral, or dorsal and palmar skin area

  II. Nerve blocked: ulnar nerve

 III. Site: 10 cm proximal to the accessory carpal bone

 IV. Needle: 22-gauge, 1-inch

  V. Anesthetic: 5 to 10 ml of 2% lidocaine

 VI. Method: the nerve is desensitized 1.5 cm deep beneath the fascia between the flexor carpi ulnaris and ulnaris lateralis muscle

VII. Use: anesthesia of part of the forelimb

MEDIAN NERVE BLOCK (Fig. 6-6)

I. Area blocked: lateral, medial, palmar, and dorsal skin areas
II. Nerve blocked: median nerve
III. Site: medial aspect of the forelimb 5 cm ventral to the elbow joint
IV. Needle: 20- to 22-gauge, 1½-inch
V. Anesthetic: 10 ml of 2% lidocaine
VI. Method: the median nerve is desensitized between the posterior border of the radius and the muscular belly of the internal flexor carpi radialis
VII. Use: anesthesia of part of the distal limb

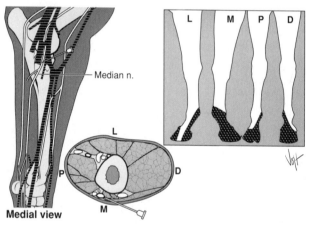

Fig. 6-6
Needle placement for median nerve block: medial and cross-sectional views. Stippled markings indicate desensitized area (*L*, lateral; M, medial; P, palmar; and D, dorsal views) after median nerve block of the left forelimb.

MUSCULOCUTANEOUS NERVE BLOCK
(Fig. 6-7)

I. Area blocked: medial, palmar, and dorsal skin area
II. Nerve blocked: cutaneous branch of the musculocutaneous nerve
III. Site: anteromedial aspect of the forelimb halfway between the elbow and carpus

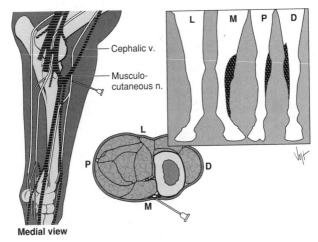

Medial view

Fig. 6-7

Needle placement for musculocutaneous nerve block: medial and cross-sectional views. Stippled markings indicate desensitized area (*M*, medial, *P*, palmar; *D*, dorsal views) after musculocutaneous nerve block of the right forelimb.

    IV. Needle: 22-gauge, 1-inch
    V. Anesthetic: 10 ml of 2% lidocaine
    VI. Method: the musculocutaneous nerve is desensitized subcutaneously, where it is easily palpated just cranial to the cephalic vein
    VII. Use: anesthesia of part of the forelimb

INTRAARTICULAR INJECTIONS

    I. General considerations
        A. Intraarticular injections require a surgical scrub to reduce the risk of introducing contaminants
        B. Use surgical gloves when performing complicated joint blocks
        C. Arthrocentesis implies aspiration of synovial fluid, but is usually done to allow for instillation of diagnostic and therapeutic agents
            1. Local anesthetic
                a. Adequate amount of local anesthetic should be administered

b. Enough time should be given for maximal effect and post-block examination
2. Saline flushes
3. Antibiotics
4. Hyaluronic acid
5. Antiinflammatory drugs

II. Common intraarticular and bursal injections at the most distal digit (Fig. 6-8)

A. Podotrochlear (navicular) bursa

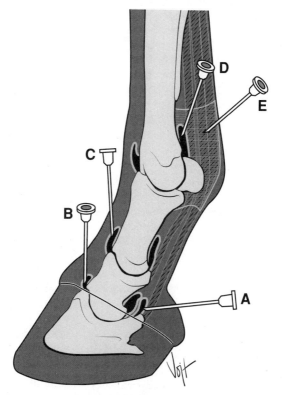

Fig. 6-8
Needle placement into **A**, podotrochlear (navicular) bursa; **B**, coffin joint; **C**, pastern joint; **D**, fetlock joint; **E**, and distal flexor tendon sheath.

B. Coffin joint
C. Pastern joint
D. Fetlock joint
E. Distal flexor tendon sheath

INTRAARTICULAR PODOTROCHLEAR (NAVICULAR) BURSA BLOCK

I. Site: podotrochlear (navicular) bursa (See Fig. 6-8, *A*)
II. Needle: 18-gauge spinal needle, 2- to 3-inch
III. Anesthetic: 2 to 5 ml 2% lidocaine
IV. Method: introduce the needle through the digital pad between the bulbs of the heel at the level of the coronary band until it strikes the bone along the midline while the limb is bearing weight; withdraw the needle until very little synovial fluid is aspirated, and then inject anesthetic

INTRAARTICULAR COFFIN BLOCK

I. Site: interphalangeal (coffin) joint (P2-P3) (See Fig. 6-8, *B*)
II. Needle: 18- to 20-gauge, 1½-inch
III. Anesthetic: 5 to 10 ml 2% lidocaine
IV. Method: insert the needle 1.5 cm proximal to the coronet approximately 2 cm lateral to the vertical center of the pastern and direct it obliquely ventral to the tendon toward the extensor process

INTRAARTICULAR PASTERN BLOCK

I. Site: interphalangeal (pastern) joint (P1-P2) (See Fig. 6-8, *C*)
II. Needle: 20- to 22-gauge, 1½-inch
III. Anesthetic: 5 to 8 ml 2% lidocaine
IV. Method: insert the needle medially or laterally to the midline on the palpable epicondyles of P2 for approximately 2.5 cm in a vertical direction

INTRAARTICULAR FETLOCK BLOCK

I. Site: metacarpophalangeal or metatarsophalangeal (fetlock) joint (See Fig. 6-8, *D*)

II. Needle: 20- to 22-gauge spinal needle, 1½-inch
III. Anesthetic: 5 to 10 ml 2% lidocaine
IV. Method: insert the needle into the lateral pouch distal to the splint bone and dorsal to the anular ligament of the fetlock to a depth of approximately 0.5 to 1 cm

DIGITAL FLEXOR TENDON SHEATH BLOCK

I. Site: digital flexor tendon sheath (See Fig. 6-8, *E*)
II. Needle: 18- to 20-gauge, 1½-inch
III. Anesthetic: 10 ml 2% lidocaine
IV. Method: insert the needle at the distal end of the splint ("button"), either medially or laterally cranial to the deep and superficial flexor tendons and caudal to the suspensory ligament

INTRAARTICULAR RADIOCARPAL BLOCK

I. Site: radiocarpal (antebrachial carpal) joint (Fig. 6-9, *A*)
II. Needle: 20-gauge, 1½-inch
III. Anesthetic: 5 to 10 ml 2% lidocaine
IV. Method: insert the needle between the radiocarpal joint space on either side of the palpable extensor carpi radialis tendon, while the carpus is flexed

INTRAARTICULAR INTERCARPAL BLOCK

I. Site: intercarpal (middle carpal) joint (Fig. 6-9, *B*)
II. Needle: 20-gauge, 1½-inch
III. Anesthetic: 5 to 10 ml 2% lidocaine
IV. Method: insert the needle between the intercarpal joint space on either side of the palpable extensor carpi radialis tendon, while the carpus is flexed

CUNEAN BURSA BLOCK

I. Site: cunean bursa on the medial aspect of the tarsus (Fig. 6-10, *A*)
II. Needle: 22-gauge, 1-inch
III. Anesthetic: at least 10 ml 2% lidocaine
IV. Method: insert the needle approximately 1.5 cm distal to the cunean tendon (medial branch of the tibialis anterior muscle)

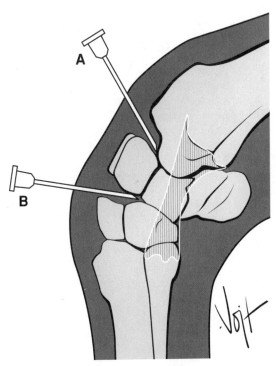

Fig. 6-9

Needle placement into **A**, radial carpal joint spaces **B**, and intercarpal joint spaces.

and advance it between the cunean tendon and the tarsal bone to penetrate the bursa from distally; at least 20 minutes are required for maximum anesthetic effect

INTRAARTICULAR TARSOMETATARSAL BLOCK

I. Site: tarsometatarsal joint at the posterior lateral aspect of the hock over the lateral head of the splint (metatarsal IV) (Fig. 6-10, *B*)

II. Needle: 22-gauge, 1-inch

III. Anesthetic: 6 to 8 ml 2% lidocaine

IV. Method: the needle is most easily inserted into the tarsometa-

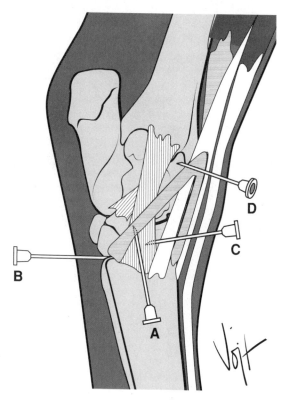

Fig. 6-10

Needle placement into **A**, cunean bursa and **B**, the tarsometatarsal joint spaces; **C**, intertarsal joint spaces and **D**, tibiotarsal joint spaces.

tarsal joint on the posterior lateral aspect of the hock proximal to the palpable lateral head of the splint; the bevel of the needle must be turned away from the bone to allow for injection of the anesthetic solution

INTRAARTICULAR INTERTARSAL BLOCK

I. Site: distal intertarsal joint on the medial aspect of the tarsus (Fig. 6-10, *C*)

II. Needle: 22-gauge, 1-inch
III. Anesthetic: 6 ml 2% lidocaine
IV. Method: insert the needle into the joint at a right angle to the skin ventral to the cunean tendon; inject local anesthetic using considerable pressure and turning the needle bevel

INTRAARTICULAR TIBIOTARSAL BLOCK

I. Site: tibiotarsal (tarsocrural) joint at the craniomedial aspect of the tibia (Fig. 6-10, *D*)
II. Needle: 18-gauge, 1½-inch
III. Anesthetic: 15 ml 2% lidocaine
IV. Method: the needle is easily inserted less than 2 cm deep into the skin and superficial capsule, 2 to 3 cm ventral to the medial malleolus of the tibia on either the medial or lateral side of the saphenous vein; inject local anesthetic after synovial fluid is recovered on aspiration

CHAPTER SEVEN

Local Anesthesia in Dogs and Cats

"Think globally, act locally."
OLIVER WENDELL HOLMES, JR.

OVERVIEW

Local anesthetic techniques can be used in selected small animals to perform surgery without the depressant effects of general anesthesia. Local anesthesia is usually administered in combination with sedation or tranquilization to produce a cooperative patient. Local analgesia techniques can also be used to produce postoperative analgesia in surgical patients. Commonly used techniques in small animals include infiltration anesthesia, nerve blocks (e.g., selected nerve blocks about the head), brachial plexus block, intravenous (IV) regional anesthesia, and continuous epidural anesthesia. Epidural opioid analgesia, intercostal nerve blocks, and interpleural analgesia provide long-lasting postoperative pain relief.

REGIONAL ANESTHESIA OF THE HEAD
(Fig. 7-1)

When combined with effective sedation of dogs that do not object to physical restraint or oral examination, the desensitization of the following nerves of the head can be routinely considered

    I. Infraorbital
   II. Maxillary
  III. Ophthalmic
  IV. Mental
   V. Mandibuloalveolar

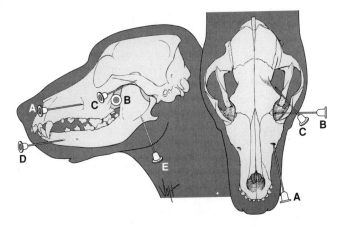

Fig. 7-1

Needle placement for nerve blocks on the head. **A**, Infraorbital. **B**, Maxillary. **C**, Ophthalmic. **D**, Mental. **E**, Mandibuloalveolar.

ANESTHESIA OF THE EYE

I. Area blocked: eye, orbit, conjunctiva, eyelids, and forehead skin

II. Nerves blocked: lacrimal, zygomatic, and ophthalmic (i.e., ophthalmic division of the trigeminal nerve)

III. Site: at the orbital fissure (see Fig. 7-1, *C*)

IV. Needle: 22- to 25-gauge, 1-inch

V. Anesthetic: 2 ml of 1% lidocaine

VI. Method: insert the needle ventral to the border of the zygomatic process at the lateral canthus of the eye; the point of the needle should be approximately 0.5 cm cranial to the anterior border of the vertical portion of the ramus of the mandible; advance the needle medial to the ramus of the mandible in a mediodorsal and somewhat caudal direction until it reaches the orbital fissure

ANESTHESIA OF MAXILLA, UPPER TEETH, NOSE, AND UPPER LIP

I. Area blocked: maxilla, upper teeth, nose, and upper lip

II. Nerve blocked: maxillary

III. Site: perpendicular portion of the palatine bone between the maxillary foramen and foramen rotundum (see Fig. 7-1, *B*)

IV. Needle: 22- to 25-gauge, 1-inch

V. Anesthetic: 2 ml of 1% lidocaine

VI. Method: insert the needle through the skin at an angle of 90 degrees, in a medial direction, ventral to the border of the zygomatic process and approximately 0.5 cm caudal to the lateral canthus of the eye; advance the needle in close proximity to the pterygopalatine fossa; local anesthetic is administered at the point at which the maxillary nerve courses perpendicular to the palatine bone between the maxillary foramen and foramen rotundum

ANESTHESIA OF UPPER LIP AND NOSE

I. Area blocked: upper lip and nose, roof of nasal cavity, and related skin ventral to the infraorbital foramen

II. Nerve blocked: infraorbital

III. Site: point of emergence of the nerve from the infraorbital canal (see Fig. 7-1, *A*)

IV. Needle: 22- to 25-gauge, 1-inch

V. Anesthetic: 2 ml of 1% lidocaine

VI. Method: insert the needle either intraorally or extraorally approximately 1 cm cranial to the bony lip of the infraorbital foramen; advance the needle to the infraorbital foramen, which can be felt between the dorsal border of the zygomatic process and the gum of the canine tooth

ANESTHESIA OF THE LOWER LIP

I. Area blocked: lower lip

II. Nerve blocked: mental

III. Site: rostral to the mental foramen (see Fig. 7-1, *D*)

IV. Needle: 22- to 25-gauge, 1-inch

V. Anesthetic: 2 ml of 1% lidocaine

VI. Method: insert the needle over the mental nerve, rostral to the middle mental foramen at the level of the second premolar tooth

ANESTHESIA OF THE MANDIBLE

I. Area blocked: cheek teeth, canine, incisors, skin, and mucosa of the chin and lower lip

II. Nerve blocked: inferior alveolar branch of the mandibular nerve

III. Site: point of entry of the nerve into the mandibular canal at the mandibular foramen (see Fig. 7-1, *E*)

IV. Needle used: 22- to 25-gauge, 1-inch

V. Anesthetic: 2 ml of 1% lidocaine

VI. Method: insert the needle at the lower angle of the jaw approximately 1.5 cm rostral to the angular process; advance the needle 1.5 cm dorsally against the medial surface of the ramus of the mandible to the palpable lip of the mandibular foramen

ANESTHESIA OF THE FOOT

I. Anesthesia of the foot may be induced by the following techniques

 A. Infiltration of the tissues around the limb with local anesthetic solution (ring block)

 B. Infiltration of the brachial plexus by local anesthetic (brachial plexus block)

 C. IV injection of anesthetic into an accessible superficial vein in a distal extremity that is isolated from circulation by placing a tourniquet on the animal's leg (IV regional anesthesia)

 D. Injection of local anesthetic into the lumbosacral epidural space (anesthesia of the hindlegs)

 E. Perineural infiltration of sensory nerves in the limbs

BRACHIAL PLEXUS BLOCK

I. Area blocked: distal foot, up to the elbow region

II. Nerves blocked: radial, median, ulnar, musculocutaneous, and axillary nerves

III. Site: medial to the shoulder joint (see Fig. 7-2)

IV. Needle: 22-gauge, 3-inch

V. Anesthetic: 10 to 15 ml of 2% lidocaine

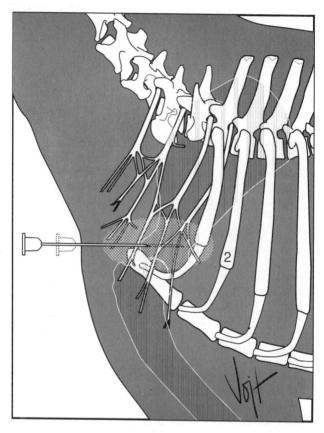

Fig. 7-2
Needle placement for brachial plexus block, lateral aspect of left thoracic limb in the dog. *2* is the second rib.

VI. Method: insert the needle medial to the shoulder joint toward the costochondral junction and parallel to the vertebral column; inject the anesthetic slowly as the needle is withdrawn; anesthesia can be obtained within 20 minutes and for 2 hours.

VII. Advantages

A. Relatively simple and safe to perform

B. Produces selective anesthesia and relaxation of the limb distal to the elbow joint

VIII. Disadvantages

A. Relatively long waiting period (15 to 30 minutes) required

B. Occasional failure to obtain complete anesthesia, particularly in fat dogs

IX. Complications

A. Toxic symptoms after intravascular administration of the local anesthetic

B. Lack of anesthesia after inadvertent intravascular injection

INTRAVENOUS REGIONAL ANESTHESIA

I. Area blocked: extremity distal to tourniquet

II. Nerves blocked: nerve endings in peripheral tissues

III. Site: any superficial vein distal to tourniquet

IV. Needle: 22-gauge, 1½-inch

V. Anesthetic: 2 to 3 ml of 1% lidocaine (without epinephrine)

VI. Method: the limb is first desanguinated by wrapping it with an Esmarch bandage; a rubber tourniquet is placed around the forearm just proximal to the elbow for thoracic limb surgery or proximal to the hock for pelvic limb surgery. The tourniquet must be tight enough to overcome blood pressure. Once the tourniquet is secured, the Esmarch bandage is unwrapped, and local anesthetic is injected with light pressure (BIER-block)

VII. Advantages

A. Safe and simple technique

B. Lack of toxicity to organs if the occlusion of blood supply is limited to 2 hours

C. Blood-free surgery site is ideal for taking biopsies and removing foreign bodies from the paws

VIII. Disadvantages: limited to 2 hours

IX. Complications

A. Shock can occur if tourniquet is left on more than 4 hours (reversible)

B. Death can occur from sepsis and endotoxemia if tourniquet is left on more than 8 to 10 hours

LUMBOSACRAL EPIDURAL ANESTHESIA

I. Indications

    A. Animals that are severely depressed, are in shock, or require immediate surgery of the rear quarters

    B. Animals that are at high risk, are aged, or in which the use of other analgesic or anesthetic agents is contraindicated

    C. To provide analgesia after abdominal surgery or surgery of the rear limbs; opioids are used

II. Specific procedures

    A. Postoperative analgesia

    B. Surgery

        1. Tail amputations

        2. Anal sac therapy or perianal surgery

        3. Rear limb lacerations or fractures

        4. Urolithiasis therapy

        5. Abdominal surgery

        6. Cesarean sections

        7. Obstetric manipulations

        8. Surgical procedures of the tail, perineum, vulva, vagina, rectum, and bladder

III. Landmarks and anatomy (Fig. 7-3)

    A. Right and left cranial dorsal iliac wings of the ilium

    B. Spinous process of the seventh lumbar vertebra and the median sacral crest

    C. Important anatomic features

        1. Shape of lumbar and sacral spinous processes

        2. Interspinous ligament

        3. Ligamentum arcuatum (ligamentum flavum)

        4. Terminal portion of the dural sac

        5. Filum terminale

        6. Intervertebral disk

    D. The spinal cord usually ends at vertebral body L6 in the dog and S1 in the cat; therefore the procedure is more hazardous when performed in the cat

IV. Equipment

    A. 2- or 4-inch, 18- or 20-gauge short beveled spinal needle with stylet (disposable needle preferred)

    B. One 2.5-ml and one 5-ml syringe

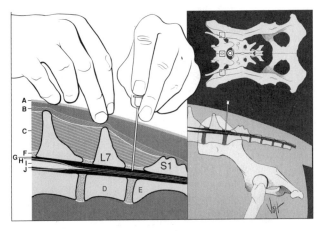

Fig. 7-3

Needle placement for lumbosacral epidural (between *L7* and *S1*) anesthesia in the dog, lateral and dorsal aspects. *A*, Skin; *B*, supraspinous ligament; *C*, interspinous ligament; *D*, seventh lumbar vertebra; *E*, sacrum; *F*, interarcuate ligament (ligamentum flavum); *G*, epidural space; *H*, dura mater spinalis; *I*, spinal cord; *J*, subarachnoid space containing cerebrospinal fluid (CSF).

    C. A thin-walled, 18-gauge, 3-inch needle is used if a polyethylene catheter is to be placed for continuous epidural anesthesia

V. Procedure

    A. Perform a surgical preparation; this is a sterile procedure

    B. Place the spinal needle perpendicular to the skin surface at the midline of the lumbosacral space; this space can be palpated halfway between the dorsoiliac wings and just caudal to the dorsal spinous process of the seventh lumbar vertebra (see Fig. 7-3)

        1. Infiltration of the area with 2% lidocaine may facilitate placement of the spinal needle

        2. Push the spinal needle ventrally in a slight cranial or caudal angle as needed

    C. Resistance is usually encountered on reaching the ligamentum flavum; A distinct "pop" is usually felt when the needle is advanced through this ligament

    D. On penetrating the ligamentum flavum, the needle is in the epidural space

       1. Needle depth may vary from ½ to 1½ inches, depending on animal size

       2. Remove the stylet and examine the needle for blood or cerebrospinal fluid (CSF); if no blood or CSF is observed, the needle should be aspirated for blood or CSF

       3. Inject 1 to 2 ml of air to check for proper needle placement

          a. If subcutaneous crepitus is felt, the needle is incorrectly placed and should be repositioned

          b. No resistance should be felt to the injection of air or local anesthetic agent

VI. Doses

    A. The dosage varies depending on the desired effect

    B. 2% lidocaine or 0.75% bupivacaine is the agent of choice; inject 1 ml of local anesthetic for each 10 pounds of body weight; this will produce anesthesia as far cranial as L2; if anesthesia is required up to T5, the dose may be increased to 1 ml of local anesthetic per 7.5 pounds of body weight

       1. A test dose of 0.5 to 1 ml of 2% lidocaine produces almost immediate dilation of the external anal sphincter, followed by relaxation and ataxia of pelvic limbs within 3 to 5 minutes

       2. Small amounts of 1:200,000 epinephrine are added to lidocaine to delay the rate of absorption and thus prolong anesthetic action

    C. Bupivacaine with epinephrine (Marcaine) produces 4- to 6-hour periods of anesthesia

VII. Continuous epidural anesthesia in dogs

    A. Procedure

       1. The procedure is similar to that previously described, except that a larger needle is used through which a catheter is passed (Fig. 7-4)

       2. Withdraw the needle, but leave the catheter in place

       3. Only ½ inch of catheter should be advanced into the epidural space

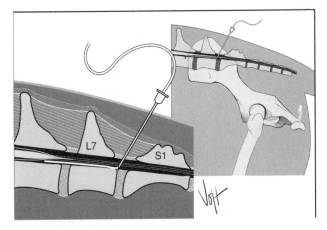

Fig. 7-4

Needle placement for continuous epidural anesthesia or opioid analagesia in the dog, shown in the lateral and dorsal aspects. *L7* and *S1* are the spinous processes of the seventh lumbar and the first sacral vertebrae.

    B. Advantages
        1. Ability to tailor the duration of anesthesia to the length of operation
        2. Route for injecting epidural opioids during and after surgery (see epidural opioid analgesia)
    C. Disadvantages
        1. Technically difficult
        2. Potential to produce damage to the spinal cord, meninges, and nerves
        3. Risk of infection
        4. Catheter-related problems (e.g. kinks, displacement, clotting with fibrin)
VIII. Factors influencing cranial level of blockade
    A. Size of patient
    B. Conformation of patient
    C. Volume of drug injected
    D. Drug mass
    E. Rate of injection

    F. Direction of needle bevel

    G. Age of patient

    H. Obesity

    I. Intraabdominal pressure attributable to presence and size of abdominal mass (e.g., pregnancy)
1. Pregnant animals generally require a medical dosage per body weight of the local anesthetic
2. The volume of the epidural space in pregnant animals is decreased because of distention of epidural veins/engorgement
3. The sensitivity of neural tissue to hormonal changes is increased

    J. Position of patient: gravity has a more definite role in the spread of subarachnoid anesthesia than in epidural anesthesia; however, with both techniques, a more rapid onset to maximal segmental anesthesia (unilateral anesthesia), a longer duration of anesthesia, and a more intensive motor blockade are achieved in the dependent side than in the upper side

IX. Proposed site of action after epidural injection (Table 7-1)

X. Possible complications

    A. Injection of local anesthetic into the vertebral sinuses
1. Vomiting, tremors
2. Decreased blood pressure caused by peripheral vasodilation
3. Convulsions
4. Paralysis

    B. Respiratory depression and paralysis in dogs and cats caused by drug overdose
1. The drug must migrate to approximately C5 or C7 to produce complete respiratory paralysis from blockade of the phrenic nerves
2. The cephalad spread of anesthesia after epidural or subarachnoid injection (of specifically prepared hyperbaric solution, e.g. "heavy nupercaine" in 6% glucose) is limited in an animal that is kept in a sitting position

    C. Temperature may fall in small animals because they are unable to shiver; the patient's rear quarters should be kept warm by wrapping them in a towel or a water blanket

TABLE 7-1
PROPOSED SITE OF ACTION AFTER EPIDURAL INJECTION

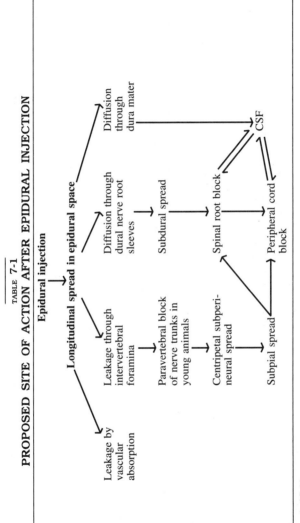

CSF, Cerebrospinal fluid.

    D. Add a sedative or tranquilizer to produce a cooperative patient

EPIDURAL OPIOID ANALGESIA

I. Indications
    A. Intraoperative analgesia
    B. Postoperative analgesia
    C. Critical care patients

II. Site of opioid injection
    A. Lumbosacral epidural space (single-dose injection) (see Fig. 7-3)
    B. Anterior lumbar epidural space (catheter technique) (see Fig. 7-4)

III. Drugs
    A. Epidural morphine (0.1 mg/kg diluted in 0.13 to 0.26 ml/kg of 0.9% NaCl solution) produces pain relief 30 to 60 minutes after injection and for as long as 10 to 24 hours
    B. Epidural oxymorphone (0.05 to 0.1 mg/kg diluted in 0.26 ml/kg of 0.9% NaCl solution) produces pain relief 20 to 40 minutes after injection and for an approximate duration of 10 to 20 hours
    C. Epidural fentanyl (1 to 10 μg/kg diluted in 0.26 ml/kg of 0.9% NaCl solution) produces pain relief 15 to 20 minutes after administration, with analgesia lasting 3 to 5 hours

IV. Advantages
    A. Relief of somatic and visceral pain is more profound and prolonged with smaller doses than the analgesia produced by comparable parenterally administered (intramuscular, IV) opioids
    B. No interference with sensory function
    C. No interference with motor function
    D. Minimal depression of the sympathetic nervous system
    E. Reversal of side effects by low-dose, IV infusion of opioid antagonists (e.g., naloxone)

V. Potential side effects (rare)
    A. Respiratory depression
    B. Urinary retention
    C. Delayed gastrointestinal motility

    D. Vomiting
    E. Pruritus
VI. Complications
    A. Respiratory depression after large doses (>1 mg/kg) of epidural morphine
    B. Catheter-related problems
        1. Catheter displacement
        2. Occlusion
        3. Infection

INTERCOSTAL NERVE BLOCKS

  I. Indications
     A. Relief of pain during thoracotomy
     B. Analgesia after thoracotomy
     C. Pleural drainage
     D. Rib fractures
 II. Nerves blocked: intercostals both cranial and caudal to the incision or injury site because of overlap of nerve supply
III. Site: intercostal spaces (R3 to R6) near the intercostal foramen (Fig. 7-5)
 IV. Needle: 22- to 25-gauge, 1-inch
  V. Anesthetic: 0.25-1 ml of 0.25% or 0.5% bupivacaine/site, with or without epinephrine 1:200,000
     A. Small dog–0.25 ml/site
     B. Medium dog–0.5 ml/site
     C. Large dog–1 ml/site
 VI. Method: insert the needle through the skin at a 90-degree angle caudal to the rib (R3 to R6) near the intervertebral foramen; inject small volumes and/or diluted anesthetic solutions into a minimum of two adjacent intercostal spaces, both cranial and caudal to the incision or injury site because of overlap of nerve supply; the total dosage should not exceed 3 mg/kg because the technique produces high blood concentrations of the anesthetic
VII. Advantages
     A. Selective intercostal nerve block is easily performed because of the proximity of each nerve to its adjacent rib
     B. The intercostal nerves can be visualized beneath the pleura during thoracotomy

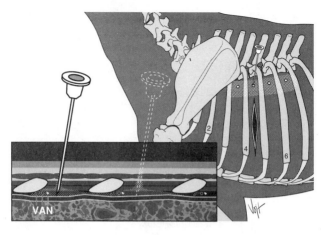

Fig. 7-5

Needle placement for intercostal nerve blocks in the dog, shown in the lateral aspect and the sagittal section. *2, 4, 6* are the second, fourth, and sixth rib; *VAN* is the intercostal vein, artery, and nerve.

    C. The technique provides consistent analgesia for 3 to 6 hours without respiratory depression

VIII. Complications

    A. Pneumothorax after faulty technique

    B. Impaired blood-gas exchange (hypercarbia, hypoxemia) in dogs with pulmonary diseases

INTERPLEURAL REGIONAL ANALGESIA

  I. Indications

    A. Relief of pain originating from the following conditions

      1. Thoracotomy

      2. Rib fractures

      3. Mastectomy

      4. Chronic pancreatitis

      5. Cholocystectomy

      6. Renal surgery

      7. Abdominal cancer

      8. Metastasis of the chest wall, pleura, and mediastinum

    II. Nerves blocked: mechanisms of pain relief are not fully understood

        A. Retrograde diffusion of local anesthetic through the parietal pleura, causing intercostal nerve block

        B. Desensitization of the thoracic sympathetic chain and splanchnic nerves

   III. Site: place a catheter into the pleural space either percutaneously or before closure of a thoracotomy (Fig. 7-6).

   IV. Equipment: 17-gauge, 2-inch, Huber-point (Tuohy) needle; medical grade silastic tubing, 5 to 10 cm, 2-mm inside diameter; sterile sets for single, continuous interpleural analgesia are available

    V. Anesthetic: approximately 1 to 2 mg bupivacaine/kg (0.5%, with or without 1:200,000 epinephrine)

   VI. Method: in a well-sedated dog, desensitize the skin, subcutaneous tissue, periosteum, and perietal pleura over the caudal border of the rib with 1 to 2 ml of 2% lidocaine, using a 22-gauge, 1-inch needle; then use the Huber-point needle to place the catheter with minimal resistance into the subat-

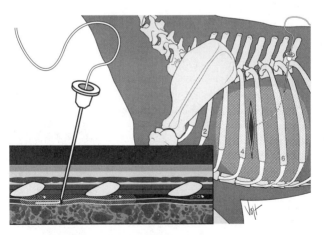

Fig. 7-6

Needle and catheter placement for interpleural regional analgesia in the dog, shown in the left lateral aspect and the sagittal section. *2, 4, 6* are the second, fourth, and sixth rib.

mospheric pleural space, 3 to 4 cm beyond the needle tip (see Fig. 7-6); withdraw the needle over the catheter and leave the catheter in place; catheter placement in the open chest is accomplished by inserting the Tuohy needle through the skin at least two intercostal spaces caudal to the incision and passing the catheter through the needle subpleurally under direct vision; inject local anesthetic over 1 to 2 minutes following negative aspiration of air or blood through the catheter; then clear the catheter with 2 ml of physiologic saline solution.

VII. Advantages
   A. The procedure is simple to perform
   B. One needlestick is needed in contrast to multiple intercostal nerve blocks
   C. Postthoracotomy pain relief lasts longer (3 to 12 hours) than analgesia produced by subcutaneous morphine (0.5 mg/kg) or selective intercostal nerve blocks with bupivacaine (0.5 ml of 0.5% bupivacaine per site)
   D. Long-term use (over several weeks) of an interpleural catheter is possible

VIII. Complications
   A. Infection
   B. Phrenic nerve paralysis or paresis; paradoxic respiration with negative intraabdominal pressure
   C. Tachyphylaxis to local anesthetic
   D. High anesthetic blood concentration
   E. Systemic toxicity after excessive doses of the local anesthetic (>3 mg bupivacaine/kg)
   F. Catheter-related complications (e.g., pneumothroax)
   G. Minimal pain relief
      1. Misplaced catheter
      2. Excessive bleeding into the pleural space
      3. Pleural effusion

CHAPTER EIGHT

Specific Intravenous Anesthetic Drugs

"To sleep: perchance to dream"
WILLIAM SHAKESPEARE

OVERVIEW

A variety of injectable anesthetic drugs can be used to induce chemical restraint and general anesthesia. Proper use of preanesthetic medication (tranquilizers, sedatives, analgesics) is imperative if anesthetic drugs are to produce the desired effect and if detrimental side effects are to be avoided. Injectable anesthetic drugs are often more convenient and economical to use than inhalation anesthetic drugs. Their principal disadvantage is that once administered, they are not immediately eliminated, although several injectable drugs (thiobarbiturates, methohexital, propofol, etomidate) have a very short duration of action.

GENERAL CONSIDERATIONS

I. All degrees of central nervous system (CNS) depression can be produced, from drowsiness and mild sedation to anesthesia and coma

II. Factors that determine rate of onset and amount of depression
   A. Anesthetic drug used
   B. Dose
   C. Route of administration (intramuscular [IM], intraperitoneal, intravenous [IV])

    D. Animal's level of consciousness (excited vs. depressed) when the drug is administered

    E. Acid-base and electrolyte balance; acidosis enhances barbiturate anesthesia

    F. Animal's cardiac output

    G. Drug tolerance

    H. Interactions with other drugs

III. Most injectable anesthetic drugs produce unconsciousness by depressing the cerebral cortex

    A. They are used to control convulsions

    B. Barbiturates increase the threshold of spinal reflexes and can be used clinically for the treatment of strychnine poisoning

IV. Routes of administration

    A. Most injectable drugs are administered intravenously; ketamine and tiletamine-zolazepam can be administered intramuscularly

    B. Sodium salts of barbiturates can be injected in a solution of up to 10%, guaifenesin in a solution of up to 10%, and chloral hydrate in a solution of up to 7%

    C. Because of the extreme alkalinity of barbiturate solutions, subcutaneous injection results in necrosis and sloughing; thiobarbiturates are not injected intramuscularly or subcutaneously

V. Dose is calculated on the basis of lean body mass (body weight minus fat)

BARBITURATE ANESTHESIA

I. Barbiturates are categorized according to their duration of action

    A. Long: many hours (8 to 12)

    B. Intermediate: several hours (2 to 6)

    C. Short: 45 minutes to 1.5 hours

    D. Ultrashort: 5 to 15 minutes

II. Official names

	APPROPRIATE DURATION OF ACTION
Phenobarbital sodium	Long
Barbital sodium	Long

Amobarbital sodium	Intermediate
Pentobarbital sodium	Short (Table 8-1)
Secobarbital sodium	Short
Thiopental sodium	Ultrashort
Thiamylal sodium	Ultrashort
Thialbarbitone sodium	Ultrashort
Methohexital	Ultrashort

III. General anesthetic actions of barbiturates

   A. Effects on the CNS

   1. CNS depression ranging from drowsiness and mild sedation to coma

   2. Response to barbiturate anesthesia

   a. Pentobarbital sodium and the ultrashort-acting barbiturates decrease cerebral blood flow (CBF), cerebral metabolic rate of oxygen ($CMRO_2$), and neuronal activity of the brain (e.g., dog); the CBF/$CMRO_2$ ratio is unchanged or increased; there are minimal changes in CSF pressure if ventilation is normal

   b. Barbiturates minimally depress arterial blood pressure (BP) and intracranial pressure and increase cerebral perfusion pressure

   c. Barbiturates are used to produce a general anesthesia (short-acting) or to induce a patient to surgical anesthesia (ultrashort-acting)

   d. Barbiturates are universally poor analgesics at subhypnotic dosages

   B. Organ system effects and responses

   1. Effects on the respiratory system

   a. Barbiturates are respiratory depressants

   (1) They depress respiratory centers in the medulla and the areas of the brain responsible for the characteristic rhythmic pattern of respiratory movement (apneustic and pneumotaxic centers)

   (2) The degree of respiratory depression is related to the dose and rate of drug administration

   b. Coughing, sneezing, hiccoughing, and laryngospasm occur frequently; these effects are caused by excessive salivary secretion and are minimized by preanesthetic medication (atropine, glycopyrrolate)

TABLE 8-1

INTRAVENOUS (mg/lb) DRUGS COMMONLY USED TO PRODUCE ANESTHESIA OF SHORT DURATION

	AGENT	HORSE	DOG	CAT	PIG	COW	GOAT
1.	Thiamylal	3-5	4-6	4-6	4-6	2-5	2-5
2.	Thiopental	3-5	4-6	4-6	4-6	2-5	2-5
3.	Etomidate		0.5-2	0.5-2	0.5-2		
4.	Propofol	4-6	2-6	2-6	2-6		
5.	Guaifenesin	30-60	20-40		20-40		30-60
6.	Chloral hydrate				6-9 g/100 lb	6-10 g/100 lb	6-10 g/100 lb
7.	Chloral hydrate (7% solution)	10 ml/100 lb*			20-30 ml/100 lb	20-30 ml/100 lb	20-30 ml/100 lb
8.	Chloropent	10 ml/100 lb				10 ml/100 lb	10 ml/100 lb
	Thiopental	2-4				2-4	2-4
9.	Ketamine			1-3	1-3		1-3
10.	Telazol		2-5	1-5	2-5	2-5	1-5
11.	Guaifenesin	20-40	15-40		15-40	20-40	15-40
	Thiopental	2-4	2-4		2-4	2-4	

No.	Drug					
12.	Guaifenesin	20-40	15-40	—	20-40	20-40
	Ketamine	0.5-0.7	0.5	—	0.3-0.5	0.3-0.5
13.	Acepromazine	—	0.1	0.2	—	—
	Ketamine	—	5.0	1-3	—	—
14.	Xylazine†	0.5	0.3	0.3	0.04	0.02
	Ketamine	0.5-1	3	1-3	1-3	1-3
15.	Xylazine	0.5	0.2	0.3	0.05	0.04
	Telazol	0.5-1	3	1-3	1-3	1-3
16.	Diazepam‡	—	0.15	0.2	0.1	—
	Ketamine	—	2-3	2-3	2-3	—
17.	Innovar-Vet	—	1 ml/30 lb	1 ml/40 lb	—	—
	Pentobarbital	1-3	1-3	1-3	—	—
18.	Xylazine, guaifenesin, ketamine	(500 ml 5% guaifenesin + 500 mg ketamine + 25 mg xylazine [ruminants]; 500 ml 5% guaifenesin + 500 mg ketamine + 500 mg xylazine [horses])				

*Sedative dose.

†Detomidine, 1-5 µg/lb intravenously, can be used in xylazine drug combinations.

‡Midazolam, 0.1-0.3 mg/lb intravenously, can be used in diazepam drug combinations.

(1) Laryngospasm is one of the common complications of barbiturate anesthesia in dogs and cats

(2) A short period of apnea frequently occurs after IV bolus administration of barbiturate

c. When respiratory arrest occurs, attention should be directed toward establishing an airway and ventilating the patient; respiratory stimulants (doxapam) may be necessary if the animal does not begin to ventilate spontaneously

2. Effects on the cardiovascular system

a. Barbiturates produce significant cardiovascular depression when administered as a bolus or in extremely large doses

b. Cardiac arrhythmias may occur

(1) Thiobarbiturates sensitize the heart to epinephrine and induce autonomic imbalance; arrhythmias, particularly ventricular extrasystoles and bigeminy can occur after thiobarbiturate administration

(2) Thiobarbiturates increase both parasympathetic and sympathetic tone; this may lead to atrial or ventricular arrhythmias; sinus bradycardia; or first-, second-, or third-degree heart block and cardiac arrest

c. Barbiturates may cause a transient drop in BP; if the patient is already in a state of surgical anesthesia, small doses of a barbiturate may cause dramatic decreases in cardiac contractility and arterial BP

(1) Barbiturates should be administered slowly and in reduced dosages to sick, debilitated, or depressed animals

(2) Concentrations greater than 4% are toxic to tissues and may injure the capillary musculature, causing capillary dilation and thrombophlebitis

(3) Induction doses of thiobarbiturates may prompt an initial increase in BP caused by tachycardia and an increase in peripheral vascular resistance caused by increases in sympathetic tone

3. Actions on the gastrointestinal (GI) tract

a. Depress intestinal motility; thiobarbiturates may depress GI tract motility initially, then increase both tone and motility

    b. Diarrhea and intestinal stasis are generally not observed at recommended dosages

4. Kidney and liver

    a. No direct effect on the kidney has been observed, unless a large dose is given, in which case a decrease in renal blood flow occurs; systemic hypotension may cause a cessation in urine production

    b. Single administrations at therapeutic doses have no effect on liver function; large doses of barbiturates may cause injury in patients with liver damage

5. Effects on the uterus and fetus

    a. Barbiturates readily diffuse across the placenta into the fetal circulation; thiopental reaches mixed fetal cord blood within 45 seconds

    b. Doses of barbiturates that do not produce anesthesia in the mother can completely inhibit fetal respiratory movements

IV. Absorption, elimination, and excretion

  A. Absorption

    1. Barbiturates are absorbed from the GI tract after oral administration

    2. IV administration

      a. Adequate provisions should be available to support respiration and circulation

      b. Short-acting barbiturates require approximately 5 to 10 minutes to produce maximal CNS effect

      c. Ultrashort-acting barbiturates reach maximal effect within 30 seconds of administration

  B. Elimination

    1. Barbiturates are eliminated by renal excretion and/or destroyed by oxidative activity of hepatic tissues

    2. The amount of active (nonionized, nonprotein-bound) drug is increased by acidosis

    3. Redistribution: ultrashort-acting barbiturates rely on redistribution of drug to lean body tissues (muscle) for their duration of action

      a. Emergence from sleep depends on shift of drug from the brain to lean body tissues

    b. Muscle and skin become saturated about 15 to 30 minutes after thiobarbiturate injection

    c. Saturation of fat may take several hours

    d. Repeated doses have a cumulative effect

    e. Extremely thin, heavily muscled animals (e.g., greyhounds, whippets) demonstrate prolonged recoveries (3 to 5 hours) from thiobarbiturate anesthesia

    f. Obesity delays drug elimination because of the high lipid solubility of barbiturates

    g. "Acute tolerance" (minimal effect with usual dose) is rarely observed following the administration of thiobarbiturates in horses and dogs; the mechanism is unknown but is probably related to the patient's level of excitement and the distribution of cardiac output; if this occurs, alternative anesthetic techniques should be used

C. Excretion

  1. Long-acting barbiturates are excreted in the urine over a period of several days; they may cause severe toxicity depression and coma when used in patients with renal disease

  2. Hepatic metabolism

    a. The barbiturates are metabolized by both hepatic and extrahepatic mechanisms

    b. Oxybarbiturates are transformed primarily by the liver

    c. Liver disease may prolong the duration of drug action; avoid using short-acting barbiturates in presence of liver disease

    d. Hypothermia and depressed cardiovascular function may prolong hepatic metabolism of barbiturates

V. Dosage and administration of specific barbiturate drugs

A. Pentobarbital sodium (Nembutal)

  1. Oral administration is neither safe nor practical for the dog or cat

  2. IV anesthetic dose varies from 3 to 13 mg/lb of body weight, depending on type and amount of preanesthetic medication; when administered as the only source of anesthesia, approximately half the anticipated dose should be injected; the rest should be administered in small increments until desired effect is reached

3. Preanesthetic drugs make the animal easier to handle and decrease the dose of barbiturates required to produce anesthesia
4. Drug may be used in combination with other anesthetics to produce surgical anesthesia
5. Complete recovery occurs in 8 to 24 hours
6. Atropine sulfate or glycopyrrolate decrease salivary secretions, the potential for laryngospasm, and vagal activity
7. The minimum lethal dose in dogs is 23 mg/lb IV
8. The anesthetic duration can be prolonged by administration of 50% intravenously; this is termed the glucose effect
9. Overdose is treated by cardiopulmonary support, respiratory stimulants, fluid therapy, alkalinizing solutions (Na^+ HCO_3^-), and diuresis

B. Thiopental sodium (Pentothal) and thiamylal sodium (Surital, Biotal)
   1. Used in a 2 to 10% solution
      a. Solution should be destroyed after being stored for 3 days at room temperature; precipitated solutions should not be used
      b. More concentrated solutions cause severe tissue damage if accidentally administered subcutaneously
      c. Subcutaneous injection causes necrosis of tissue; tissue necrosis may be minimized by infiltrating the area with saline; pain can be minimized by injecting 2% lidocaine
   2. Thiamylal is similar to thiopental, but slightly more potent (1.5 times). Therefore, it is potentially more toxic than thiopental on a mg/mg basis
   3. Given in small increments intravenously to produce anesthesia (3 to 8 mg/lb)
   4. Dose is based on lean body weight (body weight minus fat)
   5. Dose for induction and intubation is 4 to 6 mg/lb of body weight; solutions of up to 10% are used in the horse; repeated doses have a cumulative effect, resulting in prolonged recovery from anesthesia
   6. Anesthesia usually occurs in 20 to 60 seconds

7. Ventricular arrhythmias (ventricular bigeminy) may occur following induction of anesthesia

8. Apnea is associated with rapid IV injections; ventilation should be supported early in anesthesia

9. Recovery occurs in 10 to 30 minutes, but the animal may remain depressed for many hours depending on dose; repeated doses have cumulative effect

10. Overdose is best treated with continuous O_2 controlled ventilation, fluids, alkalinizing solutions, and diuretics

C. Methohexital (Brevane)

1. Drug is similar to other ultrashort-acting drugs, except its effects are not cumulative (it is rapidly metabolized)

2. Drug is preferred in sight hounds (e.g., greyhounds, whippets, borzois,) because of the prolonged effect produced by thiobarbiturates in these breeds

3. 3 to 7 mg/lb provides light anesthesia in small animals

4. Duration is 5 to 10 minutes

5. Respiratory depression and apnea are common

6. Recovery may be accompanied by pronounced involuntary excitement and convulsions (emergence delirium); CNS effects can be prevented by diazepam (0.1 mg/lb)

7. Drug is not routinely used in large animals; occasionally used in cattle

NONBARBITURATE ANESTHESIC DRUGS

I. Etomidate (Amidate)

A. A rapid-acting, ultrashort, nonbarbiturate, IV anesthetic

B. General anesthetic actions

1. Produces hypnosis (sleep), minimal analgesia at subhypnotic doses

2. Produces depression of the reticular formation of the brain stem

3. Enhances monosynaptic reflex activity, which may result in myoclonal activity

4. Decreases CBF and $CMRO_2$; increases ratio of CBF to $CMRO_2$

C. Organ system effects

1. Respiratory system

a. Brief periods of apnea may occur immediately after IV injections

       b. Tidal volume and respiratory rate are minimally affected during anesthetic maintenance; respiration may increase

  2. Cardiovascular system

       a. Produces little change in heart rate, arterial BP, and cardiac output when administered at induction dosages

       b. Cardiac contractility is mildly depressed

       c. Etomidate does not sensitize the myocardium to catecholamine-induced cardiac arrhythmias

       d. Etomidate does not produce histamine release

  3. GI system

       a. Nausea and vomiting are occasionally observed during induction and following anesthesia; these effects can be inhibited by proper preanesthetic medication

       b. GI motility is minimally affected

  4. Endocrine system

       a. An antiglucocorticoid and mineralocorticoid effect is produced; adrenocorticotropic hormone. Stimulation tests and glucose tolerance tests may be invalid

       b. Adrenocorticoid function is suppressed for 2 to 3 hours in dogs after a single IV administration of etomidate

D. Fate and elimination

  1. Rapidly distributed to the brain, heart, spleen, lung, liver, and intestine

  2. Anesthetic duration of action depends on drug redistribution and capacity; limited ester hydrolysis by the liver

  3. No cumulative effect; acquired tolerance has not been demonstrated after repeated administrations

E. Other

  1. Produces good muscle relaxation during anesthesia; involuntary muscle movements and myoclonic reactions occur during induction and recovery

  2. Does not trigger malignant hyperthermia in susceptible pigs, but predisposes susceptible pigs to a more rapid onset of malignant hyperthermia if triggered by other drugs

3. Pain may occur during IV injection
4. Decreases intraocular pressure

F. Clinical uses
   1. Short-term (5 to 10 minutes) anesthesia in the dog and cat; produces excessive muscle rigidity and seizures in horses and cattle
   2. Induction agent for general anesthesia

G. Dosages
   1. 0.25 to 1.5 mg/lb intravenously in dogs and cats
   2. The best results are obtained after sedating the animal with diazepam, xylazine, or acepromazine

II. Propofol

A. A rapid-acting, ultrashort, nonbarbiturate IV anesthetic

B. General anesthetic actions
   1. Produces sedation-hypnosis similar to that induced by the thiobarbiturates and methohexital
   2. Produces dose-dependent depression of the cerebral cortex and CNS polysynaptic reflexes; may enhance the effects of nondepolarizing neuromuscular blocking drugs
   3. Produces minimal analgesia at subhypnotic doses
   4. Anesthetic doses decrease CBF and $CMRO_2$; the $CBF/CMRO_2$ ratio is unchanged or minimally increased
   5. Possesses anticonvulsant properties similar to the barbiturates

C. Chemistry
   1. An alkylphenol poorly soluble in water
   2. Solubilized in a lecithin-containing emulsion (10% soybean oil and 1.2% egg lecithin) called Intralipid

D. Organ system effects
   1. Respiratory system
      a. Similar to thiobarbiturates
      b. Dose-dependent respiratory depression and initial periods of apnea
   2. Cardiovascular system
      a. Produces little change in heart rate
      b. Dose-dependent decreases in arterial BP caused by decreases in cardiac output and systemic vascular resistance

       c. Minimal but dose-dependent negative inotropic effect at anesthetic doses

   3. Other organ systems: effects of propofol on the liver, kidney, and GI system are secondary to changes in arterial BP and organ blood flow

E. Fate and elimination

   1. Termination of anesthetic effects and short duration of action are due to redistribution from well-perfused (vessel-rich) tissues such as the brain to muscle and fat

   2. Relatively rapid biotransformation by the liver compared to thiobarbiturates

   3. Rapidly cleared from the body by hepatic and extrahepatic metabolism compared to thiobarbiturates

   4. Noncumulative

F. Other

   1. Produces good-to-excellent muscle relaxation

   2. May cause excitement and vomiting during induction if the patient is not given preanesthetic medication

   3. May elicit pain on induction to anesthesia

   4. Alllows rapid recovery; little or no "hangover" effect

G. Clinical uses

   1. From induction to general anesthesia

   2. Maintenance of general anesthesia when combined with opioid analgesics or other sedative-analgesic drugs

H. Dosages

   1. 1 to 3 mg/lb intravenously in dogs and cats for induction

   2. 0.1 to 0.3 mg/lb/min IV infusion in dogs and cats for anesthetic maintenance; usually used with diazepam and oxymorphone or fentanyl for added muscle relaxation and analgesia; medetomidine is an excellent adjunct to propofol anesthesia

III. Chloral hydrate

A. General anesthetic actions

   1. Drug is sedative-hypnotic, depressing the cerebral cortex, resulting in hyporeflexia

   2. CNS depression believed to be due to trichloroethanol; CBF is decreased or unchanged; $CMRO_2$ is decreased

      3. Subanesthetic doses depress motor and sensory nerves and produce mild sedation

      4. Anesthetic doses produce deep sleep lasting for several hours; recovery is prolonged (6 to 24 hours)

      5. Drug is a poor analgesic at subhypnotic doses; excitement or delirium are precipitated by painful stimulation

B. Chemistry

    1. Physical properties: colorless, translucent crystals that volatilize on exposure to air

    2. Chemical properties

      a. Readily soluble in both water and oil

      b. Largely reduced to trichloroethanol in the body

      c. Bitter, caustic taste; quite irritating to the skin and mucous membranes

C. Organ system effects

    1. Respiratory system

      a. Hypnotic doses depress both respiratory rate and tidal volume

      b. Anesthetic doses markedly depress ventilation by depression of the respiratory centers; death is usually caused by progressive respiratory center depression

    2. Cardiovascular system

      a. Anesthetic doses produce depression of the myocardium (decreased contractility)

      b. Chloral hydrate potentiates vagal (parasympathetic) activity, causing bradycardia, P-R interval prolongation, and sinus arrest or atrioventricular block

      c. Supraventricular arrhythmias and transient period of atrial fibrillation have been observed after chloral hydrate anesthesia in horses

    3. GI system

      a. GI secretions and motility are increased because of the parasympathomimetic effect; diarrhea may occur following anesthesia

      b. Nausea and vomiting, salivation, and defecation are induced when chloral hydrate is given orally

    4. Liver and kidney: effects on these systems appear to be secondary to parasympathetic and cardiovascular effects

5. Uterus and fetus: chloral hydrate readily crosses the placenta

D. Absorption, fate, and excretion

1. May be administered orally, rectally, intravenously, or intraperitoneally; very irritating if given perivascularly, intramuscularly, or intraperitoneally

2. Small amount is excreted unchanged in the urine; the majority is reduced to trichloroethanol, a less potent hypnotic, and then conjugated with glucuronic acid, after which it is excreted in the urine

3. Recovery is often prolonged and characterized by a "hangover" effect

E. Clinical uses

1. Chloral hydrate is frequently used as a sedative and adjunct to surgical anesthesia in horses and cattle; the dosage for anesthesia is variable (100 to 300 mg/lb)

2. Casting harnesses or hobbles are generally necessary

3. Drug is generally used in combination with pentobarbital and magnesium sulfate

4. Pharmaceutical companies no longer supply chloral hydrate for veterinary use, but it can be obtained from chemical companies (Sigma, Aldrich)

F. Dosage

1. Sedation: 1 to 3 g/100 lb

2. Anesthesia: 6 to 10 g/100 lb

IV. Guaifenesin (glyceryl guaiacolate)

A. Chemistry

1. Physical properties: a white, finely granular powder that is soluble in water

2. Chemical properties

a. A common decongestant and antitussive also noted for its muscle-relaxant properties

b. Very similar to mephenesin chemically; mephenesin is an aromatic glycerol ether

B. General anesthetic actions

1. Blocks impulse transmission at the internuncial neurons of the spinal cord and brainstem; guaifenesin is a centrally acting muscle relaxant

2. Produces relaxation of skeletal muscles but does not affect function of the diaphragm

    3. Relaxes both laryngeal and pharyngeal muscles, thus potentiating intubation of the trachea

    4. Potentiates other preanesthetic and anesthetic agents and is compatible with them

    5. Produces excitement-free induction and recovery from anesthesia

    6. In excessive doses produces a paradoxic increase in muscle rigidity

C. Organ system effects

    1. Respiratory system

        a. Little, if any, effect on overall respiration

        b. Ventilatory rate may be increased initially; tidal volume decreases

        c. Excessive doses produce an apneustic pattern of breathing

    2. Cardiovascular system

        a. Initial mild decrease in BP, which returns to normal

        b. Myocardial contractile force and cardiac rate are relatively unchanged

    3. GI system: increases GI motility but does not abnormally affect the function of the liver or kidney

    4. Uterus and fetus: guaifenesin crosses the placental barrier, but appears to have minimal effects on the fetus

D. Absorption, fate, and excretion: excreted in the urine after conjugated in the liver to a glucuronide

E. Clinical uses

    1. Used for restraint and muscle relaxation in large and small animal species

    2. Used for short anesthetic procedures of up to 30 to 60 minutes duration

    3. Used as a 5%, 10%, or 15% solution; high concentrations (>6%) may cause hemolysis and hemoglobinuria in cattle; solutions greater than 15% cause hives, hemolysis, and apneustic breathing in horses

    4. Often made by mixing 50 g of guaifenesin with 50 g of dextrose and 1 L warm sterile water

    5. Compatible with other IV and inhalation anesthetic drugs

F. Dosage

    1. The dose varies from 30 to 70 mg/lb

2. Guaifenesin may be administered in small amounts until effective in 1 L solutions with the following agents
   a. 5% 10%, 2 g thiamylal or thiopental
   b. 5% 10%, 2.5 g pentobarbital
   c. 5% guaifenesin (500 ml); 500 mg ketamine with 20 to 50 mg xylazine for ruminants and 500 mg xylazine for horses has been used to produce total IV anesthesia
3. The margin of safety (guaifenesin alone) is three times the therapeutic dose
4. Excessive doses cause muscle rigidity and an apneustic pattern of breathing

DISSOCIOGENIC ANESTHETIC DRUGS

This group includes the arylcyclohexylamines, of which ketamine, phencyclidine, and tiletamine are members

I. Anesthesia is characterized by profound amnesia, superficial analgesia, and catalepsy
   A. Oral, ocular, and swallowing reflexes remain intact, and muscle tone generally increases
   B. Large doses of these agents produce convulsions, which can be controlled with small doses of pentobarbital, thiobarbiturates, or diazepam
II. Psychosomatic effects such as hallucinations, confusion, agitation, and fear have occurred in humans and seem to occur in animals when large doses are administered
III. Muscle rigidity can be minimized by the addition of small doses of tranquilizers, barbiturates, or benzodiazepines (diazepam)
IV. Effects are partially reversed by adrenergic and cholinergic blockade
V. Specific agents
   A. The most commonly used arylcyclohexylamine is ketamine HCl (Vetalar, Ketaset). Telazol (tiletamine-zolazepam drug combination) is used as an alternative and in aggressive animals
   B. Ketamine increases CBF and causes no change or an increase in $CMRO_2$; the $CBF/CMRO_2$ ratio increases; arterial BP and intracranial pressure increase; cerebral perfusion pressure decreases

       1. Used for restraint and minor surgical procedures

       2. Palpebral, conjunctival, corneal, and swallowing reflexes persist; nystagmus is common

  C. Telazol, a 1:1 drug combination of zolazepam (a benzodiazepine) and tiletamine, is a dissociogenic drug combination for use in all species of animals; it is very useful in exotic animals

  D. Tiletamine produces profound CNS side effects; although it possesses anticonvulsant activity, tremors, oculogyria, tonic spasticity, and convulsions occur when excessive dosages are administered

  VI. Salivation and lacrimation may become copious

 VII. Analgesia is selective, with the best results obtained in superficial pain models; visceral pain is not abolished

VIII. Muscle relaxation is poor; ketamine and other arylcyclohexylamines should be used with drugs that produce muscle relaxation to produce the best results

  IX. Animals are hyperresponsive and ataxic during recovery (a result of emergence delirium)

   X. System effects and responses

  A. Respiratory system

       1. Apneustic pattern of breathing; respiratory rate may be increased; arterial Po_2 generally falls after IV administration

       2. Possible increases in Pco_2 and decreases in arterial pH caused by the irregular pattern of breathing

  B. Cardiovascular system

       1. Increased heart rate

       2. Increased BP

       3. Decreased cardiac contractility

       4. Ketamine and other cyclohexamines minimally sensitize the heart to catecholamine-induced arrhythmias

  C. Kidney and liver

       1. Ketamine HCl is metabolized by the liver and excreted unchanged by the kidneys

       2. Ketamine should be used with caution in animals with hepatic or renal disease; ketamine can be used in cats with urethral obstruction, provided renal disease is absent or not severe and the obstruction is eliminated

XI. Dose

  A. Ketamine

    1. Cat: 2 to 15 mg/lb intramuscularly or subcutaneously; 0.5-1 mg/lb intravenously. Doses as small as 1 to 3 mg *total* are administered intravenously to sick animals and cats with urethral obstruction

    2. Dog: xylazine 0.3 mg/lb intravenously and ketamine 3 to 5 mg/lb intravenously; diazepam 0.15 mg/lb intravenously and ketamine 2.5 mg/lb intravenously

    3. Pigs: 2 to 10 mg/lb intramuscularly of ketamine may be used with thiamylal following Innovar-Vet 1 ml/80 lb intramuscularly or azaperone 1 mg/lb intramuscularly

  B. Telazol

    1. Dogs, cats, cattle, sheep, goats: 2 to 8 mg/lb intramuscularly

    2. Horses: guaifenesin (5 to 10%) until effective 0.3 to 0.5 mg/lb telazol

CHAPTER NINE

Inhalation Anesthesia

"O sleep! O gentle sleep!
Nature's soft nurse, how have I frightened thee,
That thou no more will weigh my eyelids down
and steep my senses in forgetfulness?"

WILLIAM SHAKESPEARE

OVERVIEW

Inhalational anesthetic drugs are used to produce general anesthesia. They are suitable for use in all species, including reptiles, birds, and both domestic and zoo animals. Their safe use requires knowledge, not only of their pharmacologic effects, but of their physical and chemical properties. Ideally these drugs should produce unconsciousness (hypnosis), hyporeflexia, and analgesia. The optimal inhalation anesthetic is easy to control, permits rapid induction and recovery from anesthesia, and produces no adverse side effects. This chapter outlines the basic principles of inhalation anesthesia and their use.

GENERAL CONSIDERATIONS

I. Inhalation anesthetic drugs are vapors or gases administered directly into the respiratory system

II. To produce anesthesia, they must be absorbed from the alveoli into the bloodstream and pass to the brain

III. Inhalation anesthetics are not primarily dependent on body detoxification mechanisms for the duration of clinical effect but are primarily eliminated by the lungs

IV. Because the uptake and elimination of inhalation anesthetics is relatively rapid, the depth of anesthesia can be well-controlled, but constant patient monitoring is required

PROPERTIES OF A DESIRABLE GENERAL ANESTHETIC

I. Nonirritating and free from disagreeable odors
II. Potent (produces pleasant, rapid induction and rapid recovery)
III. Produces adequate muscular relaxation and analgesia for surgical procedures
IV. Safe (potentially reversible or easily controlled)
V. Minimal to no side effects
VI. Should not promote bleeding
VII. Nontoxic to the patient and to humans
VIII. Easily and inexpensively produced
IX. Not explosive (stable during storage)
X. Compatible with other drugs

FACTORS CONTROLLING THE BRAIN TENSION OF VOLATILE ANESTHETIC (Table 9-1)

I. Factors governing the delivery of a suitable concentration of inhalation anesthetic
   A. Physical and chemical properties of the agent
      1. Vapor pressure of the agent governs the volatility of inhalation anesthesia
      2. Boiling points (other than nitrous oxide and desflurane) are higher than room temperature (70° F or 27° C)
   B. Anesthetic system
      1. The concentrations delivered to the patient vary with the type of anesthetic system, fresh gas flow rate, type of vaporizer, and other equipment
      2. Frequent inspection and maintenance is necessary to prevent malfunctions caused by factors such as leaks and sticky valves
II. Factors responsible for the delivery of inhalation anesthetic to lungs and alveoli
   A. The partial pressure of inhalation anesthetic in the brain depends on the alveolar partial pressure of anesthetic; the

TABLE 9-1

BOILING POINTS, VAPOR PRESSURES, AND VAPORIZATION OF INHALATION AGENTS

DRUG	BOILING POINT (°C)	VAPOR PRESSURE AT 20° C (mm Hg)	MAXIMUM CONCENTRATION OF VAPOR DELIVERED BY SATURATION VAPORIZER AT 20° C (%)	USEFUL RANGES OF CONCENTRATION (AGENT USED ALONE) INDUCTION (%)	USEFUL RANGES OF CONCENTRATION (AGENT USED ALONE) MAINTENANCE (%)
Volatile anesthetics					
Ether	36	443	58	10-40	3-12
Desflurane	23.5	664	87.4	8-15	5-9
Isoflurane	48	252	33	2-6	1-3
Halothane	50	243	32	1-4*	0.5-2
Enflurane	57	180	24	3-7	1-3
Methoxyflurane	105	24	3	Up to 3	0.25-1
Anesthetic gases					
Nitrous oxide	−89	39,5000 (50 atm)			
Cyclopropane	−33	4,800 (6 atm)			

*Up to 10% may be used in induction of large animals.

alveolar concentration of anesthetic is the result of: delivery of anesthetic to the lungs and uptake from the lungs; delivery to the lungs depends on: inspired concentration, and the alveolar ventilation

B. Inspired concentration
  1. Concentration effect: the greater the inspired concentration administered, the more rapid the rate of rise of alveolar concentration
  2. Second gas effect
     a. Ventilation effect: passive increase in inspired ventilation is due to rapid uptake of large volumes of a poorly blood-soluble drug (e.g., nitrous oxide) *or* smaller volumes of a highly blood-soluble drug (e.g., ether or methoxyflurane), this increase in alveolar ventilation accelerates the rate of rise of the second gas, regardless of its concentration
     b. Concentration effect: uptake of the first gas (e.g., nitrous oxide) results in shrinkage of the alveoli, thereby concentrating the second gas (e.g., halothane); and increasing its concentration gradient, which speeds its absorption
  3. A 50% to 80% concentration of nitrous oxide augments the inflow and rate of uptake of the concentration of a second gas (e.g., halothane) in the inspired mixture
C. Alveolar ventilation
  1. Generally, the greater the ventilation, the more rapid the approach of the alveolar gas concentration to the inspired gas concentration*
  2. Limited by lung volume; the larger the functional residual capacity, the longer it takes to wash in a new inhalant
  3. Excessive increases in alveolar ventilation may decrease cerebral blood flow, thus slowing induction
  4. Factors affecting ventilation
     a. Decreased breathing rate
     b. Decreased tidal volume as a result of drug-induced respiratory depression

---

*See Eger EI, editor: *Anesthetic uptake and action,* Baltimore, 1974, Williams & Wilkins.

      c. Increased dead space (anatomic and physiologic) during anesthesia, which decreases effective alveolar ventilation

      d. Effective alveolar ventilation requires a patent airway

III. Factors responsible for uptake of anesthetic from the lungs

    A. Solubility: this term describes how an anesthetic is distributed between two phases (e.g., between blood and gas, between tissue and blood); solubility is usually expressed as a partition coefficient; Ostwald's partition coefficient between blood and gas is commonly used to describe anesthetic uptake in terms of solubility

AGENT	BLOOD-GAS PARTITION COEFFICIENT (OSTWALD'S COEFFICIENT)
Diethyl ether	15.2
Methoxyflurane	13
Halothane	2.36
Enflurane	1.91
Isoflurane	1.41
Nitrous oxide	0.49
Desflurane	0.42

    A gas with a blood-gas partition coefficient of 2 has *one* volume in the alveoli per *two* volumes in the blood at equilibrium

    1. Anesthetic solubility and anesthetic uptake are not the same as potency, but they can determine the rapidity of onset of anesthetic effect

    2. The greater the blood-gas partition coefficient, the greater the uptake of anesthetic by blood; therefore the tension of anesthetic in arterial blood rises slowly for drugs that are highly soluble in blood (high blood-gas coefficients); onset of the clinical effect is contingent on the tension of anesthetic developing in the blood; very soluble drugs, such as methoxyflurane, have long induction and recovery periods because large amounts of anesthetic must be taken into the blood before the tension or partial pressure of the anesthetic rises sufficiently to produce anesthesia; clinically, slow induction may be overcome by raising the inspired concentration

to values exceeding those necessary to maintain anesthesia

3. The lower the blood-gas partition coefficient, the less soluble the drug in the blood (only small quantities are carried in the blood; thus both alveolar concentration and tension will rise rapidly), and the more rapidly the tension or partial pressure of the drug will increase in the blood; less soluble drugs such as nitrous oxide and isoflurane have relatively short induction and short-recovery periods

4. Generally, drugs with high blood-gas partition coefficients exhibit long induction and recovery times, whereas drugs with low blood-gas partition coefficients exhibit short induction and recovery times

B. Cardiac output: blood carries anesthetic from the lungs; thus the greater the cardiac output, the greater the uptake of anesthetic, the slower the rate of rise of alveolar concentration and tension, and, in excited, stressed animals, the slower the rate of induction; animals with depressed cardiac output may be induced very rapidly; changes in cardiac output have the greatest effect on the most soluble agents (e.g., methoxyflurane)

C. Alveolar-venous anesthetic tension difference: during induction, tissues remove nearly all the anesthetic brought to them; venous blood returning to the lungs contains little anesthetic, so there is maximal anesthetic uptake; as time passes, increasing tissue saturation raises the venous blood concentration, and less anesthetic is taken up in the lungs; clinically, however, anesthetic uptake is a continuous process

D. Shunts

1. Right-to-left intracardiac or intrapulmonary shunts (e.g., Fallot's tetralogy) delay induction; this effect is more important for poorly soluble agents (nitrous oxide)

2. Body shunts (left to right) may speed the rate of induction if cardiac output is low; endotoxic shock mimics a body shunt

E. Pathologic changes in alveoli: if the alveolar membranes are affected by disease resulting in exudate, transudate, emphysema, or pulmonary fibrosis, diffusion may be impaired; uptake of anesthetic is thus reduced

IV. Factors governing brain and tissue uptake of anesthetic
   A. Same as those determining uptake from the lungs
      1. Tissue–blood flow
      2. Solubility (arterial blood to tissue anesthetic tension difference)
      3. Arterial blood tissue–anesthetic tension difference
   B. The uptake by tissue is primarily dependent on blood flow to that tissue and its capillary density; tissues can be divided into four groups according to blood supply
      1. Vessel-rich group (VRG): 75% of cardiac output (e.g., brain, heart, intestine, liver, kidney, spleen)
      2. Vessel moderate group, or muscle group (MG): 15 to 20% of cardiac output (e.g., muscle, skin)
      3. Neutral fat group (FG): 5% of cardiac output (e.g., adipose tissue)
      4. Vessel-poor group (VPG): 1 to 2% of cardiac output (e.g., bone, tendons, cartilage)
   C. Tissue-blood partition coefficients vary far less than blood-gas coefficients (except for fat)
      1. Lowest is approximately 1 (nitrous oxide in lung tissue)
      2. Highest is approximately 4 (halothane in muscle tissue)
   D. Important considerations
      1. Equilibration of an anesthetic drug in the VRG is complete in 5 to 20 minutes
      2. Equilibration in the MG may take 1½ to 4 hours
      3. Arterial-tissue, partial-pressure difference, and thus uptake, decrease far more rapidly in VRG than in MG
      4. Solubility of an inhalation drug in VRG and MG may affect recovery time
      5. The fat group occupies 10% to 30% body mass and receives about 5% the cardiac output; the FG has a higher tissue solubility for inhalation anesthetics than most other tissues and thus has a greater and more prolonged capacity to absorb anesthetic; because of its low blood flow, the FG has little effect on induction of anesthesia; the FG may affect recovery time after prolonged anesthetic periods (over 4 hours)

AGENTS	FAT-BLOOD PARTITION COEFFICIENT
Diethyl ether	4.2
Methoxyflurane	61
Halothane	65
Enflurane	37
Isoflurane	48
Nitrous oxide	2.3
Desflurane	27.2

6. VPG (vessel poor group) tissues have very little effect on short duration anesthesia
7. Rubber solubility: agents such as halothane and methoxyflurane are freely absorbed into rubber components of the anesthetic system; during recovery, they are excreted back into the anesthetic circuitry
8. Methoxyflurane, halothane, isoflurane, and desflurane are stable in moist soda-lime

ELIMINATION OF INHALATION ANESTHETICS

I. By lung
   A. Inhalation anesthetics are excreted largely unchanged by the lungs
   B. The same factors that affect the rate of anesthetic uptake are important in anesthetic elimination
      1. Pulmonary ventilation
      2. Blood flow
      3. Solubility in blood and tissue
   C. As anesthetic gas washes out of the lungs, the arterial blood tension falls, followed by the tension in tissues; because of the high blood flow to the brain, its tension of anesthetic falls rapidly and accounts for the rapid awakening from anesthesia with insoluble agents such as N_2O; decreases in other tissues are progressively slower and dependent on blood flow
II. Other routes through which small quantities of inhalation anesthetic agent may be excreted are skin, milk, mucous membrane, urine
III. Biotransformation
   A. Anesthetic gases are metabolized in the body to variable degrees

   B. Metabolism is generally by hepatic microsomal enzyme
      systems; various intermediate metabolites are formed;
      these may be responsible for certain toxic effects or after-
      effects
      1. Approximately 10% to 20% inspired halothane is me-
         tabolized, compared to 50% methoxyflurane; approxi-
         mately 2.5% enflurane and 0.25% isoflurane are me-
         tabolized; less than 1% of desflurane is metabolized
      2. Toxic metabolites are primarily inorganic fluoride and
         bromide ions
IV. Diffusion hypoxia may occur at the end of anesthesia and is
    described in the discussion of nitrous oxide (see Chapter 10);
    briefly, the rapid elimination of N_2O from the blood into the
    alveoli results in the dilution of alveolar oxygen by N_2O and
    hypoxemia if ventilation is not maintained

POTENCY OF INHALATION ANESTHETICS

   I. Anesthetic potency can be expressed in several ways; one
      commonly accepted method is to measure the minimum al-
      veolar concentration (MAC) of the inhalation anesthetic
      (Table 9-2); MAC is the minimum alveolar concentration of
      an anesthetic (1 atm), that produces no response in 50% of
      patients exposed to a painful stimulus
      A. MAC is generally measured as the end-tidal concentration
         of anesthetic

TABLE 9-2

MINIMAL ALVEOLAR CONCENTRATIONS OF INHALATION ANESTHETICS IN VARIOUS SPECIES

	HUMAN	**DOG**	**CAT**	**HORSE**
Desflurane	~6	~7	~7	—
Diethyl ether	1.92	3.04	2.1	—
Methoxyflurane	0.16	0.29	0.23	0.22
Halothane	0.76	0.87	1.19	0.88
Enflurane	1.68	2.06	2.4	2.12
Isoflurane	1.2	1.3	1.63	1.31
Nitrous oxide	101.1	188-200	150	190

    B. MAC values are not vaporizer settings
    C. MAC values are used to compare the potency of anesthetics
II. MAC values vary with species and with
    A. Age–older patients require less inhalation anesthetic
    B. Temperature–hypothermia reduces MAC
    C. Administration of other CNS-depressant drugs
    D. Disease
        1. Hyperthyroidism or hypothyroidism
        2. Hypovolemia, anemia
        3. Septicemia
        4. Extreme acid-base imbalances
    E. Pregnancy
III. Studies using dogs suggest that
    A. 1 MAC produces light anesthesia
    B. 1.5 MAC produces moderate surgical anesthesia
    C. 2 MAC produces deep anesthesia

CHAPTER TEN

Pharmacology of Inhalation Anesthetic Drugs

"Sleep is pain's easiest salve, and doth fulfill
All offices of death, except to kill"

JOHN DONNE

OVERVIEW

Inhalation anesthetic drugs are pharmacologically active chemicals that cause unconsciousness, various degrees of muscle relaxation and analgesia, and changes in organ system function. Their administration requires familiarity with a variety of equipment (e.g., vaporizers, flow meters, pressure valves) needed to vaporize the anesthetic liquid and accurately deliver the anesthetic to the patient. Theoretically, the depth of anesthesia is easily controlled. This chapter outlines the pharmacologic properties and the interactions of inhalation anesthetic drugs.

GENERAL CONSIDERATIONS

I. The ability of an inhalation anesthetic to produce general anesthesia is a function of its tissue membrane effects and physiochemical properties (Table 10-1)
   A. Factors that influence anesthetic uptake and delivery to the brain include
      1. Alveolar ventilation
      2. Blood-gas partition coefficient
      3. Cardiac output
      4. Alveolar to mixed, venous anesthetic, partial pressure difference

II. Ventilation-perfusion abnormalities and hypoventilation may hinder the rate of anesthetic induction

III. Left-to-right intracardiac shunts may hinder the rate of anesthetic induction

IV. Hypothermia decreases the need for anesthesia

V. The anesthetic requirement is determined by the anesthetic system used (in circle vs. out of circle)

VI. Inhalation anesthetics produce more than unconsciousness and may markedly change organ system physiology

VII. The metabolites of inhalation anesthetics can be toxic

VIII. Familiarity with an anesthetic drug is the key to its safe and effective use

DIETHYL ETHER (ETHER)

I. Ether was once a frequently used inhalation anesthetic; it is now occasionally used in laboratory animals and to make tape sticky

II. Ether is highly flammable and explosive

III. Ether is an ideal anesthetic in some respects because it maintains respiration and minimally depresses cardiac output

IV. Ether may cause nausea and vomiting during induction and recovery

V. The signs and stages of ether anesthesia (Table 10-2) can be loosely applied to other anesthetics

    A. Stage I: the stage of analgesia (that period from the beginning of induction to the loss of consciousness)

        1. Disorientation, with normal reflexes or hyperreflexia, is the most common feature displayed

        2. Fear and subsequent release of epinephrine with increased heart rate and rapid respirations may occur

        3. Excessive salivation occurs

        4. Urine and feces may be voided

    B. Stage II: a stage of delirium or excitement, which represents the period of early loss of consciousness

        1. The hazards of stage II are struggling, physical injury, and the consequences of increased sympathetic tone

        2. Voluntary centers in the brain are depressed and abolished

TABLE 10-1

SUMMARY OF PHYSIOCHEMICAL PROPERTIES OF INHALATION AGENTS

PROPERTIES	ETHER	NITROUS OXIDE	HALOTHANE
Chemical formula	$(C_2H_5)_2O$	N_2O	$\begin{matrix} F & Br \\ \mid & \mid \\ F-C-C-H \\ \mid & \mid \\ F & Cl \end{matrix}$
Molecular weight	74	44	197.4
Boiling point (at 760 mm Hg)	36.5° C	−89° C	50.2° C
Specific gravity (g/ml)	0.72	1.53	1.87
Vapor pressure (mm Hg) (at 20° C)	443	39,500	243
Odor	Pungent, unpleasant	Sweet, pleasant	Sweet, pleasant
Preservative	Necessary	Unnecessary	Necessary (thymol)
Stability			
To metal	May react	Nonreactive	May react
To alkali	Stable (traces of aldehydes)	Stable	Slight decomposition
To ultraviolet light	Decompresses	Stable	Decomposes
Explosiveness	Explosive (in air or oxygen)	None	None
Partition coefficients	See Chapter 9		
MAC values	See Table 9-2		
Presentation at room temperature	Colorless liquid	Colorless gas (liquid under pressure)	Colorless liquid

MAC, minimum alveolar concentration.

TABLE 10-1 cont'd
SUMMARY OF PHYSIOCHEMICAL PROPERTIES OF INHALATION AGENTS

METHOXYFLURANE	ENFLURANE	ISOFLURANE	DESFLURANE
Cl F H $\mid$ $\mid$ $\mid$ H-C-C-O-C-H $\mid$ $\mid$ $\mid$ Cl F H	Cl F F $\mid$ $\mid$ $\mid$ H-C-C-O-C-H $\mid$ $\mid$ $\mid$ F F F	F Cl H $\mid$ $\mid$ $\mid$ F-C-C-O-C-H $\mid$ $\mid$ $\mid$ F H F	F F H $\mid$ $\mid$ $\mid$ F-C-C-O-C-K $\mid$ $\mid$ $\mid$ F H F
165	184.5	184.5	193.4
104.7° C	56.5° C	48.5° C	23.5° C
1.41	1.52	1.52	—
24	180	252	664
Fruity, pleasant	Ethereal, pleasant	Pleasant	Pleasant
Necessary (butylated hydroxytoluene)	Unnecessary	Unnecessary	Unnecessary
May react Stable	Nonreactive Stable	Nonreactive Stable	Nonreactive Stable
Decomposes	Stable	Stable	Stable
None	None	None	None
Colorless liquid	Colorless liquid	Colorless liquid	Colorless liquid

TABLE 10-2
STAGES OF ETHER ANESTHESIA*

STAGE OF ANESTHESIA	RESPIRATION	PUPIL	EYE MOVEMENT	ABOLITION OF REFLEXES	SOMATIC MUSCLES	PULSE RATE AND BLOOD PRESSURE (BP)
I. Analgesia	Regular	Normal	Voluntary	All present	Normal tone	Rapid pulse; elevated BP
II. Delerium	Irregular	Dilated	Involuntary	All present	Excited movement	Rapid pulse; elevated BP
III. Surgical Plane I	Increased depth, rate	Constricted	Involun-tary; fixed	Conjunctival; pharyngeal; cutaneous	Slight relaxation	Normal pulse; normal BP
Plane II	Regular rate, depth	Normal		Laryngeal; corneal; peritoneal	Moderate relaxation	Normal pulse; normal BP
Plane III	Decreased rate, depth	Slightly dilated			Marked relaxation	Rapid, normal, or slow fall in BP
Plane IV	Abdominal breathing	Moderately dilated				Slow, weak pulse; then no pulse; fall in BP to zero

*The classical stages described by A.E. Guedel.

3. During light anesthesia, the patient reacts to any sort of external stimuli with exaggerated reflex struggling

4. Respirations are generally irregular in depth and rate, and breath holding may occur

5. The eyelids are widely open, and the iris is dilated because of sympathetic stimulation

6. Reflex vomiting is common unless food has been withheld for 6 or more hours before anesthesia; defecation and urination may occur

7. The duration of stage II should be decreased if possible, but there is a maximum limit to the rate of administration of an anesthetic to avoid depressing the respiratory center

C. Stage III

1. Plane I: marked by the appearance of full rhythmic and mechanical respiration

   a. CO_2 retention during the preceding stages may double tidal volume for the first minute

   b. Preanesthetic medication directly affects the rate and volume of respiration throughout anesthesia

   c. Responses to pain are still present, and minute volumes of anesthetic are administered in direct proportion to the amount of stimulation from the operative field

   d. Cardiovascular function is only minimally affected

2. Plane II: tidal volume is usually somewhat decreased; respiratory rate may be increased or decreased; cardiovascular function is mildly depressed

3. Plane III: entrance into this plane is marked by the beginning of paralysis of the intercostal muscles

   a. The level of anesthesia is potentially dangerous

   b. Respiratory depression is marked

   c. Cardiovascular function is noticeably depressed, dependent on the specific characteristics of the anesthetic drug used

4. Plane IV: complete paralysis of intercostal muscles

   a. Passage into plane IV is marked by cessation of all respiratory effort and dilation of the pupil

b. Cardiovascular function is generally impaired, producing hypotension and decreased cardiac contractility

D. Stage IV

Respiratory arrest followed by circulatory collapse; death ensues within 1 to 5 minutes

NITROUS OXIDE

I. General anesthetic properties (see Table 10-1)
   A. A gas at room temperature, but readily compressible at 30 to 50 atm (750 psi) to a colorless liquid; returns to gaseous state when released from the cylinder into atmospheric pressure
   B. Nonflammable, but supports combustion by decomposing into nitrogen and oxygen

II. Effect on systems
   A. Nervous system
      1. Mild analgesic and anesthetic action produced by cerebrocortical depression
      2. Dangerous in excessive concentrations because of hypoxia (70% total gas flow)
   B. Respiratory system
      1. Nonirritating to the respiratory tract
      2. Does not depress cough reflex
      3. Causes only minimal respiratory depression in the presence of hypoxia; respiratory rate may increase
   C. Cardiovascular system
      1. Few side effects occur except in the presence of hypoxia
      2. Heart rate, cardiac output, and arterial blood pressure (BP) remain relatively unchanged
      3. Tachycardia may develop
      4. N_2O does not sensitize the myocardium to catecholamines
   D. Gastrointestinal system
      1. Ileus may occur secondary to gas accumulation within the gastrointestinal tract
      2. The kidney and liver are not significantly affected

E. Muscular system
  1. Does not cause muscle relaxation
  2. Does not potentiate muscle relaxants
F. Uterus and fetus
  1. Passes placental barrier
  2. May cause fetal hypoxemia

III. Absorption, fate, and excretion
  A. Crosses alveolar membranes because of its administration in relatively large inspired concentrations (40% to 75%)
  B. Speeds the uptake of inhalation anesthetics (second gas) into the blood (second-gas effect). The enhanced uptake of the second gas is caused by a N_2O-dependent increase in alveolar ventilation
  C. Diffuses into closed air cavities: N_2O is 30 times more soluble in blood than nitrogen; when N_2O is given in high concentrations (over 50%), it diffuses into air-containing cavities faster than nitrogen diffuses out; if the cavity is closed (e.g., pneumothorax, obstructed bowel, air embolism, blocked paranasal sinuses) and N_2O administered, then either the volume or pressure inside the cavity increases; volume or pressure increases until the alveolar nitrous oxide ratio is in equilibrium with the closed cavity; the relative volume increase can be calculated using the formula: $M = 100/100 - FiN_2O$; M = magnitude of volume change; FiN_2O = fraction of inspired N_2O; Example: If a patient is exposed to 50% N_2O, $FiN_2O = 50\%$; $M = 100/100 - 50 = 2$; volume increases by a factor of 2
  D. Does not combine with hemoglobin; has no value as an O_2 source nor does it form any chemical combinations in the body; carried in simple solution
  E. Eliminated through the lungs rapidly and completely in 2 minutes
  F. Diffusion hypoxia: a result of the low blood-gas partition coefficient (0.49); rapid diffusion of nitrous oxide into the alveoli at the end of anesthesia dilutes the oxygen in the alveoli; alveolar oxygen tension may be drastically reduced, especially if the patient is breathing room air; hypoxia is prevented by administering high oxygen flow rates for at least 5 to 10 minutes after discontinuing N_2O

G. Recovery is fast and devoid of unpleasant sequelae

H. Circumstantial evidence suggests some biotransformation; bone marrow depression may occur after prolonged exposure; N_2O may be teratogenic especially in females after prolonged exposure in the first trimester of pregnancy

IV. Clinical use

A. Used as an analgesic in veterinary anesthesia

B. Adds to the effect of other inhalation anesthetics; therefore less of more potent inhalants is needed to produce general anesthesia

C. Often used to supplement narcotic or inhalation anesthesia

D. To prevent hypoxia a minimum of 30% O_2 must be present

E. The patient should be denitrogenated by administering O_2 at the beginning of the anesthetic period

F. Closed-circuit (low O_2 flow) administration of N_2O is potentially dangerous because of the low flow rates of N_2O and oxygen used; high flow rates and efficient expiratory valves are essential for safe anesthesia without hypoxia

G. The ratio of N_2O to O_2 delivered by the anesthetic machine must be continually monitored; not more than 70% N_2O should be used

V. Dosages

A. Up to 70% N_2O is used

B. Maintenance concentrations are usually 50% or 66% ($N_2O:O_2 = 1:1$ or $2:1$)

C. If the patient's cardiopulmonary status deteriorates while receiving nitrous oxide, it should be discontinued

D. N_2O is not potent enough in many species to make administration of less than 40% worthwhile

HALOTHANE (FLUOTHANE)

I. General anesthetic properties (see Table 10-1)

A. Nervous system

1. Depresses central nervous system (CNS)

2. Depresses body temperature regulating centers; can cause hyperpyrexia and malignant hyperthermia in humans, pigs, horses, dogs, and cats

3. Stages of anesthesia are not the same as classic signs described for ether: pupils may be constricted at all stages, respiration may be shallow but rapid, and the abdominal muscles are relaxed only at deeper planes of anesthesia; the arterial BP may provide the best information about the depth of halothane anesthesia
4. Increases cerebral blood flow

II. Effect on organ systems
   A. Respiratory system
      1. Respirations are depressed at all levels of halothane anesthesia
      2. Tidal volume is decreased
      3. There is less ventilation at any level of $Paco_2$ than in the conscious state, but ventilation is usually adequate
      4. The response to hypercarbia is lost in deeper anesthesia, and ventilation becomes inadequate
      5. Respiratory depression is pronounced in ruminants
      6. Tachypnea may occur; the mechanism is uncertain
   B. Cardiovascular system
      1. Causes hypotension related to the depth of anesthesia
      2. Directly depresses vascular smooth muscle causing vasodilation (e.g., in cerebral, skeletal muscle and peripheral tissue) and decreasing total peripheral resistance
      3. Directly depresses myocardium, decreasing cardiac output, stroke volume, and cardiac contractility
      4. Decreases efferent sympathetic nervous system activity
      5. Cardiac rate is less affected, but is usually decreased at deeper planes of anesthesia
      6. May cause sinus node depression and ventricular arrhythmias especially if acidosis, hypoxia, or other causes of sympathetic stimulation are present
      7. Sensitizes the heart to catecholamines, occasionally producing cardiac arrhythmias
   C. Gastrointestinal system
      1. Decreases intestinal tract motility, tone, and peristaltic activity
      2. Liver: a number of reports in humans have related halothane to jaundice and fatal postanesthetic liver necrosis; biotransformation of halothane to hepatotoxic metabolites may produce hypersensitivity in a small number of

individuals; the effect is believed to be related to halothane administration in conjunction with tissue hypoxia

D. Renal system: no nephrotoxic effects have been reported other than those resulting from hypotension

E. Muscular system
   1. Relaxation is only moderate during light anesthesia
   2. Muscle-relaxing agents may be needed if pronounced muscle relaxation is required
   3. Halothane potentiates the action of nondepolarizing muscle relaxants
   4. Malignant hyperthermia in swine can occur

F. Uterus and fetus
   1. Decreases uterine tone; may decrease uterine involution postpartum
   2. Readily crosses the placental barrier

III. Absorption, fate, and excretion
   A. Absorption takes place rapidly in the lungs
   B. Up to 20% to 40% inspired halothane is metabolized by liver microsomes; trifluoroacetic acid and bromide and chloride radicals are produced and excreted in the urine for many hours to days
   C. Metabolites may persist for many days in the liver
   D. The major portion of administered halothane is excreted unchanged by the lungs

IV. Clinical uses
   A. One of the most useful anesthetics because it is nonflammable, potent, nonirritating, controllable, and relatively nontoxic
   B. Can be used in all species
   C. Accurate concentrations of halothane can be delivered from precision, thermostable or thermocompensated, calibrated vaporizers; draw-over, in-the-circle vaporizers have been used once the wick is removed
   D. Decomposes slowly when exposed to light; stored in dark bottles with thymol added as a preservative; thymol is potentially tissue toxic
   E. Can be used in rebreathing and nonrebreathing techniques

    F. Used in in-the-circle, draw-over vaporizers during "low flow" (closed system) techniques (see Chapter 13)

V. Dosage

    A. 2% to 4% at induction; careful monitoring is important to avoid overdosage

    B. Induction time is decreased if nitrous oxide is given simultaneously, because of the second-gas effect

    C. Concurrent use of nitrous oxide reduces the amount of halothane required

    D. Maintenance: 0.5% to 1.5% small animals; 1 to 2% large animals

METHOXYFLURANE (METOFANE, PENTHRANE)

I. General anesthetic properties (see Table 10-1): the vapor pressure of methoxyflurane is low; the highest concentrations that can be produced at room temperature are between 2.5% and 3%

II. Effect on organ systems

    A. Nervous system

        1. Dose-dependent CNS depression

        2. Potent CNS depressor

        3. Reticular activating system depression

        4. Excitement (delirium) may occur during mask induction (not recommended)

        5. Good muscle relaxation and analgesia

        6. Most potent inhalation anesthetic (maximum alveolar concentration [MAC] = 0.29)

    B. Respiratory system

        1. Produces more respiratory depression than halothane

        2. Ventilation may need to be assisted in order to prevent hypercarbia

        3. The rate and depth of spontaneous respiration can be used to monitor the depth of anesthesia

        4. Nonirritating to the respiratory tract

    C. Cardiovascular system

        1. Decreases cardiac contractile force (negative inotrope)

    2. Decreases cardiac contractility and cardiac output with increasing depth of anesthesia

    3. Produces mild-to-moderate hypotension in light planes of anesthesia

    4. May cause changes in heart rate (bradycardia) and rhythm

    5. Sensitizes the heart to catecholamines, but less so than halothane

D. Gastrointestinal system: decreases smooth muscle tone and motility

E. Renal system

    1. Incriminated in the production of a high-output renal failure in humans; polyuria, weight loss, and dehydration may last for days after the anesthetic period; inorganic fluoride, a metabolite, is thought to be responsible; methoxyflurane is not used in humans

    2. Acute renal failure has been reported in humans after methoxyflurane anesthesia and is frequently associated with obese patients, those with renal disease, those given concurrent nephrotoxic drugs (tetracyclines, aminoglycosides), or those undergoing extensive surgical procedures

    3. Acute methoxyflurane administration has not produced renal failure in animals, except when administered with other nephrotoxic drugs (e.g., aminoglycosides, tetracycline)

F. Muscular system

    1. Excellent muscle relaxation and analgesia at relatively low inspired concentrations

    2. Muscle relaxation is due to drug effects on the CNS (spinal cord) rather than the neuromuscular junction

G. Uterus and fetus

    1. Rapidly crosses the placental barrier

    2. Does not markedly affect motility and tone

III. Absorption, fate, and excretion

A. Absorbed and eliminated by the lung

B. Up to 50% absorbed methoxyflurane may be metabolized by the liver; metabolites include inorganic fluoride

C. Metabolites are excreted by the kidney

IV. Clinical use

    A. Good muscle relaxation is produced; potent relaxation is produced; therefore low concentrations of methoxyflurane can be used clinically for many minor surgical procedures

    B. Methoxyflurane is the most potent anesthetic, but induction is prolonged, as is recovery, because of the relatively high blood-gas partition coefficient (13)

    C. Analgesia may continue into the recovery period

    D. Accurate concentrations can be delivered by precision, heat-compensated, calibrated vaporizer; however, simple draw-over wick vaporizers can be used

    E. If nitrous oxide is used, the amount of methoxyflurane required is reduced

V. Dosages

    A. Methoxyflurane is rarely used by mask induction because of the slow onset of anesthesia and the possibility of excitement or delirium

    B. After barbiturate induction, a 2% to 3% concentration is used to induce surgical anesthesia

    C. Maintenance: 0.2% to 1%

ENFLURANE (ETHRANE)

I. General anesthetic properties (see Table 10-1)

    A. Similar to isoflurane

    B. Low blood-gas partition coefficient (1.9)

    C. Stable in moist soda lime

II. Effects on body organ systems

    A. Depresses CNS, produces involuntary muscle twitching, high-frequency spike complexes (burst suppression), and seizures at deeper levels of anesthesia

    B. Produces good muscle relaxation and analgesia

    C. Causes potent cardiorespiratory depression; the most potent negatively inotropic inhalant

    D. Minimally sensitizes the heart to catecholamine-induced cardiac arrhythmias

    E. Crosses the placenta producing fetal depression

    F. Produces minimal biotransformation; low levels of serum fluoride rarely cause renal toxicity

    G. Used in precision vaporizers
       1. Rapid induction and recovery from anesthesia
       2. MAC of approximatley 1.6%
    H. May cause malignant hyperthermia

SEVOFLURANE (not available in the United States at this time)

I. General anesthetic properties (see Table 10-1)
    A. Low blood-gas partition coefficient (0.6 to 0.7)
       1. Rapid smooth induction; rapid recovery
       2. MAC of approximately 2.4%
    B. Nonpungent
    C. Not stable in moist soda lime
II. Effects on body organ systems
    A. Depresses CNS; no convulsive activity
    B. Produces good muscle relaxation and analgesia
    C. Dose-dependent cardiorespiratory depression
       1. Respiratory depression similar to isoflurane
       2. Cardiovascular effects similar to but more desirable than isoflurane (slower heart rate, less myocardial depression)
    D. Does not sensitize the heart to catecholamine-induced cardiac arrhythmias
    E. Rapidly crosses the placenta producing fetal depression
    F. Causes minimal biotransformation; metabolized to the same extent as enflurane
    G. Used in precision vaporizers
    H. Can cause malignant hyperthermia

DESFLURANE (SUPRANE)

I. General anesthetic properties (see Table 10-1)
    A. Identical in structure to isoflurane, except that fluorine is substituted for chlorine
    B. Extremely low blood-gas partition coefficient (0.42); extremely rapid induction and recovery
    C. Less potent than other halogenated agents; MAC is approximately 7.2%

    D. Pungent; produces airway irritation provoking coughing or breath holding

    E. Requires a special electrically heated vaporizer

    F. Stable in moist soda lime

II. Effects on body organ systems

    A. Nervous system

        1. Similar to isoflurane

        2. Dose-dependent CNS depression

        3. Good muscle relaxation; enhances nondepolarizing neuromuscular blocking drugs

        4. Good analgesia

    B. Respiratory system

        1. Causes dose-dependent respiratory depression; decreases the breathing response to increases in $Paco_2$

        2. Pungent odor irritates the airway; induction to anesthesia may be difficult unless preceded by a preanesthetic drug

    C. Cardiovascular system

        1. Qualitatively and quantitatively similar to isoflurane

        2. Decreases arterial BP and cardiac contractility

        3. Sustains autonomic activity better than other inhalants

        4. Keeps heart rate relatively constant

        5. Does not sensitize the heart to catecholamine-induced cardiac arrhythmias

    D. Gastrointestinal system: decreases smooth muscle tone and motility

    E. Renal system: does not affect renal function

    F. Muscular system

        1. Produces good muscle relaxation

        2. Can cause malignant hyperthermia in swine

    G. Uterus and fetus

        1. Crosses the placental barrier; causes fetal depression

        2. Allows rapid recovery (fetus) from depression because of low blood-gas partition coefficient (0.42)

III. Absorption, fate, excretion

    A. Absorbed and eliminated by the lung

    B. Resists degradation by the liver; produces even less inorganic fluoride than isoflurane

C. Has shown no hepatotoxicity or nephrotoxicity
IV. Clinical use
   A. Induction and recovery from anesthesia is about twice as fast as with isoflurane because of the extremely low blood-gas partition coefficient (0.42) despite compartively low potency (MAC ~ 7.2%)
   B. Comparatively good muscle relaxation and analgesia is produced
   C. Pungent odor makes mask induction difficult unless appropriate preanesthetics are used
   D. Recovery may be so rapid that resedation is needed to avoid emergence delirium
V. Dosages
   A. Mask induction: 10% to 15% concentration
   B. Anesthetic maintenance: 6% to 9% concentrations
   C. Preanesthetic use, N_2O, and adjuncts to anesthesia (fentanyl) can reduce MAC

ISOFLURANE (FORANE, AERRANE)

I. General anesthetic properties (see Table 10-1)
   A. An isomer of enflurane and exceptionally stable
   B. Produces comparatively rapid induction and recovery from anesthesia
   C. Can be used in all species
II. Effects on organ systems
   A. Nervous system
      1. Generalized CNS depression
      2. Cerebral blood flow is not increased if ventilation is maintained
      3. Burst suppression is observed in moderate-to-deep surgical anesthesia
   B. Respiratory system
      1. Respiratory depression is similar to methoxyflurane; respiratory patterns may be different
      2. Tidal volume increases initially with depth of anesthesia; respiratory rate decreases; unrelated to anesthetic depth
      3. $Paco_2$ concentration increases with time, although surgical stimulation partly compensates for the respi-

ratory depression and thus prevents a large rise in $Paco_2$

C. Cardiovascular system
1. Cardiac depression is less than with halothane or methoxyflurane
2. Cardiac contractility is depressed, but cardiac output is maintained
3. Progressive vasodilation occurs with increasing depth of anesthesia, possibly because of increased muscle and skin blood flow
4. Hypotensive: mean arterial BP and peripheral vascular resistance decrease with depth of anesthesia
5. Isoflurane does not sensitize the heart to catecholamines

D. Gastrointestinal system
1. Smooth muscle tone and motility are decreased
2. No hepatotoxicity reported (metabolism is very low)

E. Renal system
No changes in renal function reported; very little metabolism to trifluoroacetic acid

F. Muscular system
1. Produces excellent muscle relaxation
2. Markedly potentiates nondepolarizing muscle relaxants
3. Can cause malignant hyperthermia in swine

G. Uterus and fetus
1. Rapidly crosses the placenta
2. Reduces uterine tone
3. Safety in pregnancy not evaluated

III. Absorption, fate, and excretion
A. Absorbed and eliminated by the alveoli
B. Primarily excreted unchanged by the lung
C. Very little biodegradation; approximately 0.25% is metabolized to inorganic fluoride (trifluoroacetic acid)

IV. Clinical use
A. Although a respiratory depressant, isoflurane is relatively inert and nontoxic and produces minimal cardiovascular effects at surgical planes of anesthesia
B. Produces fast, smooth induction and recovery in all species tested

    C. Rapid recovery may predispose some animals to emergence delirium

    D. Calibrated vaporizer is used to deliver accurate concentrations

    E. Can be used in in-the-circle, draw-over vaporizers during "low flow" (closed system) techniques (see Chapter 13)

    F. Can be used with nitrous oxide

    G. Can be used for mask induction

V. Dosages

    A. Induction: 2.5% to 4.5% usually necessary

    B. Induction is facilitated by the use of intravenous anesthesia or nitrous oxide

    C. Maintenance: 1% to 3%

CHAPTER ELEVEN

Neuromuscular Blocking Drugs

"Don't fight forces; use them."
R. BUCKMINSTER FULLER

OVERVIEW

Neuromuscular blocking drugs (NMBDs), commonly referred to as "muscle relaxants," interfere with or block neuromuscular transmission and are useful adjuncts to general anesthesia. Although they do not provide analgesia, sedation, amnesia, or hypnosis, they do stop ventilation, necessitating controlled ventilation and constant patient monitoring.

GENERAL CONSIDERATIONS

I. A primary pharmacological effect of neuromuscular blocking drugs is to produce skeletal muscle (SM) relaxation

II. NMBDs are potentiated by many intravenous (IV) and inhalation anesthetic drugs

III. Other clinically useful drugs (some antibiotics) and some toxins evoke SM weakness or paralysis

IV. Potential mechanisms of SM relaxation

    A. NMBDs interfere with cholinergic neuromuscular transmission in the peripheral somatic nervous system

    B. NMBDs enhance the activity of endogenous inhibitory mechanisms in the central nervous system, which normally modulate SM tone

  V. NMBDs are occasionally used adjunctively during anesthesia to produce controlled, transient muscle weakness
 VI. NMBDs produce no analgesia or hypnotic effect; only muscle relaxation
VII. NMBDs produce respiratory paralysis, which necessitates mechanical or manual support of ventilation
VIII. Hypothermia is an important secondary effect of prolonged SM relaxation in small animals
 IX. NMBDs are positively charged (ionized) and therefore do not pass the blood-brain barrier or cross the placenta in significant amounts
  X. Various electrical stimulators and stimulation protocols can be used to determine the degree of neuromuscular blockade

NORMAL NEUROMUSCULAR FUNCTION

  I. Release of acetylcholine (ACh) in the resting state
   A. Random, infrequent fusion of intraneuronal synaptic vesicles containing ACh with membranes of the unmyelinated nerve terminal
   B. Random, infrequent release of ACh packets
   C. Random ACh release causes mini-endplate potentials at the postsynaptic muscle membrane, which are insufficient to evoke muscle contraction
 II. Action potential (AP)–dependent ACh release
   A. AP causes large depolarization in nerve terminals of α-motor neurons
   B. Depolarization and extracellular Ca^{++} causes nearly simultaneous fusion of many ACh-containing vesicles with the terminal nerve membrane (Fig. 11-1)
   C. Release of many ACh packets evokes a large endplate potential, leading to muscle contraction
III. Combination of ACh with postjunctional receptors
   A. Receptors on the muscle endplates are nicotinic, type IV cholinergic receptors

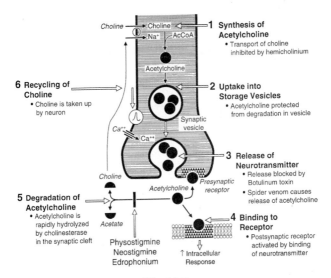

Fig. 11-1

Release of acetycholine from neurons at the neuromuscular junction.

  B. Strength of muscle contraction is proportional to the number of receptors activated by ACh
IV. Hydrolysis of ACh, reuptake of choline, synthesis and packing of ACh
  A. The duration of ACh activity at any cholinergic synapse is limited by the action of acetylcholinesterase (ACh esterase); ACh → acetic acid + choline at synaptic cleft
  B. Choline produced by hydrolysis of ACh is taken up by the nerve terminals and resynthesized into ACh; choline + acetyl CoA ↔ ACh (choline acetyl transferase) at nerve terminal membrane
  C. ACh is packaged into vesicles or stored freely in the cytoplasm of the nerve terminals

MECHANISMS OF SKELETAL MUSCLE RELAXATION EVOKED BY INTERFERENCE WITH NORMAL PERIPHERAL NEUROMUSCULAR FUNCTION

I. At presynaptic site
   A. Inhibition of ACh synthesis (e.g., hemicholinium blocks choline uptake)
   B. Inhibition of ACh release
      1. Calcium deficiency, Mg^{++} increase
      2. Procaine
      3. Tetracyclines and aminoglycoside antibiotics
      4. Some β-blockers
      5. Botulinum toxin
II. At postsynaptic site
   A. Persistent *depolarization* with an agonist that has longer duration of action than ACh (e.g., succinylcholine chloride)
   B. Competitive block of ACh receptors causing *nondepolarizing* blockade (e.g., curare, pancuronium)

TYPES OF NEUROMUSCULAR BLOCKS

I. Phase I block: depolarizing block (succinylcholine)
II. Phase II block: nondepolarizing block (pancuronium)
III. Mixed block: any combination of I and II
IV. Dual block: excessive amounts of depolarizing agents producing phase II block
V. Nonacetylcholine block (procaine, botulinum, decreased Ca^{++}, increased Mg^{++}, increased K^+, decreased K^+)

SEQUENCE OF MUSCLE RELAXATION

I. Oculomotor m. → palpebral m. → facial m. → tongue and pharynx → jaw and tail → limbs → pelvis m. → caudal abdominal m. → cranial abdominal m. → intercostal m. → larynx → diaphragm
   A. The sequence of motor blockade is highly variable in clinical patients
   B. Motor activity to the limbs may appear to return (twitching, jerking) before the diaphragm is fully functional

II. Intercostal and diaphragmatic muscles are thought to be affected last
III. Recovery is generally in the reverse order of paralysis
IV. It is possible but difficult to titrate the specific neuromuscular blocking drug to paralyze the muscles of the eye yet maintain diaphragmatic function

SPECIFIC NEUROMUSCULAR BLOCKING DRUGS
(Tables 11-1, 11-2)

I. Depolarizing drugs act like ACh
   A. Succinylcholine chloride (Sucostrin, Anectin, Quillicine, Suxamethonium)
   B. Decamethonium bromide (Syncurine)
II. Nondepolarizing drugs; competitive blocking drugs
   A. d-Tubocurarine chloride (curare, Metubine)
   B. Gallamine triethiodide (Flaxedil)
   C. Pancuronium bromide (Pavulon)
   D. Vecuronium bromide (Norcuron)
   E. Atracurium besylate (Tracrium)
   F. Mivacurium (Mivacron)
   G. Doxacurium (Nuromax)
   H. Pipecuronium (Arduan)

CLINICAL DIFFERENTIATION BETWEEN DEPOLARIZING AND NONDEPOLARIZING DRUGS

I. Depolarizing
   A. First: transient muscle fasciculations caused by asynchronous depolarization
   B. Second: paralysis caused by prolonged depolarization of the motor endplate
   C. Paralysis is not reversed by anticholinesterase drugs
   D. Paralysis is terminated by metabolism of the NMBD by pseudocholinesterase
II. Nondepolarizing
   A. No muscle fasciculation occurs before muscle paralysis and there is no depolarization of motor endplate; the animal gradually relaxes or "fades"

TABLE 11-1
DOSE OF NEUROMUSCULAR BLOCKING ANESTHETICS WITH SIDE EFFECTS
AND CONTRADICTIONS

AGENT	SPECIES	DOSE IV (mg/lb)	DURATION OF ACTION (minutes)	SIDE EFFECTS	CONTRAINDICATIONS
Succinylcholine chloride	Dog	0.1	1-10	Little cardiovascular effect; muscarinic effect—bradycardia; nicotinic effect—hypertension, increased intraocular pressure; hyperpyrexia	Organophosphate anthelmintics, chronic liver disease, malnutrition, high-K glaucoma, penetrating eye injury
	Cat	0.5	2-3		
	Pig	0.5			
	Horse	0.04	1-10		
Gallamine triethiodide	Dog	0.5	15-20	Tachycardia, 10%-20% of which in dogs is caused by antimuscarinic (atropine-like) effect; transient decrease in arterial blood pressure in cats is caused by ganglionic blockade	Renal dysfunction
	Cat	1-2			
	Horse	0.5			
d-Turbocurarine chloride	Dog	0.2	10-20	Hypotension caused by release of significant quantities of histamine; vagal blockade in dogs, which precludes routine use in veterinary medicine	Renal dysfunction
	Cat	0.2			
	Pig	0.15			
Pancuronium bromide	Dog	0.02	15-20	Negligible	
	Cat				
	Pig	0.05			
Vecuronium*	Dog	0.006-0.1	10-15	Negligible	Liver or kidney disease
Atracurium*	Cat	0.03-0.05	10-15	Negligible	

*Clinical pharmacodynamics and pharmacokinetics are not thoroughly documented in animals.

TABLE 11-2

AUTONOMIC EFFECTS OF NEUROMUSCULAR BLOCKING DRUGS

DRUG	AUTONOMIC GANGLIA	CARDIAC MUSCARINIC RECEPTORS	HISTAMINE RELEASE
Succinylcholine	Stimulated	Stimulated	Slight
Decamethonium	None	None	None
d-Tubocurarine	Blocks	None	Moderate
Gallamine	None	Blocked strongly	None
Pancuronium	None	Blocked weakly	None
Atracurium	None	None	Slight
Vecuronium	None	None	None
Mivacurium	None	None	Slight
Doxacurium	None	None	None
Pipecuronium	None	None	None

    B. Effects can be partially reversed by anticholinesterase drugs (see Fig. 11-1)
       1. Neostigmine
       2. Pyridostigmine
       3. Edrophonium
III. Onset of effect
    A. Rapid (<1 min): succinylcholine
    B. Medium (1 to 2 min): mivacurium, atracurium, vecuronium
    C. Slow (3 to 5 min): doxacurium, pancuronium
IV. Duration of Effect
    A. Ultra-short (1 to 3 min): succinylcholine
    B. Short (5 to 10 min): mivacurium, atracurium
    C. Intermediate (10 to 20 min): vecuronium
    D. Long (20 to 40 min): doxacurium, pancuronium, pipecuronium
V. Speed of antagonism by anticholinesterases
    A. Rapid (<1 min): mivacurium
    B. Medium (1 to 2 min): atracurium, vecuronium
    C. Slow (3 to 5 min): doxacurium, pancuronium

VI. Metabolism
  A. Hoffman elimination: atracurium
  B. Plasma cholinesterase: succinylcholine, mivacurium
  C. Liver: vecuronium, pancuronium, pipecuronium

DEPOLARIZING BLOCKING DRUGS

I. Mechanism of action
  A. Persistent depolarization alone may result in neuromuscular block because of Na^+ inactivation, which prevents electrical impulse generation
  B. Dual block: prolonged exposure of ACh membrane receptors to large doses of depolarizing drugs (ACh, succinylcholine, C-10) reduces the ability of these drugs to cause conductance changes; the reason for this is uncertain

II. Indications
  A. Diagnostic or surgical procedures requiring a short duration of muscle relaxation
  B. Facilitation of endotracheal intubation in humans and primates
  C. Cesarean sections
  D. Fracture reductions

III. Contraindications with depolarizing drugs
  A. Patients with liver disease—pseudocholinesterase produced in the liver
  B. Chronic anemia—acetylcholinesterase partly located on red blood cell membrane
  C. Chronic malnutrition—reduced enzyme concentrations
  D. High K^+ (burns, massive muscle trauma, digitalis therapy) depolarizing blockers may exacerbate hyperkalemia
  E. Organophosphates (anthelmintics)—organophosphates are acetylcholinesterase inhibitors
  F. Glaucoma, penetrating eye injury—contraction of the extraocular muscles may result in expulsion of tissues within the globe

IV. Specific depolarizing drugs: succinylcholine, decamethonium (see Table 11-2)
  A. Succinylcholine: adverse effects
    1. Muscle soreness: reason unknown, probably related to muscle fasciculations and K^+ release before paralysis

2. Histamine release
3. Cardiovascular effects
   a. Potential for bradycardia
   b. The more common response is tachycardia and hypertension caused by sympathetic stimulation
4. Hyperkalemia: caused by increased efflux of K^+ from endplate region of skeletal muscle
5. Some patients have a deficiency of plasma cholinesterase; in these patients, neuromuscular block may be prolonged
6. Genetic anomaly in which plasma cholinesterase is replaced by an atypical cholinesterase may prolong drug effects; differentiation is possible with dibucaine, which inhibits normal plasma cholinesterase 80% and atypical cholinesterase only 20%
7. Malignant hyperpyrexia: manifested by a severe, rapid rise in temperature, which may be accompanied by marked muscle ridigity
   a. Usually occurs when using succinylcholine and halothane together
   b. Treat with 100% O_2, rapid cooling, sodium bicarbonate to control acidosis, and dantrolene sodium (1 to 2 mg/lb)

B. Decamethonium (Syncurine)
1. Basically identical to succinylcholine except
   a. Does not release histamine
   b. Is not metabolized by plasma cholinesterase, thereby prolonging the duration of action
   c. Does not undergo metabolism; excreted by the kidney unchanged; not used renal disease

NONDEPOLARIZING BLOCKING DRUGS
(see specific NMBDs)

I. Mechanism of action
Competitive blocking drugs: compete with ACh for postsynaptic receptors, thereby reducing the depolarization caused by ACh

II. Indications
A. Same as depolarizing drugs

B. High-risk cases as part of a balanced anesthetic technique with narcotics, inhalation, or other analgesic drugs

C. Ocular surgery

D. Control of ventilation at any time

III. Specific nondepolarizing drugs (see Table 11-2)

A. Tubocurarine

1. Curare was used by South American Indians to poison the tips of arrows
   a. Infrequently used in veterinary medicine
   b. Not used in dogs because of histamine release
2. Poor oral absorption
   a. Usually administered intravenously
   b. Effective intramuscularly
3. Ganglionic blockade can occur with high doses
4. Releases histamine, which can cause
   a. Vasodilation and hypotension (probably main cause of hypotension with tubocurarine)
   b. Increased bronchial and salivary secretion
   c. Bronchospasm, which may precipitate an asthmatic attack
5. Synergism
   a. Tubocurarine should be used carefully in the presence of streptomycin, neomycin, and polymyxin, which tend to block neuromuscular transmission
      (1) By a Mg^{++}-type presynaptic block
      (2) By a curariform postsynaptic block
   b. High CO_2 enhances block

B. Gallamine triethiodide (Flaxedil)

1. No histamine release or ganglionic block at clinically effective dosages
2. Selective blockade of parasympathetic innervation of the heart
   a. Questionable ganglionic block; questionable block of muscarinic receptors in heart
   b. Causes tachycardia and occasionally hypertension

C. Pancuronium (Pavulon)

1. No histamine release or ganglionic block; no catecholamine release or inhibition
2. Effects are enhanced by inhalation anesthetics
3. Major portion is excreted unchanged in urine

    4. Tachycardia is occasionally seen following administration

D. Vecuronium (Norcuron)
  1. Developed in an attempt to produce a competitive NMBD with short onset and duration and to eliminate the tachycardia seen occasionally with pancuronium
  2. Eliminated in bile (40%), through kidneys (15%)—a potential advantage in patients with compromised renal function
  3. Minimal cardiovascular effects; no histamine release; no ganglionic block

E. Atracurium (Tracrium)
  1. Developed as a rapid-onset and duration-competitive NMBD; can be administered by infusion
  2. pH and temperature-dependent degradation (Hoffman elimination); therefore a potential benefit is that biologically mediated metabolism and elimination by the liver and kidneys are not needed
  3. Some histamine release at high dosages
  4. Occasionally decreases heart rate and arterial blood pressure (BP)

F. Mivacurium
  1. Slight histamine release
  2. Rapid clearance by plasma cholinesterase
  3. Occasional decrease in arterial BP

G. Doxacurium
  1. No histamine release
  2. Low clearance eliminated by the kidney
  3. Minimal cardiovascular effects

H. Pipecuronium
  1. No histamine release
  2. Low clearance eliminated by the kidney
  3. Minimal cardiovascular effects

FACTORS THAT MAY INFLUENCE NEUROMUSCULAR BLOCKADE (Table 11-3)

I. Temperature
  A. Hyperthermia antagonizes competitive blockade, but enhances and prolongs depolarizing blockade

TABLE 11-3

FACTORS ALTERING INTENSITY OF DEGREE AND DURATION OF MUSCLE RELAXATION

FACTOR	DEPOLARIZING AGENT	NONDEPOLARIZING AGENT
Tranquilizers	↑	↑
Volatile anesthetic agents	↑	↑
Decreased body temperature	↑	↑
Decreased cardiac output/kg bodyweight	↓	↓ (Gallamine)
Increased age	↑	↑
Antibiotics		
Streptomycin	↑	↑
Neomycin	↑	↑
Kanamycin	↑	↑
Organophosphates	↑	—

↑, increase; ↓, decrease; —, no effect.

    B. Hypothermia prolongs nondepolarizing neuromuscular blocking drugs

  II. Acid-base balance (Table 11-4)

    A. Respiratory acidosis augments nondepolarizing neuromuscular blockade

    B. Inadequate reversal of nondepolarizing drugs causes depressed ventilation and respiratory acidosis, which enhances the blockade (vicious cycle)

 III. Fluid and electrolyte imbalance

    A. Hypokalemia and hypocalcemia potentiate nondepolarizing drugs

    B. Dehydration increases the plasma concentration of a normal dose of a nondepolarizing drug, augmenting its effect

    C. High Mg blood levels enhance both depolarizing and nondepolarizing neuromuscular blocking drugs

 IV. Other Drugs

    A. The following antibiotics potentiate nondepolarizing drugs: neomycin, streptomycin, gentamicin, kanamycin, paromomycin, viomycin, polymyxin A and B, colistin, tetracycline, lincomycin, clindamycin

TABLE 11-4

THE EFFECT OF ALTERATIONS IN ACID-BASE BALANCE ON MAGNITUDE AND DURATION OF NEUROMUSCULAR BLOCKADE

ACID-BASE	SUCCINYL-CHOLINE	D-TUBOCURARINE	GALLAMINE	PANCURONIUM
Respiratory acidosis (PaCO$_2$ 60-170)	↓	↑		↑ or —
Respiratory alkalosis (PaCO$_2$ 13-30)	↓	↓ or —	↑	↓ or —
Metabolic acidosis (pH 7.05-7.2)	↑	↑ or —	↓	NE
Metabolic alkalosis (pH 7.6-7.7)	—	↑ or	↑	NE

↑, increase; ↓, decrease; —, no effect; NE, no effect.

ANTICHOLINESTERASE DRUGS

I. Reversal of neuromuscular block

   A. Anticholinesterase drugs such as edrophomium, physostig-mine, pyridostigmine, and neostigmine can be used together with or without anticholinergic drugs

   1. Atropine is used to block the undesirable muscarinic ef-fects of anticholinesterase drugs; muscarinic effects in-clude increased bronchial and salivary secretions and bradycardia

   2. This regimen is ineffective against a depolarization block; in fact, it exacerbates the block because of addi-tional depolarization by excess ACh

   3. This regimen may be effective when depolarizing, block-ing drug is producing a phase II block

   B. Reverse with 0.02 mg/lb neostigmine combined with 0.01 mg/lb atropine (average dose); do not repeat the neostigmine dose more than three times

C. Edrophonium dose is 0.25 mg/lb IV; may be repeated up to five times

D. Complete reversal may take 5 to 45 minutes

CENTRALLY ACTING SKELETAL MUSCLE RELAXANTS

I. Guaifenesin (see Chapter 8)
   A. Mechanism of action is poorly understood but probably relates to depression of transmission through spinal polysynaptic pathways, which normally maintain SM tone
   B. No effect on cerebral arousal
      1. Mild sedation
      2. Variable, mild analgesia
   C. Clinical use: significantly reduces dose of induction drug required to produce recumbency
   D. Dosage and route of administration
      1. 25 mg/lb or to ataxic effect by IV infusion
         50 mg/lb for recumbency by IV infusion
      2. Typically administered as a 5% solution
II. Benzodiazepines (see Chapter 2)
   Mechanism of skeletal muscle relaxant activity is probably related to ability to activate benzodiazepine receptors, activate chloride channels, and potentiate gamma amino butyric acid, a CNS inhibitory neurotransmitter

CHAPTER TWELVE

Anesthetic Toxicity, Oxygen Toxicity, and Drug Interactions

"Can we ever have too much of a good thing?"
DON QUIXOTE DE LA MANCHA

OVERVIEW

All drugs that produce chemical restraint and anesthesia have the potential to produce cytotoxic effects. These toxic effects, if allowed to continue or if sufficiently severe, can jeopardize the patient's life. Toxicity occurs when drugs are administered by persons who are either unfamiliar with the pharmacologic properties of a drug or who have insufficient knowledge regarding the means to counteract the toxic effects of the drug. Inhalation anesthetic drug toxicity is cause for concern in patients and operating room personnel. All inhalation anesthetics are central nervous system (CNS) depressants. When these agents are used, waste anesthetic vapors should be scavenged to minimize personnel exposure and reduce the potential for harmful side effects. Oxygen can be both beneficial and detrimental, depending on the tension of the oxygen and the duration of exposure. Drug interactions underscore the importance of obtaining a comprehensive history and preliminary physical examination.

GENERAL CONSIDERATIONS

I. All drugs used to produce chemical restraint and anesthesia are potentially toxic. Toxicity is caused by

175

    A. Inhibition of nervous system activity

    B. Alteration of normal physiology and depression of cardiopulmonary function

    C. Inhibition of enzyme systems

    D. Direct cytotoxic effects

    E. Differences in species' sensitivity to drugs

    F. Idiosyncratic reactions

II. The toxic manifestations of drugs used to produce chemical restraint and anesthesia are generally reversible

III. Many drugs used to produce chemical restraint and anesthesia can be antagonized

    A. Opioids by narcotic antagonists such as naloxone

    B. Xylazine by α_2-antagonists such as yohimbine, tolazoline, and atipamazole

    C. Nondepolarizing muscle relaxants by acetylcholinesterase inhibitors such as neostigmine and edrophonium

    D. Benzodiazepines by the antagonist flumazenil

    E. General anesthetic–induced depression can be antagonized by analeptics, such as doxapram, 4-aminopyridine, and yohimbine

IV. Waste gas scavenging minimizes the potential danger of drug-induced toxicity

V. Drug interactions may markedly potentiate or inhibit the actions of drugs used for chemical restraint and anesthesia

VOLATILE ANESTHETICS

I. The anesthetic molecule, per se, is nontoxic; however volatile anesthetics are not completely inert and are metabolized to varying degrees (except for nitrous oxide)

    A. Metabolites are believed to be responsible for drug toxicity

    B. Chloride, bromide, and fluoride metabolites have been reported

II. Metabolism of inhalation anesthetics occurs primarily in the liver; metabolites are excreted predominantly by the kidneys

III. Volatile anesthetics are amazingly uniform in distribution, except in areas high in fat, in the thymus, and in the adrenal gland

IV. Three general mechanisms of tissue injury are associated with inhaled anesthetics

A. Toxic intracellular accumulation of metabolites

B. Initiation of immune responses caused by hapten formation

C. Destructive free radical chain reactions initiated by reactive intermediate products of metabolism

V. Normal metabolic functions are affected as long as anesthetic is present; at normal metabolic rates, no toxic side effects may occur; however some individual animals may have metabolic rates far below normal, which may augment toxic effects

A. Animals in shock

B. Hypothermic animals

VI. Metabolism of all inhalation anesthetics may be increased following the administration of enzyme-inducing agents (i.e., phenobarbital)

VII. Several inhalation anesthetic agents have demonstrated teratogenicity in mice when administered chronically or at high concentrations; further investigations are needed to clarify the importance of these findings and their relationship to other animals and humans

VIII. Materials that are properly prepared, stored, and used have not led to any known catastrophes attributable to contaminants; toxic impurities can be and have been caused by human error

A. Cylinders of nitrous oxide (N_2O) have been mislabeled as nitrogen dioxide (NO_2)

B. Improper storage can lead to decomposition of initially pure anesthetics

C. Halogenated compounds are unstable in light

TOXICOLOGY OF ANESTHETIC DRUGS

I. Halothane toxicity

A. Halothane sensitizes the myocardium to catecholamine-induced dysrhythmias

B. Halothane predisposes some animals to hyperpyrexia and malignant hyperthermia

C. Halothane is extensively metabolized

1. Major metabolites

a. Trifluoracetic acid

         b. Fluoride ion

         c. Chloride ion

         d. Bromide ion

    2. Prolonged exposure to subanesthetic concentrations increases metabolism

D. Hepatotoxicity

    1. Many halogenated hydrocarbons are hepatotoxic

    2. Degree of halogenation increases the incidence of toxicity

    3. Hepatic necrosis is believed to be caused by toxic effects of the fluoride or bromide molecules released after halothane metabolism by the liver

    4. Toxic effects are potentiated by halothane-induced, decreased liver perfusion

    5. The National Study of Hepatic Necrosis was unable to identify any unique or consistent lesion resulting from halothane administration

E. Toxicity to halothane

    1. Is dose related

    2. Increases with multiple use

    3. Thymol preservative in commercially prepared halothane is potentially toxic to both the liver and the kidney; however, it is present in minute quantities

II. Methoxyflurane toxicity

A. The primary metabolites of methoxyflurane metabolism

    1. Fluoride ions; all patients recovering from methoxyflurane anesthesia have elevated inorganic fluoride levels

    2. Dichloroacetic acid

    3. Methoxyfluroacetic acid (fluoride and oxalic acid)

    4. Carbon dioxide

B. Renal and liver failure may occur following methoxyflurane anesthesia in the dog, particularly if the animal is receiving other potentially nephrotoxic drugs (tetracyclines, aminoglycosides)

C. Nephrotoxicity

    1. Fluoride ions are excreted by the kidney and are known nephrotoxins that can cause tubular injury

    2. The degree of renal injury is dose related

3. Adequate fluid replacement should be provided to ensure maximum excretion of fluoride ion

4. Tetracyclines may impair renal function, leading to renal failure

5. Both high- and low-output forms of renal failure may occur

6. Clinical studies in normal dogs have not proven renal dysfunction after clinical dosages of methoxyflurane

D. Recommendations

1. Methoxyflurane should be avoided in the aged and markedly obese patient, especially those with impaired renal function

2. Tetracycline or aminoglycoside antibiotics should not be administered concurrently with methoxyflurane

III. Isoflurane, enflurane, sevoflurane, desflurane toxicity

A. Metabolism is slow and minimal

1. Defluorination of isoflurane and desflurane does not result in clinically significant concentrations of serum fluoride ions

2. Metabolism of enflurane and sevoflurane results in higher fluoride concentrations, but seldom reach the threshold for nephrotoxicity

B. Desflurane resists degradation by the liver

C. All agents predispose some animals to malignant hyperthermia

D. Future evaluation of these agents clinically and in the laboratory may reveal additional concerns

IV. Nitrous oxide toxicity

A. Nitrous oxide is not metabolized in vivo

B. It undergoes a physiochemical reaction with vitamin B_{12}

1. Resulting in megaloblastic bone marrow changes and neurologic disease

2. Indirectly inhibiting deoxyribonucleic acid synthesis resulting in reproductive disorders

C. Toxic effects appear after relatively long-term exposure (>10 hrs)

D. Clinical use is not associated with any direct toxic effects

1. Diffusion hypoxia and diffusion into closed cavity spaces are discussed in Chapter 10

V. Barbiturate toxicity
   A. In general, clinical use of barbiturates is not known to display any direct cellular toxic manifestations
      1. Barbiturates stimulate liver microsomal enzymes and may alter the metabolism of other drugs
      2. Some seemingly normal animals appear to be sensitive to the cardiorespiratory depressant effects of barbiturate anesthetics; this clinical observation is probably due to inadvertent overdosage but may be due to idiosyncracy (although unlikely)
      3. Thiobarbiturates increase the susceptibility to the development of ventricular arrhythmias
VI. Propofol toxicity
   Intravenous (IV) infusions administered for greater than three consecutive days result in significant Heinz body production, lethargy, anorexia, and diarrhea in normal cats
VII. Local anesthetic toxicity
   A. In general, the proper administration of local anesthetics causes little or no deleterious effects to tissues
   B. Toxic reactions primarily affect the CNS and cardiovascular system
      1. Acidosis and hypoxia potentiate toxicity
      2. Sensitivity is increased by rapidity of injection
   C. CNS toxicity
      1. Dose necessary to produce CNS toxicity is usually less than the dose that causes cardiovascular collapse
      2. Excessive levels of agents such as lidocaine can cause hypotension, anxiety, tremors, convulsions, or coma
   D. Cardiotoxicity
      1. Rapid IV injection of more potent local anesthetics, such as bupivicaine, may cause cardiovascular collapse
      2. Ventricular dysrhythmias and fatal ventricular fibrillation result
      3. Resuscitation is more difficult following bupivicaine
      4. Pregnant animals may be more sensitive
VIII. Narcotic, ataractic, and cyclohexamine toxicity
   A. These drugs produce little or no toxic effects on the dif-

ferent organ tissues when administered in anesthetic dosages

B. Deleterious side effects
   1. Narcotics
      a. Most common are hyperexcitability, respiratory depression, and bradycardia
      b. Anaphylactic reactions
      c. Blood dyscrasias, thrombocytopenia
   2. Ataractics
      a. Phenothiazine tranquilizers
         (1) Noted for their sympatholytic and hypotensive effects
         (2) Rarely cause extrapyramidal behavioral changes and bradycardia
      b. Butyrophenone tranquilizers can cause aggressive behavior and, rarely, excitement
      c. Benzodiazepines; propylene glycol, a preservative and diluent for diazepam, may cause bradycardia and cardiac arrest
      d. α_2-Agonists cause marked respiratory depression and bradycardia
   3. Cyclohexamines
      a. Produce an apneustic pattern of ventilation and increased arterial P_{CO_2}, resulting in respiratory acidosis
      b. Prolonged recovery from anesthesia may occur following the administration of Telazol to cats and pigs

WASTE ANESTHETIC GAS POLLUTION

I. Waste anesthetic gases are the portion of fresh gases delivered through the anesthetic system that are not inhaled or absorbed by the patient

II. Pollution and exposure of staff occur when anesthetic waste gases leak into the environment

III. Health concerns
   A. Adverse effects associated with chronic exposure to trace levels of waste gases include increased incidence of spontaneous abortion, birth defects, neoplasia, hepatic and re-

nal disease, neurologic disturbances, hematopoietic changes, infertility, and pruritus
1. Individuals at highest risk
   a. Persons with preexisting hepatic or renal disease
   b. Persons with immune system compromise
   c. Women in the first trimester of pregnancy
B. Anesthetics incriminated
  1. Nitrous oxide
  2. Halothane
  3. Methoxyflurane
  4. Enflurane
  5. Isoflurane
C. Epidemiologic studies, animal studies, and human volunteer studies reveal conflicting evidence
  1. To date, no proof of a direct cause-and-effect relationship between exposure to waste gases and disease is available
  2. Overall evidence implies a potential hazard
IV. Regulations regarding waste anesthetic gas levels
A. Standards for maximum allowable concentrations have been established by the National Institute for Occupational Safety and Health
B. Recommended acceptable levels
  1. Volatile agents used alone: less than 2 ppm
  2. Volatile agents combined with nitrous oxide: less than 0.5 ppm
  3. Nitrous oxide: less than 25 ppm
  4. Levels are time-weighted averages over the span of surgical procedure(s)
C. These standards are used by the Occupational Safety and Health Administration when inspecting veterinary hospitals
V. Monitoring for waste gas levels
A. Continuous sampling
  1. Instantaneous point sampling in many areas
  2. Immediate results
  3. Expensive equipment
B. Instantaneous (Grab) sampling
  1. Room air aspirated into a container and sent to a laboratory for evaluation

    2. Delayed results

    3. Results may not reflect overall exposure

    4. Inexpensive and easy to do

  C. Time-weighted average sampling

    1. Samples absorbed by a collection device over a period of time

    2. Delayed results

    3. Best indication of overall exposure

    4. Inexpensive and easy to collect

VI. Collection and removal of waste gases

  A. Scavenging is the collection and removal of waste gases from the anesthetic system and the workplace (Fig. 12-1)

  B. Scavenging systems are comprised of the following major components

    1. Pressure relief valve (pop-off)

      a. Collects excess gases for conduction to removal system

      b. May need to be modified or replaced for leak-free connection to transfer tubing

      c. In nonrebreathing circuits waste gases are collected from the reservoir bag

    2. Interface

      a. Serves to protect breathing circuit and patient from excessive positive or negative pressures

      b. Located between the pop-off valve and the disposal system

      c. Open interfaces contain no valves and are open to the atmosphere

        (1) Best suited for use with high-flow active evacuation systems

        (2) Must have reservoir to buffer pressure differences

        (3) Safety depends on number of vents

        (4) Economical and easily made

      d. Closed interfaces contain mechanical pressure relief valves

        (1) Best suited for use with low-flow active or passive evacuation systems

        (2) Positive-pressure relief valve protects system from pressure buildup if line is occluded

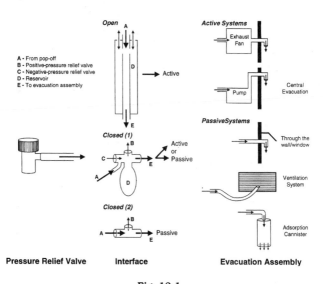

A - From pop-off
B - Positive-pressure relief valve
C - Negative-pressure relief valve
D - Reservoir
E - To evacuation assembly

Pressure Relief Valve   **Interface**   **Evacuation Assembly**

Fig. 12-1
Different methods of scavenging waste anesthetic gases.

      (3) Negative-pressure relief valve required for use with active evacuation system
      (4) Does not require a reservoir, except when active evacuation used
      (5) More costly, but safer and more versatile

  3. Evacuation systems
    a. The evacuation system moves the collected waste gases to a remote area for release
    b. Passive evacuation systems
      (1) The flow of gases is controlled by ventilation
      (2) Gases are exhausted into a nonrecirculating ventilation system, directly out into the atmosphere or through an adsorption device
      (3) Inexpensive and easy to install
      (4) Inefficient and a potential hazard to the patient because of potential resistance to exhalation
    c. Active evacuation systems
      (1) Mechanical flow-inducing devices

        (2) Consist of a central vacuum system or a dedicated fan or pump

        (3) Negative pressure produced requires an interface with a negative pressure relief valve

        (4) More costly and complex than passive systems

        (5) More effective than passive systems

    4. Transfer tubing

       a. Connects the different components of the system

       b. Tubing should be resistant to kinking, easily differentiated from the breathing circuit, and able to transfer high flows

       c. Tubing for passive systems should be as short and wide as practical

VII. Additional control methods

   A. Pressure check all breathing circuits and machines for leaks (see Chapter 14)

   B. Use agent-specific bottle cap adaptors when filling vaporizers to avoid spillage, and fill at the end of the work day when fewer people are present

   C. Use low flow or closed-system techniques whenever possible

   D. Check endotracheal tube cuff before use and be sure it is adequately inflated during use

   E. Avoid chamber and mask inductions; when they cannot be avoided, use tight-fitting mask and attach scavenger tubing to chamber

   F. Ventilate areas where inhalation anesthesia is commonly used and areas where animals are recovering; remain at least 3 feet from recovering patient's head

   G. Do not turn on vaporizer until patient is connected to the circuit

   H. When disconnecting patient from breathing circuit, turn off flowmeter and vaporizer, occlude Y piece, and evacuate remaining gas in system into scavenger

   I. Wear a half-mask respirator if waste gases cannot be avoided

   J. Inform all employees of potential risks associated with waste gas exposure and emphasize measures to reduce exposure

OXYGEN TOXICITY (HYPEROXIA)

I. Tolerance to oxygen
  A. Exposure of animals to increased oxygen tensions (>40%) at atmospheric pressures for prolonged periods (>24 hr) causes metabolic derangements resulting in pulmonary dysfunction; changes include decreases in vital capacity, lung compliance, minute ventilation, respiratory rate, ph, arterial oxygen partial pressure, total lung volume, and carbon dioxide-diffusing capacity.
  B. Animals show considerable variation in the susceptibility to oxygen toxicity
  C. The rate of onset of the disease process is proportional to the inspired tension of oxygen and the duration of exposure
  D. Reductions in vital capacity and pulmonary compliance are the best criteria for identifying onset of toxicity
II. Mechanisms of pulmonary oxygen toxicity
  A. Although oxygen is necessary for the production of energy and survival of all aerobic cells, it is also a cellular poison
    1. Cellular injury results from the metabolic processing of oxygen itself
    2. The majority of oxygen entering the body is metabolized to create adenosine triphosphate and enzymatically reduced to form water
    3. Free radicals are active products of this process: superoxide anion (O_2^-), the hydroxyl radical (OH^-), and hydrogen peroxide (H_2O_2)
    4. Elevated levels of these products released when increased tensions of oxygen are administered are thought to be the cause of biologic membrane damage related to oxygen toxicity
    5. Interaction of free radicals with side chains of membrane lipids results in the formation of lipid peroxides, which inhibit many enzyme activities and further byproducts that can create holes in cell membranes
    6. Damaged membranes leak fluids into extracellular spaces

       7. Inflammation and phagocytosis occurs, producing additional free radicals

III. Lesions

  A. Pulmonary responses to increased oxygen tension

    1. Low doses of oxygen (25% to 60%) are associated with proliferative changes in endothelium and epithelium and permanent widening of the interstitium caused by increased collagen and elastin fiber deposition

    2. Exposure to high concentrations (>60%) of oxygen for more than 12 hours results in

      a. Pulmonary capillary endothelial congestion and hyaline accumulation, type 1 epithelial cell death

      b. Enhanced alveolar epithelial permeability

      c. Interstitial and alveolar edema

      d. Atelectasis; increased shunting

      e. Intraalveolar hemorrhage

    3. Bronchiolar epithelium is also damaged to a lesser degree

  B. Erythrocyte hemolysis

  C. Multiorgan damage (retinal, hepatic, renal, and myocardial)

IV. Signs of toxicity

  A. Early signs

    1. Restlessness

    2. Coughing

    3. Anorexia and lethargy

    4. Dyspnea

  B. Late signs

    1. Respiratory insufficiency

    2. Cyanosis

    3. Frothy or bloody fluid from mouth

    4. Asphyxia

V. Conditions contributing to toxicity

  A. General rate of metabolism has been found to affect the response to oxygen toxicity

  B. Hyperthyroidism and elevations of adrenocortical hormones hasten toxicity

  C. The depression of cellular activity by anesthesia decreases susceptibility to oxygen toxicity

    D. Preexisting pulmonary disease and hypoxia may help protect against rapid onset

    E. Increased susceptibility may result from extremes in humidity, hypercapnia, acidosis, hyperthermia, and pulmonary edema

VI. Recommendations

    A. Do not overreact to the use of oxygen

        1. Hypoxia is commonly associated with anesthesia and hypoventilation, and the damage it causes occurs rapidly

        2. Pulmonary injury from oxygen is uncommon, and onset is slow

        3. Early symptoms are fully reversible on termination of oxygen administration

    B. There are no known contraindications to the use of pure oxygen for brief periods or in emergencies; in the normal lung, no significant toxicity develops in breathing pure oxygen for 12 hours or less

ANESTHETIC DRUG INTERACTIONS

I. Physiochemical interactions: combining two or more drugs in solution may result in a chemical incompatibility; unless you are certain there is not incompatibility, do not combine drugs

II. Some known incompatibilities

    A. Blood or blood products with any solution other than saline

    B. Acidic drug with basic drug

        1. Thiobarbiturate plus lidocaine

        2. Sodium bicarbonate with calcium-containing solutions

III. Pharmacokinetic interactions: interactions affecting absorption, distribution, or elimination of a drug

    A. Protein-binding effects

        1. Phenylbutazone displacing thiobarbiturates from binding sites, resulting in relative barbiturate overdose

        2. Decreased protein binding caused by hemodilution of IV fluid administration

B. Alterations in biotransformation
   1. Phenobarbital enhances liver microsomal enzyme activity
   2. Organophosphates inhibit plasma cholinesterase, prolonging duration of action of ester-linked local anesthetics and depolarizing muscle relaxants
   3. Cimetidine and chloramphenicol reduce hepatic microsomal enzyme activity, thus prolonging duration of action of some drugs
   4. Epinephrine prolongs local anesthetic duration of action, and hyaluronidase increases area of local anesthetic spread

IV. Pharmacodynamic interactions: the actions of a drug on a particular organ system or on the body as a whole can be altered by concurrently administered drugs
   A. Agonist-antagonist interactions
      1. Narcotic agonists-antagonists
      2. α_2-Agonists: yohimbine/tolazoline
      3. Nondepolarizing muscle relaxants–cholinesterase inhibitors
      4. Benzodiazepines: flumazenil
      5. Autonomic receptor agonists-antagonists
   B. Other alterations in pharmacodynamics
      1. Arrhythmogenicity of halothane in presence of catecholamines
      2. Enhancement of halothane-catecholamine arrhythmias by certain drugs, such as barbiturates, xylazine, or ketamine
      3. Decrease in digitalis-induced arrhythmias by halothane
      4. Acepromazine and epinephrine reversal
      5. Aminoglycoside antibiotics prolong effects of muscle relaxants
      6. Tetracyclines enhance nephrotoxicity of methoxyflurane

CHAPTER THIRTEEN

Anesthetic Machines and Breathing Systems

"Give the tools to him that can handle them."
NAPOLEON BONAPARTE

OVERVIEW

A variety of equipment is needed to administer inhalation anesthetic drugs. Volatilizing the anesthetic, delivering it safely to the patient, and minimizing environmental pollution require the use of relatively sophisticated and, at times, cumbersome devices. Regardless of their seeming complexity, most inhalation anesthetic delivery systems have similar designs, many common features, and the same ultimate goal—the delivery of oxygen and safe anesthetic concentrations to the patient and the removal of carbon dioxide. This chapter provides a functional description of the anesthetic machine, breathing circuits, and ancillary equipment for delivery of inhalation anesthesia.

GENERAL CONSIDERATIONS

Although seemingly different in design and appearance, most anesthetic machines contain the same components. The anesthetic machine reduces the pressure of stored oxygen and nitrous oxide and precisely mixes these gases with potent inhalation anesthetics for delivery to the patient through a breathing system.

ANESTHETIC EQUIPMENT

I. Compressed gases, generally, are oxygen and nitrous oxide; occasionally helium and air are used; they come in color-coded cylinders of varying size (see Table 13-1)

    A. Cylinders should be handled carefully

        1. Never leave an unattended cylinder sitting upright

           a. Store E cylinders in a rack

           b. Secure H cylinders to the wall or a transport cart with a chain

        2. Be aware that a cylinder may explode if dropped because it is under high pressure

        3. Open valves slowly and completely

        4. Crack cylinder valve (open and shut quickly) before attaching to machine to remove dust from port

        5. Install the fresh gasket supplied with each freshly filled cylinder

    B. Most machines have a hanger yoke for direct attachment of one or more E cylinders; hanger yokes and E cylinders are keyed with a pin index safety system that prevents inadvertent connection of the cylinder to the wrong gas yoke on the machine

    C. Centralized oxygen sources usually use G or H cylinders, which are more economical

        1. H cylinders require a separate pressure regulator

TABLE **13-1**
COMPRESSED GASES

		CYLINDER SPECIFICATION (LITERS, STP)			
		E	**G**	**H**	
AGENT	**COLOR**	**(4 in × 30 in)**	**(8 in × 55 in)**	**(9 in × 55 in)**	**FILLING PRESSURE (psi)**
Oxygen	Green	655	5,290	6,910	2,200
Nitrous oxide	Blue	1,590	12,110	14,520	750
Carbon dioxide	Gray	1,590	4,160		800
Helium	Brown	500	4,350	5,930	1,650

STP, Standard temperature and pressure; *psi,* pounds per square inch.

(thread size and connection are coded for different types of gas)

2. These cylinders are attached to the machine by a length of high-pressure hose connected to the Diameter Index and Safety System (DISS) fitting of the machine

3. Alternatively the high pressure hose is connected to a special yoke-block connector that attaches to the pin index system in the hanger yoke

4. Oxygen is present within the cylinder only as a gas and its pressure is proportional to gas volume

5. Nitrous oxide is present within the cylinder as a liquid and a gas; pressure within the tank is constant at 750 psi; when all liquid is gone, the pressure rapidly falls

D. Oxygen generators can be installed for central gas supply; they concentrate oxygen from room air to 90% to 95% O_2

II. Hanger yoke
Site of E-cylinder attachment

A. Pin index system configuration avoids improper cylinder connection

B. Brass filter prevents particulate contamination of machine

C. Gauge measures cylinder pressure

D. Check valve prevents transfilling of cylinders or cylinder into pipeline supply

III. Pressure-reducing valves (pressure regulators) reduce the variable pressure of the gas within the cylinder to a constant pressure of approximately 50 psi

A. Providing constant pressure at the flowmeter

B. Allowing a wider range of flowmeter settings for increased sensitivity

C. Ensuring that flowmeter does not have to operate at high pressures

D. Most anesthetic machines have pressure regulators built in to reduce tank pressure from E cylinders

IV. Oxygen "failsafe" system

A. If oxygen supply is interrupted, nitrous oxide and any other gas flow is automatically interrupted

B. An audible oxygen supply failure alarm is also included on some machines

V. Flowmeters

A. A flowmeter controls the rate at which a particular gas is delivered to the fresh-gas outlet; the most common is the rotameter; it contains a ball or bobbin that rises within the tube to a height proportional to the flow of gas through the tube; the ball or bobbin is read at its widest diameter

B. Ideally the oxygen flowmeter should be the last in a series of flowmeters (a hypoxic gas mixture is less likely to develop if a flowmeter tube is cracked)

C. Avoid excessive torque when closing flowmeters, since this may score the valve seat

D. Flowmeters are gas specific; an N_2O flow tube should not be substituted for an O_2 tube or vice versa

E. Through a manifold, individual gas flows are combined downstream of the flowmeters; from here gases move to an out-of-circuit vaporizer or directly to the common gas outlet

VI. Oxygen flush valve

A. Deliver oxygen into the system at 35 to 75 L/min

B. Generally bypasses the vaporizer and delivers oxygen directly to the common gas outlet

C. Serves to dilute the anesthetic gases in the system

VII. Common gas outlet: the point-of-exit from the machine for oxygen, nitrous oxide, and vaporizer (out-of-circuit) output; has a 15 mm connector

VIII. Anesthetic vaporizers

A. Vaporizers volatilize liquid anesthetics and deliver clinically useful concentrations of anesthetic vapor to the common gas outlet or to the breathing circuit if the vaporizer is included therein

B. Vaporizers used out of the circle (VOCs)

1. Variable bypass construction (i.e., inlet gas flow is split between the bypass and vaporization chamber); splitting ratio is determined by the desired output and the specific anesthetic

2. Precision-type instruments

  a. Deliver precise anesthetic concentrations independent of temperature and flow rate; check manufacturer's specifications concerning limits of temperature and flow compensation at different flow rates
  b. Can change anesthetic concentration relatively rapidly
  c. Are expensive
3. Specific VOCs
  a. Halothane vaporizers
    (1) Fluotec Mark II, III (Cyprane, Matrix)
    (2) Fluotec IV and V (Ohmeda), available only on newer machines for use in humans
    (3) Vapomatic (old Foregger Fluomatic) (A. M. Bickford)
    (4) Vapor and Vapor 19.1–Halothane (Drager)
    (5) Ohio Vaporizer for Halothane (Ohmeda)
  b. Methoxyflurane vaporizers
    (1) Pentec Mark II (Cyprane, serviced by Fraser Harlake)
    (2) Pentomatic (Foregger)
    (3) Vapor-Methoxyflurane (Drager)
  c. Enflurane vaporizers
    (1) Enfluratec (Cyprane, serviced by Ohmeda)
    (2) Enflurane Vapor 19.1 (Drager)
    (3) Ohio Vaporizer for Enflurane (Ohmeda)
  d. Isoflurane vaporizers
    (1) Ohio Vaporizer for Isoflurane (Ohmeda)
    (2) Vapor 19.1 (Drager)
    (3) Fortec and Fortec 4, also sold as Isotec (Cyprane, serviced by Ohmeda)
    (4) Isoflurane can be used in halothane vaporizers, provided vaporizer is completely drained and wick is thoroughly dried
  e. Vaporizers used for various inhalation agents (measured flow, nonagent specific)
    (1) Vernitrol (Ohio Medical)
    (2) Copper Kettle (Foregger)
    (3) A separate flowmeter controls carrier gas flow through vaporizer

(4) Components needed to calculate vaporizer flowmeter setting
  (a) Vapor pressure (depends on agent and temperature)
  (b) Desired total gas flow
  (c) Desired anesthetic percent

(5) A slide rule is provided by the manufacturer to easily calculate flow rate through the vaporizer; an exception is the Metomatic 980, an old veterinary machine; it is a vernitrol with specific calibration marks for methoxyflurane that should not be used for any other anesthetic

f. Maintenance
  (1) Vaporizers should ideally be sent to the manufacturer yearly for cleaning and recalibration
  (2) Alternatively they should be serviced whenever the control dial becomes "sticky" or whenever the dial setting does not match clinical perception

C. Vaporizers in the circle (VIC) (also called draw-over vaporizers); animal's breathing pushes gas through vaporizer and volatizes anesthetic
  1. Output depends on
    a. Specific anesthetic
    b. Temperature
    c. Flow through vaporizer
    d. Vaporizer construction
    e. Location of vaporizer in breathing circuit
  2. Variation in respiration alters flow through the vaporizer, thus affecting the concentration of anesthetic delivery; output increases with increasing ventilation
  3. Calibration marks on top of vaporizer are not synonymous with percentage
  4. Relatively inexpensive
  5. Types
    a. Ohio No. 8 Vaporizer (Pitman-Moore); wick must be removed when using with halothane or isoflurane
    b. Stephens Universal (Henry Schein); wick must

be removed when using with halothane or isoflurane

c. Others: Goldman, EMO, McKesson, Rowbotham

6. Maintenance: wick should be allowed to dry weekly to rid system of excess water vapor

ANESTHETIC BREATHING SYSTEMS

I. Purpose
   A. Delivery of anesthetic gases safely, inexpensively, and with adequate oxygen
   B. Removal of carbon dioxide by one of three methods
      1. Dilution
      2. Nonrebreathing valve systems are no longer used since disadvantages outweigh advantages
      3. Carbon dioxide absorbents
II. Classification of systems
   A. Open (nonrebreathing)
      1. Open drop or cone (Fig. 13-1)
      2. Insufflation: anesthetic gas and oxygen are delivered to airway with high flow rate through a small-diameter catheter
      3. Induction chamber: typically used for induction of small, difficult-to-handle animals
      4. Features
         a. No reservoir
         b. No or slight rebreathing of expired gases
         c. Carbon dioxide removal by dilution
      5. Advantages
         a. Low cost of equipment
         b. Minimal or no rebreathing of expired gases by patient
         c. Minimal resistance to breathing
      6. Disadvantages
         a. Wasteful because so much anesthetic is vaporized
         b. Difficult to control anesthetic concentration delivered; requires relatively high flows to prevent dilution with room air
         c. No ventilation method
         d. Difficult or impossible to scavenge waste gas

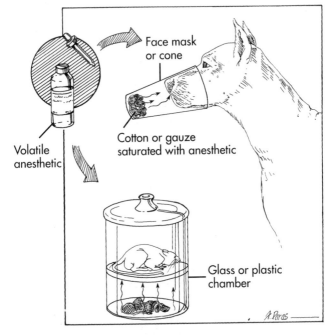

Fig. 13-1
Open system. Gauze or cotton is saturated with anesthetic and placed in a cone or chamber from which the animal breathes.

  e. Vaporization of anesthetic depends on room temperature (open drop)
B. Mapleson (nonrebreathing) systems rely on relatively high, fresh gas flow rate (Table 13-2) to remove carbon dioxide; the following classifications are based on location of fresh gas inlet and opening (or valve) for exit of exhaled gas
  1. Types
    a. Rees modification of Ayre's T piece (Fig. 13-2) (Mapleson F: fresh gas enters near the patient and exits from the reservoir bag)
    b. Bain circuit (Fig. 13-3) (modified Mapleson D: fresh gas enters circuit near bag, but in coaxial design de-

RECOMMENDED OXYGEN FLOW RATES FOR ANESTHETIC SYSTEMS

Closed circle	2-3 ml/lb/min O_2*
Semiclosed circle	5-20 ml/lb/min O_2†
Mapleson systems	
Magill system	Equal to minute ventilation (spontaneous respiration only)
Ayre's T piece	0.5-4 L/min‡
Bain circuit	100-150 ml/lb/min
Insufflation	100-150 ml/lb/min

*Cannot use nitrous oxide in a closed circle.
†If using nitrous oxide, add to the O_2 flow.
‡Indicates total flow rate for nonrebreathing.

Ayres Y-or T-piece system

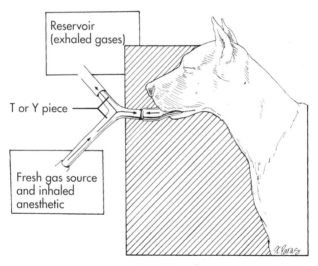

Fig. 13-2

Mapleson F (Ayres T piece). Low resistance method of delivering anesthetic and oxygen. High, fresh gas flow rates are used to minimize or eliminate the rebreathing of exhaled gas. Exhaled gas flows through corrugated tubing into a rebreathing bag. Excess gas is vented through an opening in the bag.

Bain circuit

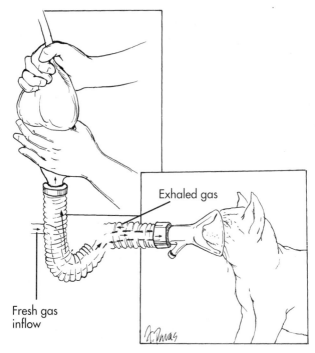

Fig. 13-3
Modified Mapleson D Bain circuit. Functions similarly to Ayres T-piece
system. It minimizes equipment dead space and facilitates warming of the
inspired gases.

        livers it near patient, and exhaled gas passes around
        fresh gas line to exit near bag)
    c. Magill system (Fig. 13-4) (modified Mapleson A:
       fresh gas enters near bag and exhaled gas exits
       through a pop-off valve located near the patient)
       (1) Efficient during spontaneous ventilation
       (2) Very inefficient during controlled ventilation
  C. Rebreathing systems allow rebreathing of exhaled gases
    minus carbon dioxide; amount of rebreathing depends on
    fresh gas flow rate

1. Circle system (Figs. 13-5 and 13-6)
   a. Components
      (1) Pop-off (pressure relief) valve
         (a) Allows the release of excess pressure from the system; the volume of gas in excess of the animal's minute oxygen consumption is vented from the system
         (b) Fitted with spring-loaded or variable orifice; modern valves usually "pop-off" or open when pressure exceeds 0.5 to 1 cm H_2O; as valve is tightened down, more pressure is required to open valve
         (c) Fitted with orifice for scavenging; excess vacuum applied to valve by scavenger can evacuate the breathing system
      (2) Carbon dioxide absorbent canister
         (a) Removes carbon dioxide from the expired gases
         (b) Capacity should be one to two times tidal volume (5 ml/lb)
         (c) absorbent used is either soda-lime or barium hydroxide-lime; Na^+, K^+, Ca^{++}, and Ba^{++} hydroxide reacts with exhaled CO_2 and water to form carbonate; heat is liberated, pH decreases
         (d) Uses 4- to 8-mesh, granule-size soda-lime
         (e) Absorbent has a pH color-change indicator (ethyl violet) that turns blue on consumption; the indicator may revert to original color when allowed to rest; should be changed after 6 to 8 hours of use, depending on fresh gas flow rates and size of the animal
      (3) Two unidirectional flow valves minimize apparatus dead space by preventing exhaled gas from being rebreathed before it passes through the absorbent canister

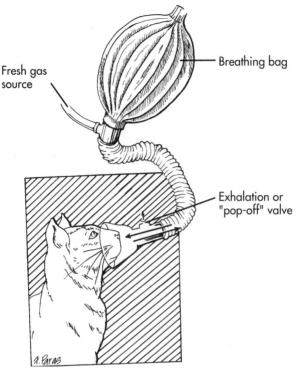

Fig. 13-4

Mapleson A Magill system. Low, fresh gas flow rates can be used during spontaneous ventilation because of the presence of a pop-off valve near the patient that preferentially exhausts alveolar gas.

    (4) Vaporizer (in or out of the circle; see Figs. 13-5, 13-6)

    (5) Rebreathing bag (reservoir bag) in the following sizes

        <15 lb = 1 L

        >15<40 lb = 2 L

        >40<120 lb = 3 L

        >120<300 lb = 5 L

        >300 lb = 35 L (large-animal system)

    (6) Pressure manometer

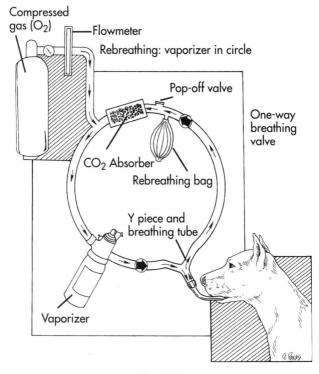

Fig. 13-5
Anesthetic circle system with the vaporizer in circle.

        (a) Monitors pressure within breathing system
        (b) Typically calibrated from -30 to $+50$ cm H_2O
     (7) Corrugated breathing tubes and Y piece
        (a) Generally 1 m long and 22 mm diameter
        (b) Longer tubes are used when machines cannot be located near patient's head
        (c) Shorter tubes with small diameter (13 mm) are used for animals <10 lbs
        (d) Large animal tubes are 50 mm diameter
  b. Advantages
     (1) Relatively low gas flow rates can be used (economical and minimize pollution)

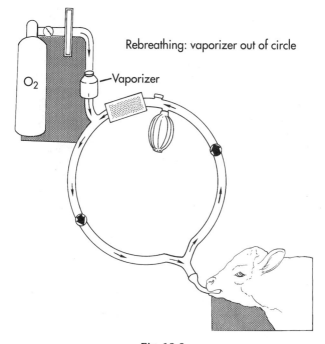

Fig. 13-6
Anesthetic circle system with the vaporizer out of circle.

        (2) Carbon dioxide–absorbent canister is located away from patient, as opposed to to-and-fro system

        (3) Ventilation is readily observed and controlled by reservoir bag

        (4) Minimal heat loss and airway drying

        (5) Absence of abrupt fluctuations in anesthetic depth

   c. Disadvantages

        (1) System is bulky

        (2) Parts may be rearranged or may malfunction

        (3) Resistance to gas flow is greater than with Mapleson systems; conventional circle systems should not be used in animals <5 lbs

        (4) Some components are difficult to clean

(5) Cross-infection of patients is possible; bag and hoses should be disinfected after each use

2. To-and-fro systems (Fig. 13-7); exhaled gas passes through the absorbent into the reservoir bag and during inhalation returns through the absorbent to the animal

   a. Same components as circle system minus the unidirectional valves

   b. Heat accumulates in the system because the carbon dioxide canister is attached near the endotracheal tube; alkaline dust from carbon dioxide absorbent may be inhaled

   c. Canister dead space increases with time because of exhaustion of absorbent near the patient

   d. Advantages

      (1) Low resistance and efficient carbon dioxide absorption

      (2) Portable

      (3) Easily cleaned and disinfected

   e. Disadvantages

      (1) Cumbersome because apparatus is near animal's head

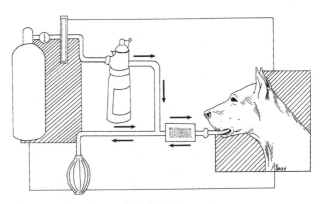

Fig. 13-7

The to-and-fro anesthetic system maximizes carbon dioxide removal and helps maintain body temperature.

   (2) Different-sized canisters needed for different-sized animals
   (3) Possible inhalation of alkaline dust
3. Fresh gas flow rates for rebreathing systems (Table 13-2)
   a. Minimum flow rate equals minute oxygen consumption
      (1) Approximately 2 to 3 ml/lb/min
      (2) Because volume of fresh gas delivered = (equals) patient uptake, volume of system will not change, and pop-off valve can remain closed
      (3) Advantages of closed system
         (a) Minimal pollution
         (b) Economical
         (c) Breathing system warmth and humidity maximized
      (4) Disadvantages
         (a) Difficult to rapidly change concentration with VOC
            • VOC can't be used with closed-system flow rate for first 10 to 20 minutes because anesthetic uptake is too great
            • VIC can be used with closed-system flow rates from the beginning of anesthesia
         (b) System volume must be more closely monitored
         (c) Increased CO_2 absorbent use
         (d) N_2O can't be used without an oxygen monitor in the system
   b. Flow rates in excess of 2 to 3 ml/lb/min require open pop-off valve (semiclosed)
III. Veterinary anesthetic machines
   A. Relatively few machines are currently manufactured for veterinary use
      1. Matrix: several small-animal machines and one large-animal machine
      2. Bickford: several small-animal models
      3. J. D. Medical: several large-animal machines with ventilators

       4. Stephens anesthetic machine: in-circle vaporizer for small animals
       5. Bowring Engineering (United Kingdom): to-and-fro, circle systems, large and small animal
       6. Minerve (France): small- and large-animal machines
       7. DRE: small-animal machine

  B. Veterinary machines no longer manufactured
       1. Dupaco compact 78: small-animal machines
       2. North American Drager Narkovet: small- and large-animal machines
       3. Pitman-Moore 970, 980, and Vetaflex-5
       4. Summit Hill: several small-animal systems and one large-animal system

  C. Human anesthesia machines (used) are available through most anesthesia equipment dealers

IV. Cleaning and disinfection

  A. Breathing hoses and reservoir bags should be cleaned and disinfected following each use
       1. Wash with hot soapy water and rinse
       2. Soak in cold disinfectant solution such as Nolvasan or Cidex and thoroughly rinse
       3. Clean anesthetic machine external surfaces daily with spray cleaner
       4. Occasionally disassemble dome valves and absorbent canister and wipe dry

  B. Gas or steam autoclaving is not necessary unless gross contamination is present

V. Anesthetic machine check (Table 13-3)

  A. Verify proper machine function before each anesthesia; some checks should be performed daily, others before each use
  B. Consult owners' manual for manufacturer's recommendations

TROUBLESHOOTING ANESTHETIC EQUIPMENT PROBLEMS

I. Rebreathing bag empty
  A. Flow rate too low or flowmeter control knob turned off
  B. System leak

TABLE 13-3

GENERIC ANESTHESIA MACHINE AND BREATHING CIRCUIT CHECK

1. Inspect machine
   a. Fill vaporizers, tighten filler caps, turn off vaporizers
   b. Fill CO_2 canister, and confirm that absorbent is functional
   c. Confirm proper function of unidirectional valves in circle—with surgical mask inhale and exhale through Y piece*
2. Confirm oxygen supply and failsafe
   a. Check cylinder pressure
   b. Turn on N_2O cylinder and flowmeter; turn O_2 cylinder off; N_2O float should drop to zero; reopen O_2 cylinder*
3. Verify proper flowmeter functions—bobbin or float should move freely throughout length of tube*
4. Check breathing circuit
   a. Proper, tight connections
   b. Occlude Y piece, close pop-off valve, pressurize circuit to 30 cm H_2O; check for total leak of <250 ml/min; open pop-off valve and confirm release of pressure
5. Check waste gas scavenging system*
   a. Confirm that scavenging system is connected to pop-off valve
   b. Turn on vacuum pump or verify patency of passive system
6. Check ventilator function*
   a. Verify connection to breathing circuit
   b. Check for leaks according to manufacturer

*Need only be performed daily.

1. Gasket on carbon dioxide cannister improperly installed
2. Hole in rebreathing bag or tubing
3. Leak in endotracheal tube cuff
4. Waste-gas scavenging system using active suction improperly regulated
5. Water drain near carbon dioxide absorbent canister is open

II. Rebreathing bag overly distended (positive pressure in circuit)
   A. Pop-off valve inadvertently left closed
   B. Flow rate too high in closed system
   C. Waste-gas scavenging system improperly regulated
III. Patient seems "light"
   A. Vaporizer empty
   B. Excessive carbon dioxide buildup

    1. Exhausted carbon dioxide absorbent

    2. Sticky unidirectional valve

C. Vaporizer needs service

    1. Water buildup on wick

    2. Recalibration necessary

D. Patient receiving hypoxic gas mixture

   Nitrous oxide flowmeter set too high relative to oxygen flow

CHAPTER FOURTEEN

Ventilation and Mechanical Assist Devices

"You don't need a weatherman to know which way
the wind blows."

BOB DYLAN

OVERVIEW

One of the most crucial aspects of providing safe general anesthesia is the maintenance of normal ventilation. Normal ventilation is defined as the maintenance of arterial carbon dioxide levels within normal limits (35 to 40 mm Hg). Generally, respiratory effort can be verified by observing the movements of the patient's chest and abdominal wall. Although these movements may be regular and give the appearance of satisfactory gas exchange, they do not ensure adequate movement of air in and out of the lungs. Adequate gas exchange can be provided by inflating the lungs to a predetermined pressure or predetermined volume by manually squeezing a rebreathing bag on an anesthetic machine or using a mechanical ventilatory-assist device. High-frequency ventilation of patients is a unique procedure based on the principle that diffusion is the primary means by which fresh gases are delivered to peripheral airways and gas exchange sites.

GENERAL CONSIDERATIONS

I. Artificial ventilation can do more harm than good if improperly used

II. Anyone attempting artificial ventilation should be thoroughly familiar with normal cardiopulmonary physiology and blood gas interpretation

III. Generally, mechanical ventilatory-assist devices do no more than compress a rebreathing bag to inflate the lungs; they are an extra pair of hands

IV. The use of artificial ventilation should be considered in patients who are not breathing adequately

V. Blood gas determinations are the best test of ventilatory adequacy

SOURCES OF RESPIRATORY INADEQUACY

I. Depression of respiratory centers
   A. Drug induced
      1. Anesthetic
      2. Drug toxicities
   B. Metabolic
      1. Acidosis
      2. Coma
      3. Toxic metabolites (endotoxins)
   C. Physical
      1. Head trauma (increased intracranial pressure)
      2. Chest trauma
      3. Severance of nerves
      4. Nerve trauma (edema)
II. Inability to adequately expand the thorax
   A. Pain (splinting of chest)
   B. Chest trauma
   C. Thoracic surgery
   D. Abdominal distention
   E. Muscle weakness
   F. Obesity
   G. Bony deformities of the chest wall
   H. Positioning
      1. Weight of viscera may impede expansion
      2. Abdominal compression may impede expansion
   I. Neuromuscular blocking drugs (NMBDs)
III. Inability to adequately expand the lungs
   A. Pneumothorax (especially tension pneumothorax)
   B. Pleural fluid
   C. Diaphragmatic hernia

D. Thoracic surgery
E. Neoplasia
F. Pneumonia
G. Atelectasis
H. Positioning
IV. Acute cardiopulmonary arrest
V. Pulmonary edema or insufficiency

MANAGEMENT OF VENTILATION IN ANESTHESIA

I. Anesthetics are respiratory depressants; thus ventilation may need to be assisted if hypoventilation occurs
II. Special indications for artificial ventilation in anesthesia
   A. Thoracic surgery
      1. Controlled respiration minimizes extraneous chest wall movements, thus aiding the surgeon
      2. With the chest open, the patient cannot adequately expand the lungs (pneumothorax)
   B. Neuromuscular blockers: clinical doses of NMBDs, which produce muscular relaxation, also paralyze the diaphragm and intercostal muscles
   C. Prolonged anesthesia (>90 min), especially in the horse
   D. Trauma
      1. Flail chest
      2. Diaphragmatic hernia
   E. Central nervous system trauma
   F. Drug overdose

PHYSIOLOGIC CONSIDERATIONS

I. Pulmonary system
   A. Normal lungs are well ventilated by a variety of different pressures, volumes, and flow rates (Fig. 14-1)
   B. During spontaneous ventilation, the portions of the lung in closest contact with moving surfaces (i.e., the peripheral lung field) receive the greater volume of inspired gases
   C. During artificial ventilation, the pressure gradient induced inflates the peribronchial and mediastinal areas of the lung;

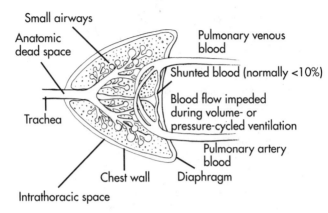

Fig. 14-1

Lung volume and airway pressure can augment or impede blood flow through the lung.

the peripheral segments remain relatively hypoventilated; pressure or volume ventilation increases airway diameter and thus anatomic dead space, further reducing alveolar ventilation

D. Positive-pressure ventilation results in marked reduction in lung compliance and progressive decline in lung volume, which can lead to atelectasis and hypoxemia
  1. Airway closure can occur
  2. Increased lung water reduces compliance
  3. Distribution of ventilation is altered
  4. Volume-cycled ventilators compensate for worsening lung mechanics to a greater degree than do pressure-cycled ventilators (by ensuring delivery of a constant volume); pressure-cycled ventilators must be reset to compensate for "stiffened" lungs (periodic "sighs" are important)

II. Cardiovascular system (Table 14-1)
  A. During spontaneous ventilation, the subatmospheric pressure within the thorax augments venous return; this subatmospheric pressure is reduced (made more negative) during inspiration by downward movement of the diaphragm

TABLE 14-1

CARDIOVASCULAR SYSTEM: EFFECTS OF BREATHING AND INTERMITTENT POSITIVE-PRESSURE VENTILATION

	PHASE OF CYCLE	INTRATHORACIC PRESSURE	RIGHT VENTRICLE FILLING	RIGHT VENTRICLE CARDIAC OUTPUT	TOTAL THORACIC BLOOD VOLUME	LEFT VENTRICLE FILLING	LEFT VENTRICLE CARDIAC OUTPUT
Normal breathing	Inspiration active	(5 cm of H_2O)	↑	↑	↑	↓	↓
	Expiration passive	↑ (−2 cm H_2O)	↓ When compared to normal inspiration	↓	↓	↑ Due to venous return	↑
IPPV	Inspiration passive	↑ (15–20 cm H_2O)	↓ (Peripheral venous pressure ↑)	↓	↓	↑ from lung for 3–5 beats, then ↓	↑ (↓ if IPP prolonged)
	Expiration generally passive	↓ To atmospheric pressure	↓ When compared to previous positive pressure inspiration	↑ If expiration is long enough, i.e., ≥ inspiration	↑	↓	↓

IPPV, intermittent positive-pressure ventilation; Ipp, intermittent positive pressure.

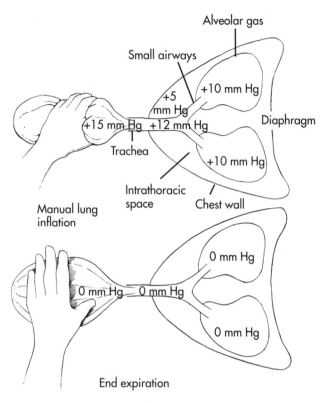

Fig. 14-2

Manual lung inflation produces a positive pressure in the lung and thoracic cavity, which impedes lung blood flow and lowers cardiac output.

B. During artificial ventilation, the pressure in the trachea and lung is transmitted to the thoracic cavity, thus impeding venous return and potentially decreasing cardiac output (Fig. 14-2; see also Fig. 14-1)

C. Artificial ventilation decreases arterial blood pressure and thus cardiac output in any of the following instances
   1. Average airway pressure consistently >10 mm Hg
   2. Low circulating blood volume caused by dehydration, anemia, blood loss

      3. Impaired sympathetic nervous system activity caused by anesthesia, local anesthetics, shock

   D. Artificial ventilation decreases pulmonary blood flow and therefore may lead to ventilation-perfusion abnormalities

   E. Circulatory changes during artificial ventilation are caused by prolonged increases in mean airway pressure and decreased CO_2

IV. Important normal values to remember

   A. Tidal volume (V_T): the amount of gas exchanged in one respiratory cycle

      1. 5 ml/lb in small animals (less than 400 pounds)

      2. 3 to 4 ml/lb in large animals (more than 400 pounds)

      3. Ventilator bellows volume is usually increased by 1 to 2 ml/lb over V_T during intermittent positive-pressure breathing (IPPV) to compensate for the increased positive pressure–induced volume of the breathing hoses and conducting airways

   B. Minute volume (V^m): the volume of gas exchanged in 1 minute

      1. Dependent on V_T and breaths per minute (BPM):

$$V_T \times BPM = V^m$$

   C. Adequate inflation of the lungs of a normal animal requires approximately 15 to 20 cm H_2O pressure; lung compliance (volume/pressure/kg) is important in determining the pressure required to inflate the lung

   D. The spontaneous ventilatory cycle

      1. Inspiration (I) is active

         a. 1 second in small animals

         b. 1.5 to 3 seconds in large animals

   E. Guides to adequate mechanical artificial ventilation in the normal patient

      1. V_T (under normal conditions)

         a. Up to 7 ml/lb in small animals

         b. Up to 6 to 7 ml/lb in large animals

      2. Pressures

         a. 15 to 20 cm H_2O in small animal species with normal lungs, and 20 to 30 cm H_2O in large animal species with normal lungs

      b. During open-chest procedures or in the presence of "stiff" or mechanically inhibited lungs, pressure must be increased

  3. I/E (inspiration/expiration) ratios

      a. 1:2 to 1:4.5 in small animals

      b. 1:1 to 1:4.5 in large animals

  4. Inspiratory times

      a. Less than 1.5 seconds in small animals

      b. Less than 3 seconds in large animals (typically 2 seconds in a 1000-lb horse)

      c. Observation of chest wall movements is a helpful indication of lung inflation

CLASSIFICATION OF VENTILATORS

I. Volume preset (Fig. 14-3)

  A. A gas or gas mixture is delivered to a preset volume by the ventilatory-assist device

  B. Advantages

    1. Delivers a known V_T regardless of the pressure imposed

      a. Most volume-cycled ventilators are equipped with a blow-off safety valve to prevent the development of extremely high pressure (>60 cm H_2O)

      b. Delivers a constant volume despite changes in compliance and resistance of the lungs during anesthesia

    2. Relatively simple machine

  C. Disadvantages

    1. High airway pressures may develop

    2. Volume ventilators do not compensate for small leaks in the system; eliminating them requires an airtight system; a major leak prevents the patient from receiving an adequate V_T

  D. Piston or bellows-type ventilator delivers a predetermined volume

II. Pressure preset (Fig. 14-4)

  A. A gas or gas mixture is delivered by a ventilatory-assist device during the inspiratory phase until the system reaches a preset pressure

Volume-cycled Ventilation

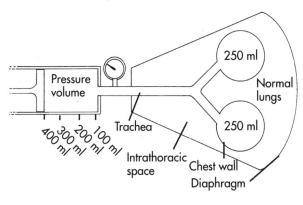

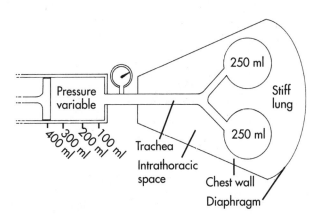

Fig. 14-3

Volume-preset ventilators deliver a predetermined volume irrespective of
the pressure developed.

Pressure-cycled Ventilator

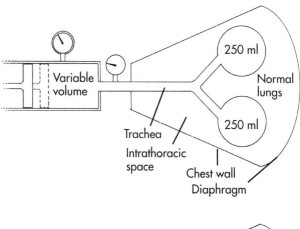

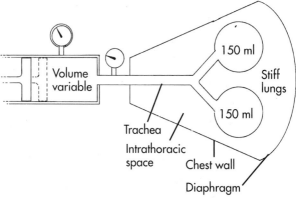

Fig. 14-4

Pressure-preset ventilators deliver a predetermined pressure irrespective of the volume delivered.

B. Advantages
1. High safety factor; a high pressure will not develop unless preset by the operator
2. Compensates for small leaks; large leaks prolong inspiratory time

C. Disadvantages
1. Volume delivered is variable and depends on the following
   a. Lung compliance
   b. Airway resistance
   c. Number of functional alveoli
   d. Pressure within the thorax
2. Measurement of tidal volume may be difficult if ventilator is not equipped with bellows or respirometer
3. Pressure may need to be increased during a procedure to maintain adequate V_T

III. Time cycled: most volume-preset ventilators can be adjusted to limit the volume delivered through a combination of adjustments to the I:E ratio, frequency or respiratory rate (f), and inspiratory flow rate

IV. Volume-preset ventilators classified by bellows movement during expiration
A. Ascending: preferred design since leaks are easily identified
B. Descending: bellows falls during expiratory phase

MODES OF OPERATION OF VENTILATORY-ASSIST DEVICES

I. Assist mode: patient triggers the ventilatory device by initiating an inspiratory effort

II. Controlled mode
A. Operator sets the desired respiratory rate
B. Ventilator is insensitive to the patient's inspiratory efforts
C. If the patient resists controlled ventilation ("bucks" the ventilator), severe cardiopulmonary embarrassment may occur

III. Assist-controlled mode: a minimal respiratory rate is set by the operator, which the patient may override by initiating spontaneous ventilatory efforts at a faster rate

TERMS USED FOR VARIABLE MODES OF OPERATION DURING MECHANICAL VENTILATION

I. **IPPV** (intermittent positive-pressure ventilation): positive pressure maintained only during inspiration

II. **CPPV** (continuous positive-pressure ventilation): mechanical ventilation with positive pressure maintained during inspiration and at lower pressure or expiration

III. **PNPV** (positive/negative–pressure ventilation): positive pressure during inspiration and negative pressure during expiration

IV. **PEEP** (positive end-expiratory pressure): used to open small airways following lung trauma or pulmonary edema

V. **ZEEP** (zero end-expiratory pressure): normal passive expiration

VI. **NEEP** (negative end-expiratory pressure): used to hasten expiration

VII. **CPAP** (continuous positive airway pressure): spontaneous breathing with positive pressure during both inspiratory and expiratory cycles

VIII. **IMV** (intermittent mandatory ventilation): breaths supplied by ventilator in addition to normal negative pressure breaths supplied by the patient

VENTILATORS COMMONLY USED IN VETERINARY MEDICINE

Most ventilators used during general anesthesia connect to the anesthesia breathing system where the rebreathing bag attaches; other free-standing ventilators are used without a breathing circuit.

I. North American–Drager Large and Small Animal Anesthetic Ventilator

A. Classification: Volume-preset ventilator; descending bellows

1. Volume is adjusted by raising and lowering bellows support to appropriate level

2. Pressure manometer indicates the pressure within the system

B. Controls

1. On/off switch

2. Frequency is adjusted to beats/min
3. Flow is adjustable; inspiratory flow rate determines inspiratory time
4. I:E ratio is adjustable from 1:1 to 1:4.5
5. Adjustment of flow rate, I:E ratio, and F determines delivered volume
6. Operates only in the control mode

C. Pop-off valve
   1. Manual pop-off valve of breathing system must be closed during ventilator use
   2. Automatic pop-off closes with the inspiratory cycle

II. Bag-in-a-barrel type ventilator, generally powered by a Bird pressure-cycled ventilator (J. D. Medical anesthetic machine)

A. Classification: pressure-preset ventilator; descending bellows

B. Large-animal ventilator
   1. Bag or bellows in a cylinder is compressed by the flow generated by a modified Bird Mark 7 ventilator
   2. Volume is indicated on the chamber encasing the bellows
   3. The pressure and f can be adjusted to give the desired volume

C. Mode
   1. Assisted: the sensitivity can be adjusted so that the patient can trigger the machine
   2. Controlled: the value of sensitivity can be increased so that the patient cannot trigger the machine
   3. Assist-controlled: the operator can control the minimum number of breaths delivered; the patient can also trigger ventilator operation

D. Controls
   1. Inspiratory pressure
      a. Usually set at 20 to 30 cm water
      b. Adjusted to give the desired tidal volume
   2. Expiratory time
      a. Controls respiratory rate by controlling time between breaths
      b. Rate usually set at 6 to 10 breaths/min for the horse

3. Flow rate (adjust to an inspiratory time of 2 seconds for the horse)
4. Air mix: pull air mix knob to OUT position
   a. Set at 50% to conserve oxygen
   b. Does not affect oxygen supply to the animal
5. Sensitivity
   a. Governs ability of the animal to trigger the ventilator
   b. Numbers are merely a rough guide to indicator of position

III. Metomatic (Ohio) veterinary ventilator (small-animals only)
   A. Classification: volume-preset ventilator; descending bellows; pressure limited
   B. Controls
      1. Tidal volume
         a. Controlled by adjustable knob
         b. Indicated on the front of the bellows
      2. Inspiratory flow rate
         a. Controls inspiratory time
         b. Adjusted to be equal to or less than expiratory time
      3. Expiratory time
         a. Controls rate by controlling length of expiratory phase
         b. Usually 6 to 12 breaths/min
      4. Inspiratory hold
         a. Holds ventilator at peak pressure; used to eliminate atelectasis
         b. Can cause cardiovascular embarrassment if the chest is closed
      5. Inspiratory pressure
         a. Can limit maximal pressure
         b. Reduces possibility of extreme pressure being placed on the chest
      6. Inspiratory trigger effort
         a. Governs ability of animal to initiate inspiration
         b. Minimal trigger effort setting allows ventilator to be used in assist or assist-control mode

7. Expiratory flow rate
   a. Governs rate of fall of the bag and therefore expiration
   b. Adjusted to regulate impedance to expiration

IV. Bird Mark 7 and Mark 9 ventilators
   A. Classification: pressure preset ventilator; volume delivered is controlled by the pressure developed unless machine is equipped with a bellows
   B. Bird must be equipped with a bag-in-a-barrel or a bellows to be used as an anesthetic system
   C. Controls
      1. Inspiratory pressure
         a. Controls peak pressure
         b. Normally set at 20 to 30 cm water
      2. Sensitivity
         a. Controls ability of animal to trigger the machine
         b. Low numbers; easily triggered
         c. High numbers; difficult to trigger
      3. Inspiratory flow rate
         a. Controls inspiratory time
         b. Set equal to or less than expiratory time
      4. Expiratory time
         a. Controls respiratory rate by controlling expiratory time
         b. Respiratory rate normally 6 to 12 breaths/min
      5. Air mix
         a. Varies percentage of inspired oxygen from 50% (knob out) to 100% (knob in)
         b. Negative pressure: (Bird Mark 9 only) allows the operator to produce NEEP

V. Mallard Medical Microprocessor controlled large animal anesthesia ventilator (Fig. 14-5)
   A. Classification: ascending bellows; time cycled, microprocessor controlled
   B. Controls
      1. Inspiratory flow rate is adjustable between 10 and 600 L/min
      2. Respiratory rate
      3. Inspiratory time

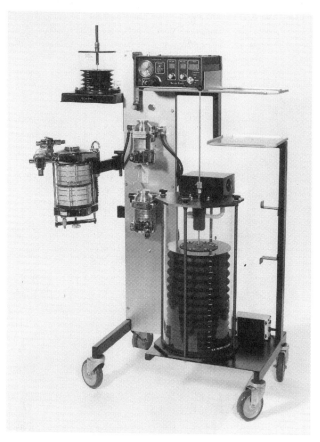

Fig. 14-5
Mallard anesthesia ventilator system.

C. Volume and pressure delivered and inspiratory flow rate are a function of adjustments in the I:E ratio.
D. Ventilator bellows connects to rebreathing bag port of large animal circle system
E. PEEP capability

VI. Engler ADS 1000
  A. Microprocessor controlled
  B. Can be used with a vaporizer for anesthesia or without vaporizer
  C. Nonrebreathing circuit principle of operation
    1. No CO_2 absorbent necessary
    2. No conventional anesthesia breathing circuit necessary
  D. Machine automatically selects ventilation parameters based on patient weight
  E. PEEP capability

VII. Hallowell EMC 2000-Volume Preset Small Animal Ventilator
  A. Ascending bellows
  B. V_T adjustable from 0 to 3000 ml

HIGH-FREQUENCY VENTILATION (HFV)

I. HFV is a relatively new form of mechanical ventilation in which f is greater than 1 Hz (hertz) and V_T is less than anatomic dead space; generally one of three modes is used
  A. High-frequency, positive-pressure ventilation: f = 1 to 2 Hz; positive pressure maintained throughout the respiratory cycle
  B. High-frequency jet ventilation: f = 2 to 7 Hz; a small cannula is used to deliver jets of gas into the airway
  C. High-frequency oscillating ventilation: f = 6 to 40 Hz; bias flow of fresh gas entrained by oscillating the column of gas

II. Potential uses include acute respiratory distress syndrome, hyaline membrane disease, bronchopleural fistula, pulmonary contusion

WEANING THE PATIENT OFF THE VENTILATOR

The initiation of spontaneous respirations following controlled ventilation can be hastened by

I. Decreasing the rate of controlled respiratory frequency
II. Decreasing anesthetic depth
III. Reversing neuromuscular blockade
IV. Antagonism of opioid induced respiratory depression
V. Patients ventilated long-term require a more sophisticated approach to weaning from a ventilator (e.g., use of IMV)
VI. Physical manipulation: rolling the patient, twisting an ear, pinching a toe
VII. Respiratory stimulants: doxapram administration, 0.1 to 0.3 mg/lb intravenously

HAZARD PREVENTION

I. Always be prepared to convert the anesthesia system back to nonventilator mode in case of unforeseen ventilator problems; keep rebreathing bag near the ventilator
II. Verify proper ventilator function before use; follow manufacturer's recommendations
   A. Verify that all controls are operational
   B. Leak test
      1. Ascending bellows: fill bellows using O_2; flush valve on anesthesia machine; occlude ventilator delivery hose and maintain bellows in ascended position
      2. Descending bellows: fully contract bellows; occlude ventilator delivery hose and keep bellows fully contracted

CHAPTER FIFTEEN

Patient Monitoring During Anesthesia

"You see only what you look for,
You recognize only what you know."
MERRIL C. SOSMAN

"Diligence is the mother of good fortune."
MIGUEL DE CERVANTES

OVERVIEW

A variety of sophisticated and complex technical equipment is available for monitoring the patient's status during chemical restraint and anesthesia. These machines record the electroencephalogram, the electrocardiogram (EKG), and the electromyogram and facilitate their interpretation. Other monitors measure arterial and central venous pressure (CVP), record and audibly transmit heart sounds, record peripheral blood flow, and measure arterial and venous oxygen and carbon dioxide tensions and arterial or capillary blood oxygen saturation (pulse oximetry). End-expired samples of respiratory gases can be measured for oxygen/carbon dioxide content as well as inhalation anesthetic concentration. All the monitoring equipment in the world, however, cannot replace an educated, attentive anesthetist.

GENERAL CONSIDERATIONS

I. A patient's physiology and homeostasis are altered by drugs used during anesthesia and by the pathophysiologic processes of disease

II. Intraoperative, physiologic patient monitoring optimizes anesthetic procedures by
   A. Allowing for informed, flexible responses to changes in patient status; tracking physiologic variables facilitates early response to changing conditions
   B. Providing a data base for any subsequent anesthetic procedures on the same animal

III. Prerequisites for intraoperative monitoring
   A. Knowledge of pharmacodynamics, toxicity, and pharmacokinetics of anesthetic drugs and adjuncts
   B. Working understanding of normal physiology and pathophysiology
   C. Thorough, accurate knowledge of the patient's preoperative physiologic status
   D. Availability of a convenient system for recording observations (anesthetic record)

BASIC PRINCIPLES

I. Monitor the functions of changeable body systems
   A. Formulate monitoring plan based on preoperative assessment of the case
      1. Specific procedure
      2. Specific disease
      3. Specific monitoring equipment
      4. Anticipated duration of anesthesia
   B. Intraoperative decisions are based on comparisons of observed-to-predicted responses (i.e., Are observed responses qualitatively and/or quantitatively appropriate to the case? Are measured variables within normal limits?)

II. Monitor more than one body system and more than one parameter per body system if possible
   A. Weighing integrated responses rather than fragments of information increases the likelihood of correct assessment
   B. Tracking the individual variables facilitates an early response

III. Use monitoring techniques that are specific, accurate, and complementary
   A. Use simple, reliable techniques (e.g., visual inspection, palpation, auscultation)

    B. Check instrument calibrations frequently; instruments may provide specific data, but inaccurate information may be confusing, distracting, and misleading

    C. Never totally depend on only one piece of monitoring equipment

IV. Noninvasive vs. invasive techniques

    A. Noninvasive (indirect) techniques

       1. Information gathered by observing readily apparent variables (e.g., counting respiratory rate) and/or noninvasive diagnostic testing (e.g., EKG)

       2. Advantages

          a. Techniques are simple, reliable, and informative

          b. Patient is not placed at risk for complications secondary to the monitoring technique

       3. Disadvantages

          a. Certain potentially useful physiologic variables cannot be monitored noninvasively

          b. Inaccurate information (highly variable) is sometimes gathered when a noninvasive technique (e.g., blood pressure (BP)) is substituted for a more invasive procedure to determine the same parameter

    B. Invasive (direct) technique

       1. Information gathered by placing instruments inside the body (e.g., intravascular pressure catheters)

       2. Advantages

          a. Physiologic data base is increased

          b. Many techniques are simple to perform, accurate, and reliable

          c. Often a direct measurement of a physiologic variable is provided rather than a derived value

       3. Disadvantages

          a. Patient at risk for secondary complications depending on technique, e.g.

             (1) Sepsis

             (2) Direct tissue damage

             (3) Inflammation with subsequent tissue damage

             (4) Acute perturbation of tissue function (e.g., cardiac dysrhythmias)

          b. Some techniques require elaborate or expensive instrumentation

PHYSIOLOGIC CONSIDERATIONS

I. Homeostasis
   A. Schematic representation (Fig. 15-1)
   B. Monitoring (Tables 15-1 and 15-2)
      1. Responses observed
         a. Individual organ systems
         b. Integrated responses
      2. Invasive monitoring techniques may evoke added responses
II. Individual organ systems
   A. Central nervous system (CNS)
      1. Observe reflex activity to monitor degree of CNS depression
         a. Eye reflexes

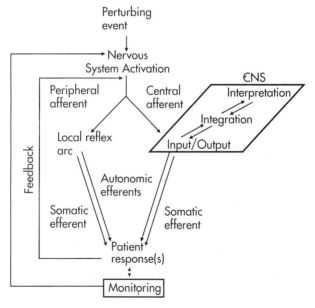

Fig. 15-1

Schematic representation of information transfer in homeostasis. CNS, Central nervous system.

(1) Palpebral
(2) Corneal
(3) Nystagmus
(4) Lacrimation
b. Jaw tone
c. Anal reflex
d. Pedal reflex

TABLE 15-1

AMERICAN SOCIETY OF ANESTHESIOLOGISTS STANDARDS FOR BASIC INTRAOPERATIVE MONITORING*

Standard I. Qualified Anesthesia Personnel

Qualified anesthesia personnel shall be present in the room throughout the conduct of all general anesthetics, regional anesthetics,
and monitored anesthesia care.

**Standard II. Oxygenation, ventilation, circulation, and temperature
shall be continually evaluated.**

Oxygenation	1. Oxygen analyzer for inspired gases
	2. Observation of patient
	3. Pulse oximetry
Ventilation	1. Auscultation
	2. Observation of patient
	3. Observation of reservoir bag
	4. End-tidal carbon dioxide analysis
Circulation	1. Continuous display EKG
	2. Heart rate and blood pressure recorded every 5 minutes
	3. Evaluation of circulation
	Auscultation of heart sounds
	Palpation of pulse
	Pulse plethysmography
	Pulse oximetry
	Intraarterial pressure tracing
Temperature	1. Core temperature
	Thermistors, thermocouple, thermometer
	2. Skin temperature
	Thermistor, liquid crystal thermometer

*Approved Oct. 21, 1986, and last amended on Oct. 23, 1990, to become effective
Jan., 1, 1991.
EKG, Electrocardiogram.

TABLE 15-2
COMMONLY MONITORED PARAMETERS AND POTENTIAL CAUSES OF ABNORMAL RESPONSES

Heart rate

Tachycardia	Pain, hypotension, hypoxemia, hypercarbia, ischemia, acute anaphylactoid reactions, anemia, drug effects (e.g., thiobarbiturates, ketamine, catecholamines), fever, hypokalemia
Bradycardia	Hypertension, elevated intracranial pressure, surgically induced vagal reflexes (e.g., visceral stretch responses), hypothermia, hyperkalemia, myocardial ischemia/anoxia, drug effects (e.g., xylazine, narcotics)

Respiratory rate and pattern

Tachypnea	Pain, hypoxemia, hypercarbia, hyperthermia, true or paradoxical CSF acidosis, drug effects (e.g., doxapram)
Apnea	Hypothermia, recent hyperventilation (especially while breathing O_2- enriched gases), musculoskeletal paralysis (pathologic or pharmacologic), drug effects (e.g., ketamine, thiobarbiturates, propofol)

Arterial blood pressure

Hypotension	Relative or absolute hypovolemia, sepsis, shock, drug effects (e.g., thiobarbiturate boluses, inhalation anesthetics)
Hypertension	Pain, hypercarbia, fever, drug effects (e.g., catecholamines, ketamine)

Corneal reflexes*

Hyperactive	Pain, hypotension, hypoxemia, hypercarbia, drug effects (ketamine)
Hypoactive	CNS depression, e.g., excessively deep anesthesia, acidosis, hypotension

*Pertains to horses and ruminants only; not useful in pigs, dogs, and cats.
CSF, Cerebral spinal fluid; *CNS*, Central nervous system.

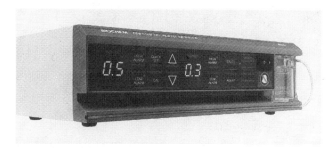

Fig. 15-2

Monitor that measures end-tidal concentration of halothane or isoflurane to ensure that proper anesthetic concentrations are being delivered to the patient.

  2. Observe for movement
  3. Quantitative electroencephalography
   a. Invasive
   b. Records and averages brain activity
   c. Correlates to depth of anesthesia
   d. Prohibitively expensive
  4. End-tidal concentration of anesthetic drugs can be monitored and correlated to anesthetic depth (Fig. 15-2)
 B. Respiratory system (see Tables 15-1 and 15-2; Figs. 15-3 to 15-5)
  1. Noninvasive measurements
   a. Respiratory frequency
   b. Respiratory pattern
   c. Changes in tidal volume, noted by observing thorax and rebreathing bag
   d. Esophageal or precordial stethoscope
   e. Pulse oximetry (see Fig. 15-5, *A*)
    (1) Measures pulse rate and functional oxygen saturation (Sao_2)
    (2) A spectrophotoelectric device applied directly to nonhaired skin over a pulsating vascular bed; light absorbance of oxygenated vs. reduced hemoglobin detected and percentage of saturated hemoglobin are displayed numerically

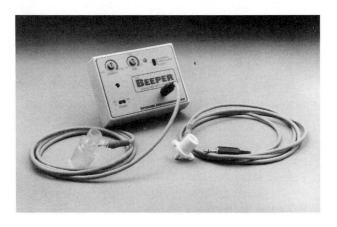

Fig. 15-3
Monitors which detect breathing frequency may be activated by changes in airway temperature (exhaled air is warmer).

    (a) Inaccurate in the presence of carboxyhemo-globin or methemoglobin
    (b) The pulsatile signal is reduced by hypotension, hypothermia, and altered vascular resistance, which limits Sao_2 determination
  f. Transcutaneous oxygen measurement: small probe with Clark-type oxygen electrode is attached to nonhaired skin; skin under probe heated to constant temperature and oxygen partial pressure of blood below probe is measured and numerically displayed
    (1) Pao_2 values depend on arterial oxygenation and peripheral perfusion
    (2) Not yet fully evaluated in all domestic species
    (3) Inhalation anesthetic drugs may interfere with accurate recording
    (4) Can cause skin burns
  g. Analysis of inspired oxygen concentration
  h. Analysis of inspired or expired carbon dioxide (see Fig. 15-5, *B*) concentration (capnography)
  i. Spirometry
2. Invasive measurements

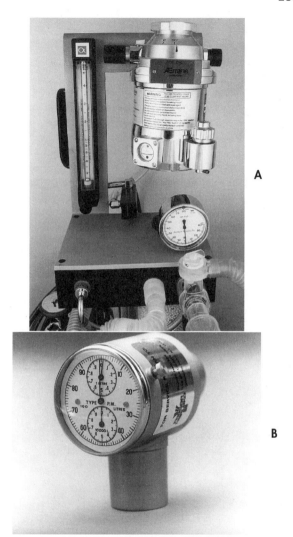

Fig. 15-4
Respiratory monitors used in anesthesia practice. **A,** P-N pressure gauge used to monitor inspiratory pressure during ventilation. **B,** Ventilometer used to measure tidal volume and minute volume.

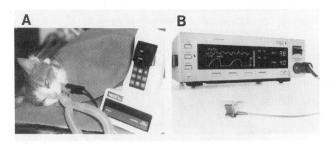

Fig. 15-5

A, Noninvasive, portable, battery-operated pulse oximeter for determining the oxygen saturation of hemoglobin (SpO_2) and **B,** capnograph for determining end-tidal carbon dioxide.

    a. Hematocrit (packed cell volume percentage) and/or hemoglobin concentration

    b. Arterial and/or venous blood gas analysis (see Chapter 16)

    c. Oximetry (oxygen saturation)

    d. Blood pH analysis

C. Cardiovascular system (see Tables 15-1, 15-2)

  1. Heart rate

    a. Range of normal heart beats, by species

      (1) Dog: 70 to 180

      (2) Cat: 145 to 200

      (3) Horse: 30 to 45; foal up to 80

      (4) Cow: 60 to 80

      (5) Sheep, goat: 60 to 90

      (6) Pig: 60 to 90

    b. Limits of heart rate during anesthesia (values outside these limits indicate that cardiovascular function may be impaired)

      (1) Dog: <60, >200

      (2) Cat: <100, >260

      (3) Horse: <28

      (4) Cow: <48

      (5) Sheep, goat: <60

    c. Techniques for monitoring heart rate

      (1) Direct palpation

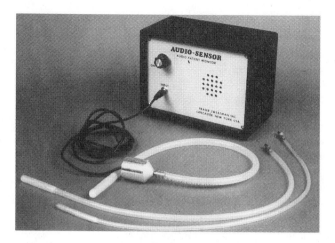

Fig. 15-6
Esophageal catheters, which are attached to a stethoscope or audio monitor to hear heart sounds.

      (a) Dog: femoral, dorsal pedal, digital, and lingual arteries; precordium
      (b) Cat: femoral artery, precordium
      (c) Cow, sheep, and goat: auricular, digital, coccygeal, and dorsal metatarsal arteries
      (d) Horse: facial, transverse facial, dorsal metatarsal, and palatine arteries
      (e) Pig: femoral and auricular arteries
    (2) Indirect method uses esophageal stethoscope (Figs. 15-6 and 15-7)
- Coupled to earpieces or to electronic amplifier
- Advantages: inexpensive; can detect abnormalities in rhythm as well as rate; can monitor breath sounds
- Disadvantages: difficult to use for surgeries involving head

  d. Peripheral pulse amplifiers
    (1) Applied over peripheral pulse; audible beep heard with each pulse

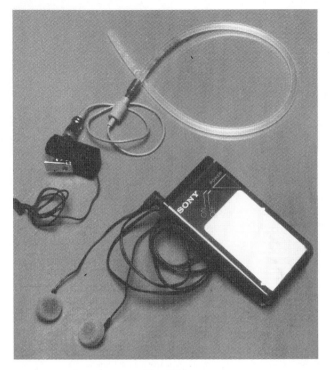

Fig. 15-7
Esophageal stethoscopes, which are attached to a transmitting device giving the anesthetist more freedom of movement.

      (2) Advantages: inexpensive
      (3) Disadvantages: prone to electrical interference; difficult to keep in place
   e. Ultrasonic Doppler device
      (1) Doppler crystal applied over peripheral pulse; sound of blood flow amplified
      (2) Advantages: can also be used to estimate systolic BP; detects abnormalities in rhythm as well as rate
      (3) Disadvantages: expense
   f. EKG and EKG/R-wave amplifier

(1) Direct visualization of EKG, or sound amplifier that beeps with each R wave

(2) Advantages: direct visualization of EKG allows interpretation of cardiac rhythm

(3) Disadvantages: expense; EKG activity can continue to look and sound normal in absence of mechanical activity (electromechanical dissociation)

g. Reasons for abnormal heart rates

  (1) Bradycardia

    (a) Drugs: narcotics, xylazine, anticholinesterases

    (b) Excessive anesthetic depth

    (c) Hyperkalemia

    (d) Preexisting heart disease

    (e) Vagal reflex (intubation, oculocardiac reflex)

    (f) Terminal stages of hypoxemia

    (g) Hypothermia

  (2) Tachycardia

    (a) Drugs: ketamine, thiobarbiturates, anticholinergics, sympathomimetics, pancuronium, gallamine

    (b) Hypokalemia

    (c) Hyperthermia

    (d) Inadequate anesthetic depth

    (e) Hypercarbia and hypoxemia

    (f) Anemia, hypovolemia

    (g) Hyperthyroidism, pheochyromocytoma

    (h) Anaphylaxis

2. Perfusion

a. A function of arteriovenous (AV) BP difference and local vasomotor tone

b. Assessment

  (1) Capillary refill time

    (a) Normal: <1 to 2 seconds

    (b) Assess on oral or vulvar mucous membranes

  (2) Urine production

    (a) Palpation of bladder

    (b) Urinary catheterization

    (c) Dog and cat: 1 to 2 ml/kg/hr

3. Central venous pressure (CVP) is obtained by measur-

ing the mean right arterial pressure; awareness of the CVP value and monitoring its changes can be important in some clinical situations (Fig. 15-8)

a. Range of normal values
   (1) 0 to 4 cm H_2O: standing, awake animals
   (2) 2 to 7 cm H_2O: anesthetized small animals
   (3) 15 to 25 cm H_2O: anesthetized large animals
b. Indications
   (1) Monitoring fluid therapy

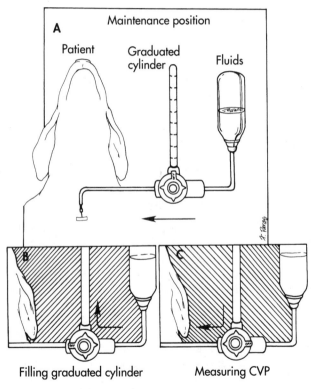

Fig. 15-8
A, CVP monitoring. **B,** A graduated cylinder at or below the level of the heart is filled with saline. **C,** The cylinder is then opened to the patient.

    (2) Assessing cardiac output
       (a) Shock
       (b) Heart failure
       (c) Anesthesia

c. Physiological significance
    (1) Right atrial pressure is a balance between
       (a) Cardiac output: ability of the heart to suck blood out of the right atrium
       (b) Venous return: tendency for blood to flow from the peripheral veins back into the right atrium

d. Primary factors affecting CVP
    (1) Blood volume
       (a) Increase in circulating blood volume may cause an increase in CVP, as in
         • Renal retention of fluid in chronic heart failure
         • Overzealous intravenous (IV) fluid administration
       (b) Decrease in effective circulating blood volume may cause a decrease in CVP, as in
         • Acute hemorrhage
         • Dehydration
         • Strangulation, obstructive lesions causing vascular congestion and sequestration of blood or body fluids
           ○ Cat: intussusception of small bowel
           ○ Dog: gastric dilatation/volvulus
           ○ Horse: large colon torsion
           ○ Cow: abomasal torsion
    (2) Vascular tone
       (a) Regulated by the sympathetic nervous system and local tissue factors
       (b) Markedly altered by various anesthetic agents
       (c) Venous dilation may cause CVP to decrease because of peripheral pooling of blood and decreased venous return
       (d) Arteriolar dilation may cause CVP to increase because of decrease in total periph

leral resistance to cardiac output (CO), allowing more rapid flow of blood from arterial to venous side of circulation

(3) Cardiac contractility
  (a) Regulated by the autonomic nervous system
  (b) Affected by venous return; increased venoconstriction increases contractility
  (c) Decreased by most anesthetic agents
  (d) Decreases may cause CVP to increase because of the decreased effectiveness of the heart as a pump

(4) Heart rate
  (a) Regulated by the autonomic nervous system
  (b) CVP may decrease acutely with sudden elevation of the heart rate
  (c) CVP may increase with sustained extreme tachycardias because of inadequate cardiac filling during shortened diastole
  (d) Severe bradycardia, AV conduction disturbances, and arrhythmia may result in an increased CVP because of the decrease in cardiac output

(5) External cardiac factors
  (a) Intrathoracic pressure
    • Elevations in intrathoracic pressure impede venous return; decreases in intrathoracic pressure facilitate venous return
    • An elevation in intrathoracic pressure is accompanied by an elevation in CVP, impediment of venous return, and lowered CO
    • Factors affecting intrathoracic pressure
      ○ Cyclic changes during normal respiration
      ○ Positive-pressure ventilation
      ○ Pneumothorax
      ○ Opening thoracic cage to the atmosphere
      ○ Diaphragmatic hernia

       ○ Thoracic neoplasia or pulmonary disease
       ○ Fluid in the thorax
- (b) Intrapericardial pressure
    ○ Cardiac tamponade
    ○ Congenital pericardial herniation
    ○ Ventricular filling is decreased or eliminated
- (c) Body position
    ○ Alterations in body position can cause changes in vascular hydrostatic pressure
    ○ Primarily a factor in large animal species (CVP may drop 10 to 15 cm H_2O when a horse is rolled from dorsal to lateral recumbency)

e. Clinical values of CVP
- (1) Three common clinical situations to be considered
  - (a) Reduced blood volume, cardiac function normal: ↓CVP ↓CO
  - (b) Expanded blood volume, cardiac function normal: ↑CVP ↑CO
  - (c) Normovolemic patient, cardiac function decreased: ↑CVP ↓CO
- (2) Clinical approach to low CVP
  - (a) Reduced effective circulating blood volume
  - (b) Patients in whom there is a relative or absolute hypovolemia should receive appropriate IV fluid until the CVP approaches the upper limit of normal range
    - The function of the heart can be assumed to be adequate if the fluid administration is accompanied by signs of adequate peripheral perfusion
      - ○ Urine output
      - ○ Strong pulses
      - ○ Pink mucous membranes
      - ○ Capillary refill: 2.5 seconds
    - If fluid administration is accompanied by signs of inadequate perfusion, increas-

ing metabolic acidosis, and pulmonary edema, further treatment should be directed toward improving cardiac function

    (3) Clinical approach to elevated CVP

        (a) Generally indicates hypervolemia or myocardial depression/heart failure

- Danger of pulmonary edema exists
- Metabolic acidosis due to poor perfusion of peripheral tissues may result

        (b) Clinical history may indicate reason for elevated CVP

- Iatrogenic cause: excessive fluid administration
- Primary cardiac disease
- Generalized drug-induced myocardial depression

        (c) Treat the patient in one or more of the following ways

- Decrease or stop IV fluid administration
- Administer drugs to improve cardiac function (dobutamine)
- Prescribe diuretic (furosemide)

  f. Hazards of CVP measurement

    (1) Impaired blood clotting caused by excessive heparinization of the fluid-filled catheter

    (2) Thrombophlebitis

    (3) Septicemia

    (4) Air embolism

    (5) Vascular endothelial damage or puncture

        (a) Extravascular migration

        (b) Cardiac tamponade

    (6) Improper placement; inaccurate data collection

  g. Equipment

    (1) IV catheter of sufficient length to reach the great veins in the chest (preferably the right atrium)

    (2) CVP manometer kit (see Fig. 15-8)

        (a) Homemade

- Three-way stopcock
- Graduated cylinder or pipette
- Connecting tubes

       (b) Commercially available
- Baxter
- Abbott

       (c) Appropriate fluids and a fluid administration set

  h. Procedure (see Fig. 15-8)

    (1) Thread a fluid-filled IV catheter into the right jugular vein (toward the heart)

    (2) Flush the catheter with saline

    (3) Attach fluid connecting tubes to the IV catheter

    (4) Attach a three-way stopcock and graduated cylinder

    (5) Attach the fluid administration line to the other port of the three-way stopcock

    (6) Suspend the graduated cylinder or pipette so that the three-way stopcock is below the animal's heart base; draw an imaginary line parallel to the floor between the animal's heart base and the cylinder; this marks the point of zero pressure on the cylinder

       (a) The animal's heart base is marked by the sternum when the animal is in lateral recumbency

       (b) The heart base is marked by the point of the shoulder when the animal is standing or in dorsal recumbency

    (7) Let the fluid run through the system at the calculated flow (5 ml/lb/hr) until ready to record CVP

  i. Use of manometer (see Fig. 15-8)

    (1) Turn the three-way stopcock so that the fluid line is open to the graduated cylinder

    (2) When the cylinder has filled, turn the stopcock so that the cylinder is open to the patient

    (3) The fluid column will fall to the level of the CVP

    (4) After taking the reading, open the patient line to the fluid, and administer fluids at the prescribed rate

4. Arterial BP

a. Noninvasive
  (1) Oscillometric method (Fig. 15-9)
    (a) Air-filled cuff is placed around peripheral limb (small animal, foal) or base of tail (large animal); air is gradually released from the cuff, and changes in oscillations at systolic, mean, and diastolic pressures are detected and electronically displayed
    (b) Advantages: easy to use; determines heart rate as well as systolic, mean, and diastolic BP
    (c) Disadvantages: may not be absolutely accurate but should accurately reflect trends; accuracy dependent upon cuff size; inaccurate at low BPs; expensive
  (2) Ultrasonic Doppler apparatus (Fig. 15-10)
    (a) Doppler crystal placed over peripheral artery
      • Dog: digital, dorsal pedal
      • Horse: coccygeal

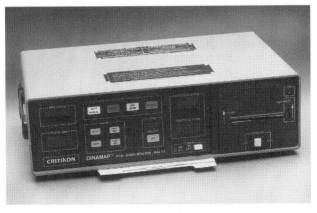

Fig. 15-9
Oscillometric peripheral pulse monitor, which is used to monitor pulse rate and blood pressure.

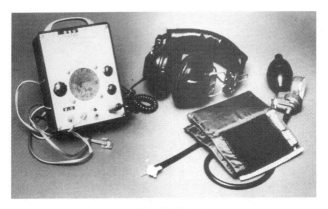

Fig. 15-10
An electronically activated Doppler crystal senses blood flow, which can
be audibly broadcast and used to monitor blood pressure.

    (b) Place inflatable cuff with aneroid gauge
     proximal to Doppler crystal; inflate cuff un-
     til pulse sound stops, then slowly deflate un-
     til pulse is first heard; this corresponds to
     systolic BP as displayed on aneroid gauge
    (c) Advantages: relatively inexpensive; can
     count pulse rate and detect abnormalities in
     pulse rhythm
    (d) Disadvantages: accuracy related to many
     factors; cuff size must be matched to limb
     circumference; measures systolic pressure
     only; inaccurate at low BPs
  b. Invasive
   (1) The technique of invasive arterial pressure
    monitoring provides an accurate quantitative
    value of the pulse pressure and a qualitative rep-
    resentation of the pulse waveform; this informa-
    tion reflects the hemodynamic state of the pa-
    tient and the effects of various drugs and/or
    treatments; BP is not an indicator of CO (Figs.
    15-11, 15-12)
    (a) Indications

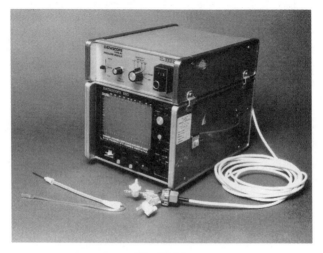

Fig. 15-11
Invasive blood pressure recording system illustrating a pressure transducer
for sensing pressure and oscilloscope for observing pressure waveforms.

- Detection of systemic arterial hypertension or hypotension
- Monitoring of hemodynamic effects of drugs
- Verification of heightened or diminished pulse pressures
- Monitoring of arterial blood gases

(2) Physiologic significance

(a) BP = lateral force per unit area of vascular wall
- Expressed clinically in millimeters of mercury (mm Hg)
- Pressure at the level of the right atrium is the zero reference level

(b) BP is needed to propel blood through high-resistance vascular beds; vascular beds of heart, brain, and kidney offer highest resistance; the mean pressure required to perfuse these organs is approximately 60 mm Hg

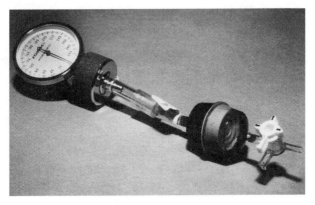

Fig. 15-12
A small blood filter attached to a three-way stopcock and then to a sphyg-momanometer—an inexpensive method of monitoring mean arterial blood pressure.

    (c) Systemic BP oscillates above and below a mean pressure
- Maximum pressure = systolic
- Minimum pressure = diastolic
- Systolic-diastolic pressure = pulse pressure; major determinant of palpable pulse strength
- Mean pressure: major determinant of perfusion pressure to most organs of the body
- Normal values (Fig. 15-13)
  Systolic: 110 to 160 mm Hg
  Diastolic: 70 to 90 mm Hg
  Mean: 80 to 110 mm Hg

    (d) The pulse waveform does not represent a fluid wave; rather, it is a pressure wave; the pressure pulse travels much faster through the arterial tree than the blood flow; the pressure pulse reaches peripheral arterioles 200 to 300 ms after the onset of ventricular ejection

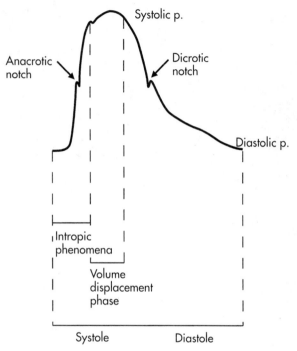

Fig. 15-13
Characteristics of the arterial pressure waveform.

(e) Components of the pressure pulse (see Fig. 15-13)
- Early systolic events: inotropic component
- Midsystolic events: volume displacement phase
- Events of late systole and diastole: runoff and reflection

(f) Inotropic component: anacrotic rise or the steep ascending limb of the pressure pulse
- Acceleration transient: the force caused when aortic valves open and the high

pressure (energy) intraventricular blood is combined with the blood within the aorta, which is at near zero velocity

- Ejection pulse: continued upstroke resulting as stroke volume is ejected into aortic root
- Steepness of the anacrotic rise is a qualitative indicator of myocardial contractility

(g) Volume displacement phase: the abrupt phenomenon of the inotropic component is sustained by continuing ejection of stroke volume from the ventricle

- Pressure continues to rise as long as flow into the vascular segment exceeds the volume of fluid leaving it
- Anacrotic notch is a discontinuity between the inotropic component and the sustained volume displacement curve
- Volume displacement phase may determine the maximum systolic pressure if stroke volume is large relative to peripheral runoff

(h) Late systole and diastole: as the rate of runoff exceeds the volume input to the aorta, the pressure declines

- Dicrotic notch is a sharp deceleration of blood flow at closure of aortic valves; peripherally the dicrotic notch is an artifact of reflection
- Undulations on the diastolic decline are caused by resonant waves in the great vessels and reflections of energy from the periphery

(i) There is an increase in pressure pulse amplitude with increasing distance from the aortic arch (Fig. 15-14)

- Distensibility of peripheral arteries progressively decreases, resulting in an increased pulse wave

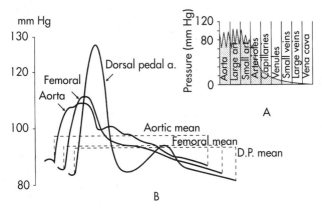

Fig. 15-14

Effects of distance from the aortic arch on the arterial blood pressure waveform.

- The mean pressure is relatively unchanged along the arterial circulation
(3) Primary factors affecting the arterial pressure
  (a) Pressure = CO × total peripheral resistance (TPR)

$$BP = CO \times TPR$$

  - Factors increasing stroke volume or cardiac output favor an increase in arterial pressure
  - Factors increasing total peripheral resistance favor an increase in arterial pressure
  (b) The inotropic component of the pulse pressure curve is modulated by three factors
    - Preload—related to venous return
    - Afterload—related to arterial pressure and peripheral resistance
    - Heart rate
  (c) Decreases in the inotropic component may reflect
    - Myocardial depression caused by
      ○ Pathology

- ○ Anesthesia
- ○ Decreased β-adrenergic stimulation
- Decreased venous return
  - ○ Relative or absolute hypovolemia
  - ○ Venodilation
  - ○ Positive-pressure ventilation
- Decreased peripheral resistance
  - ○ Decreased sympathetic tone
  - ○ Anesthesia
  - ○ Endotoxin

(d) Volume displacement and the amplitude and duration of the pressure pulse reflect a balance between
  - Volume and rate of ejection fraction, which is related to venous return and contractility
    - ○ Small stroke volume yields narrow systolic peak and a precipitous downstroke
    - ○ Large stroke volume yields broad systolic peak with ramplike diastolic component
  - Rate of runoff to the periphery, which is governed by changes in peripheral resistance
    - ○ Dicrotic notch occurs high on the pulse pressure curve with adequate stroke volume and low peripheral resistance
    - ○ Dicrotic notch occurs a few millimeters above the lowest diastolic value if the rate of runoff is rapid

(e) Late systole and diastole reflect the rate of runoff to the periphery and reflection from the periphery
  - High peripheral resistance diminishes forward flow and increases reflection, creating a horizontal diastolic element
  - Substantial volume displacement toward the periphery when vascular resistance is

               low forms a diastolic tracing resembling an oblique but fairly steep ramp

    (f) Pulse pressure curves (Fig. 15-15)

        • Myocardium initiates explosive systolic peak under the influence of a positive inotrope (see Fig. 15-15, *A*); small stroke volume suggested by rapid downstroke in volume displacement phase

        • Discontinuation of halothane and dopamine (see Fig. 15-15, *B*): phenylephrine causes increased tone in arterial and venous vessels; decreased rate of ejection; dicrotic notch has moved upward on the descending limb of the systolic curve; this suggests a greater flow state

  (4) Clinical value of arterial pressure monitoring

    (a) Depth of anesthesia

        • The effects of anesthetic drugs on cardiac output and peripheral resistance can markedly affect BP

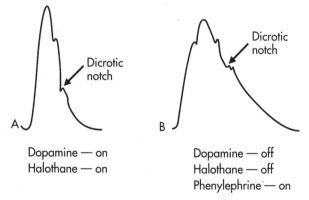

Fig. 15-15

Effects of **A,** peripheral artery vasodilation and **B,** vasoconstriction on the arterial blood pressure waveform.

    ○ Light plane of anesthesia: animal responds to painful stimulus by an increase in sympathetic tone and sudden elevation of BP

    ○ Profound anesthetic depression: loss of homeostatic reflexes and impairment of myocardial function; decline in mean BP, prolonged anacrotic rise, and decreased pulse pressure

(b) Adequacy of fluid therapy

Narrow volume displacement phase may indicate need to volume-expand the patient; marked discrepancy in the appearance of a pulse-pressure curve before and after assisted ventilation often indicates a need for rapid IV fluid administration (Fig. 15-16)

(c) Maintenance of peripheral perfusion pressure

    • Prevention of tissue ischemia and subsequent metabolic acidosis relies on normal arterial oxygen values and mean BPs of greater than 60 mm Hg

      ○ If mean BP is less than 60 mm Hg, treatment may include

        Rapid IV fluid administration

        Decreased depth of anesthesia

        Initiation of positive inotrope therapy

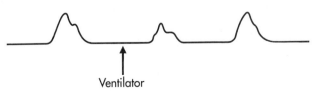

Ventilator

Fig. 15-16

Changes in arterial blood pressure waveform caused by assisted ventilation.

○ Potential sequelae to inadequate tissue perfusion

Postoperative rhabdomyolysis in the horse

Acute renal failure in all species

Cardiac arrhythmias in all species

Shock

(d) Assessment of ventilatory status: arterial blood gases, available through the arterial pressure line, are ideal for determining adequacy of ventilation (see Chapter 16)

(5) Hazards of invasive arterial pressure monitoring

(a) Hematoma formation

(b) Air embolization

(c) Arterial thrombosis and occlusion (rare)

(d) Infection (rare)

(e) Formation of AV fistula or aneurysm (rare)

(6) Equipment and procedure

(a) Intraarterial catheter with three-way stopcock

(b) Pressure sensing device

- Pressure transducer and oscilloscope
- Mercury manometer
- Aneroid gauge (see Fig. 15-12)

(c) Procedure

- Cannulate a peripheral artery aseptically with the arterial catheter

○ Dog

Dorsal pedal artery

Femoral artery

○ Ruminants

Caudal auricular artery

Coccygeal artery

Common digital artery

○ Horse

Facial artery

Transverse facial artery

Dorsal metatarsal artery

- Flush the catheter with heparinized saline; always aspirate first to prevent air embolism

- Attach the pressure transducer while stopcock is closed to the artery
- Open the transducer to air to establish the baseline (zero) reference pressure with the transducer at the level of the right atrium
- Open the arterial line to the pressure transducer; pulse-pressure curve should be displayed at this point
- Reading pressures
  - Systolic pressure: uppermost point of the pulse-pressure curve
  - Diastolic pressure: lowermost point of the pulse-pressure curve
  - Mean pressure (determined automatically by most monitoring devices); calculated by dividing the difference between systolic and diastolic pressure by 3 and adding the product to the diastolic pressure
- After removing the arterial catheter, place manual pressure on the site of cannulation for 5 minutes to prevent hematoma formation

D. Musculoskeletal system (see Chapter 11)
  1. Skeletal muscle tone
  2. Quality of elicited reflexes
  3. Peripheral nerve stimulation (Figs. 15-17, 15-18); used to assess quality of skeletal muscle responses during onset and reversal of neuromuscular blocking agents; observed reversal responses may not correlate well with actual return of functional muscle strength and adequacy of breathing

III. Thermoregulation
  A. Body temperature regulation is an integrated process involving the following body systems or organs
    1. Central nervous system
    2. Cardiovascular system
    3. Musculoskeletal system

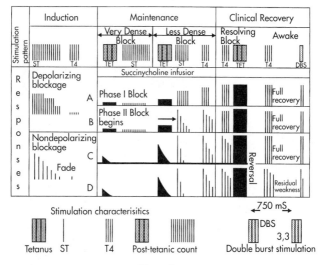

Fig. 15-17

Assessing neuromuscular function. Diagram simulates the clinical responses observed following neuromuscular stimulation. Stimulation patterns are depicted in the upper panel. (*ST,* Single twitch; *T4,* Train of four; *TET,* Tetanus; *DBS,* Double burst-stimulation.) The following four situations are demonstrated by the letters: *A,* The normal use of a succinylcholine infusion; *B,* The development of a phase II block; *C,* A nondepolarizing blockade that is reversed with full recovery; and *D,* A nondepolarizing blockade that demonstrates residual weakness.

(From Barash PG, Cullen BK, Stoelting RK: *Clinical anesthesia,* ed 2, Philadelphia, 1992, JB Lippincott, p. 763).

    4. Respiratory system
    5. The liver
  B. Abnormalities of thermoregulation during anesthesia
    1. Hypothermia
      a. Heat loss in excess of production
      b. Most often encountered in small animals because of their larger surface area to body mass ratio
      c. Potential causes
        (1) CNS depression
        (2) Vasodilation

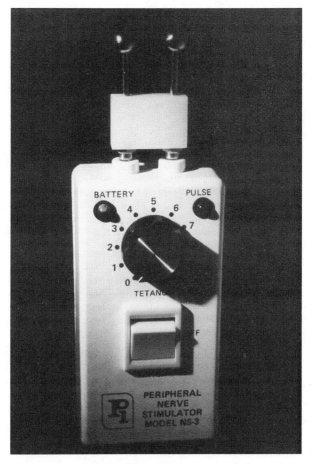

Fig. 15-18

One of a variety of peripheral nerve stimulators available to test the adequacy of neuromuscular blockade.

        (3) Reduced heat production by skeletal muscle

        (4) Other iatrogenic causes

          (a) Cold IV fluids

          (b) Open body cavities

  2. Hyperthermia

        (a) Heat production exceeding loss

        (b) Iatrogenically produced in response to specific drug combinations in certain species

        (1) Drugs: halothane, isoflurane, succinylcholine, and ketamine

        (2) Species

          (a) True malignant hyperthermia syndrome occurs in humans, pigs, and dogs

          (b) Isolated reports of increased body temperature during anesthesia also reported in horses and cats

  C. Body temperature monitoring during the anesthesia and postoperative periods should be considered an integrated response involving the specific species, drugs, and each of the body systems listed (Fig. 15-19)

IV. Integrated responses (see Table 15-2)

  A. Body systems do not exist as separate entities in vivo

  B. Observed responses represent the outcome of a series of events involving simultaneous input and output of many systems, leading to combined autonomic and somatic responses (see Fig. 15-1)

  C. Integrated responses to diseases, surgical stress, and anesthetic-induced depression of certain functions are modulated by the autonomic nervous system and the adrenal medulla

    1. Sympathetic tone mediates "fight-or-flight" responses to any stress

      a. Causes of increased sympathetic tone

        (1) Pain

        (2) Hypotension

        (3) Hypoxemia

        (4) Hypercarbia

        (5) Ischemia

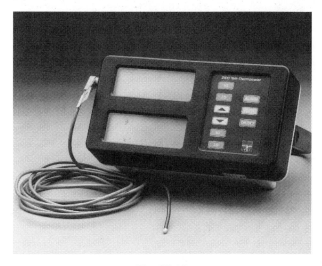

Fig. 15-19
Digital-display temperature monitoring device.

    2. Parasympathetic tone may change as part of an integrated reflex
      a. Vagovagal
      b. Vagophrenic
      c. Vagal efferent (baroreceptor)
  D. Correct interpretation of isolated responses requires understanding of integration and ability to work backwards from the observation to its probable cause
  E. Acute intervention in the care of anesthetized patients should be justified on the basis of
    1. A set of monitored observations
    2. Rational selection of alternative approaches to achieve desired physiologic goals
    3. The anticipated patient responses to the procedure

CHAPTER SIXTEEN

Acid-Base Balance and Blood Gases

"The management of a balance of power
is a permanent undertaking, not an exertion
that has a foreseeable end."

HENRY KISSINGER

OVERVIEW

The diagnosis of acid-base disorders hinges on the interpretation of changes in blood pH, P_{CO_2}, and HCO_3^- concentration. Very simply, changes in pH signal either an increase in hydrogen ions (acidosis) or a decrease (alkalosis). The associated changes in carbon dioxide and bicarbonate concentration help determine the precise cause for the pH change. Evaluation of a patient's acid-base status is useful in the diagnosis of disease processes and the formulation of therapy. Electrolyte abnormalities are frequently associated with, and may be responsible for, acid-base disorders, further emphasizing the importance of a basic understanding of pH, P_{CO_2} and HCO_3^- regulation.

GENERAL CONSIDERATIONS

I. Definitions
   Acid: A substance that can donate hydrogen ion (H^+)

   Example: $H_2CO_3 \rightarrow H^+ + HCO_3^-$

   Actual bicarbonate: The amount of bicarbonate (HCO_3^-), expressed in mEq/L of plasma
   Base (B): A substance that can accept hydrogen ion (H^+)

Examples: $OH^- + H^+ \rightarrow H_2O$
$HCO_3^- + H^+ \rightarrow H_2CO_3$

Base excess (BE): The amount of base above or below the normal buffer base, expressed in mEq/L, in blood; positive values (+) reflect excess of base (or deficit of acid), and negative values reflect a deficit of base (or excess of acid)

Buffer: a mixture of substances in a solution that resists or reduces changes in hydrogen ion concentration (changes in pH); important buffers in the body include hemoglobin and bicarbonate

BUFFERS IN WHOLE BLOOD	% BUFFERING
Hemoglobin and oxyhemo-globin	35
Organic phosphate	3
Inorganic phosphate	2
Plasma proteins	7
Plasma bicarbonate	35
RBC bicarbonate	18
Total	100

Free water: Water without electrolytes (pure H_2O); increases in free water can cause dilution acidosis; decreases in free water can cause contraction alkalosis

Partial pressure: The pressure an individual gas exerts on a column of mercury; expressed in mm Hg; see the following example of gaseous components of air

GAS	FRACTIONAL CONTENT (%)	PARTIAL PRESSURE (mm Hg)
Nitrogen (N_2)	78.084	593.44
Oxygen (O_2)	20.948	159.2
Argon (Ar)	0.934	7.1
Carbon dioxide (CO_2)	0.031	0.24
Others	0.003	0.02
Total	100	760 (atmospheric pressure)

pH: The negative log of the hydrogen ion (H^+) concentration; the pH is inversely proportional to the H^+ concentration

Examples: $(H^+) = 0.000001 = 1 \times 10^{-6}$ pH = 6.0
          $(H^+) = 1 \times 10^{-7}$ pH = 7.0
          $(H^+) = 1 \times 10^{-8}$ pH = 8.0

P_{tot}: Total protein; increases in P_{tot} (weak acids) can cause metabolic (nonrespiratory) acidosis; decreases in P_{tot} cause metabolic alkalosis

Strong ions: Salts that are completely dissociated in water (e.g., Na^+, K^+, Cl^-)

Strong ion difference (SID): The difference in all the positive and negative strong ions; normally ($Na^+ + K^+ - Cl^-$); increases in SID usually cause metabolic (nonrespiratory) alkalosis; decreases in SID usually cause metabolic (nonrespiratory) acidosis.

Total CO_2 content: The amount of carbon dioxide gas extractable from plasma; total CO_2 consists of

HCO_3 (95% the total CO_2
      is HCO_3)
Carbonic acid ($H_2CO_3^-$)
Carbon dioxide

II. Many factors influence a patient's acid-base balance
   A. Species
   B. Diet (carnivorous vs. herbivorous)
   C. Physical status
   D. Temperature
   E. Concentration of "strong" ions or salts that completely dissociate in water (e.g., Na^+, K^+, Cl^-, lactic acid)
   F. Total protein
III. Normal cellular metabolism continuously produces hydrogen ions, which are regulated and eliminated by the lungs, kidneys, and gastrointestinal system so as to maintain an extracellular pH of approximately 7.4
   A. The kidneys eliminate hydrogen ions by excreting fixed acids
   B. The lungs reduce plasma hydrogen-ion concentration by eliminating carbon dioxide
   C. The gut participates in regulating pH by modulation of acid (HCl), base (Na^+, HCO_3^-), and water excretion.
IV. Substances within the body referred to as buffers help minimize changes in pH
V. Determination of pH and blood gases are useful in determining patient acid-base status during anesthesia
VI. When interpreting the absolute values of a patient's pH and

blood gases, the patient's clinical history and physical status should be considered

FORMATION AND ELIMINATION OF ACIDS AND BASES IN ANIMALS

I. The waste products of oral intake or metabolism are mostly acidic substances that release hydrogen ions

A. Volatile acid: an acid that produces a gas

$$H_2CO_3 \rightarrow H_2O + CO_2$$

B. Nonvolatile or fixed acids: acids that cannot be converted to gas
1. Lactate + H^+
2. Sulfate + H^+
3. Phosphate + H^+

II. The pathways for acid removal include the kidney, lung, and gastrointestinal tract

Input →	Oral intake	Metabolism and oral intake	Aerobic metabolism
	↓	↓	↓
	HCO_3^- +	$H^+ \leftrightarrow H_2CO_3 \leftrightarrow H_2O + CO_2$	
	↓	↓	↓
Output	Kidney	Kidney	Lung
		Gastrointestinal tract	

This is the carbonic acid equation or CO_2 hydration equation and is the basis for explaining acid-base kinetics in the body.

A. High-protein diets (cat, dog, pig, human)
1. H^+ excess is derived from oxidation of neutral sulfur in these amino acids
   a. Methionine
   b. Cystine
   c. Cysteine

B. Diets high in plant material and grain have HCO_3^- excess from salts in
   a. Fatty acids (acetate, proprionate)
   b. Citrate (fruits)
   c. Gluconates

Example: $$H_2CO_3 \leftrightarrow H^+ + HCO_3^-$$

$$
\begin{array}{c}
\quad H \quad\; O \\
\quad | \quad\;\; || \\
H - C - C - O - Na^+ + 2O_2 + H^+ \rightarrow 2CO_2 + 2H_2O + Na^+ \\
\quad | \\
\text{(sodium acetate)} \qquad\qquad\qquad \text{Lung}
\end{array}
$$

Metabolizable salts of fatty acids yield HCO_3^- after metabolism

    C. Based on primary dietary intake

        1. Carnivores have acid urine or excess acid to excrete

        2. Herbivores have alkaline urine or an excess base to excrete

    D. Dietary and metabolic intake of acid or base equals the urinary and respiratory output, thereby maintaining the pH of the body fluids near 7.4

    E. Many approaches to the diagnosis and treatment of acid-base disorders are based on the following Henderson-Hasselbach equation

        1. $CO_2 + H_2O \overset{CA}{\leftrightarrow} H^+ + HCO_3^-$ (carbonic anhydrase [CA])

        2. $K_1 = \dfrac{[CO_2] + [H_2O]}{[H_2CO_3]}$

           $K_2 = \dfrac{[H^+] + [HCO_3^-]}{[H_2CO_3]}$

        3. $\dfrac{K_2}{K_1} = \dfrac{[H_+] + [HCO_3^-]}{[CO_2] + [H_2O]} = K_3$

        4. Given: $[CO_2] = \alpha \times P{co_2}$ ($\alpha = 0.0301 -$ solubility coefficient)

        5. $\dfrac{K_3 \times \alpha P{co_2}}{[HCO_3^-]} = (H^+)$

        $-\log (H^+) = pH;\; -\log K_3 = pK$

        pK is that pH at which 50% of an acid or a base is in the ionized state; The pK of the acid (pK_a) H_2CO_3 is 6.1

        6. $-\log K3 - \log \alpha P{co_2} + \log [HCO_3^-] = -\log [H^+]$

        $pH = pK_a + \log \dfrac{[HCO_3^-]}{\alpha P{co_2}}$: Henderson-Hasselbach equation

    F. In the body: pH = 7.4, $pK_a = 6.1$, $P{co_2} = 40$ mm Hg

1. $pH = pK_a + \log \dfrac{[HCO_3^-]}{\alpha P_{CO_2}}$

2. $7.4 = 6.1 + \log [HCO_3^-] - \log \alpha P_{CO_2}$

3. $1.3 = \log [HCO_3^-] - \log \alpha P_{CO_2}$

4. Antilog $1.3 = \dfrac{[HCO_3^-]}{0.0301 \times 40}$ antilog $1.3 = 20$

   $(HCO_3^-) = 20 \times 0.0301 \times 40 = 24$ mEq/L

ARTERIAL OXYGENATION

I. Normal gas partial pressures (expressed mm Hg) during inspiration in ambient air, conducting airways, terminal alveoli, and arterial and mixed venous blood*

	AMBIENT AIR	CONDUCTING AIRWAYS	TERMINAL AVEOLI	ARTERIAL BLOOD	MIXED VENOUS BLOOD
P_{O_2}	156	149	100	95	40
P_{CO_2}	0	0	40	40	46
P_{H_2O}	15†	47	47	47	47
P_{N_2}	589	564	573	573	573
P total	760	760	760	755	706

II. The inspired oxygen-arterial tension (F_{IO_2}) relationship
  A. Relationship between F_{IO_2} and P_{AO_2}

$F_{IO_2}\%$	PREDICTED IDEAL P_{AO_2} (mm Hg)
20	95-100
30	150
40	200
50	250
80	400
100	500

  B. The alveolar gas equation

  $$P_{AO_2} = P_{IO_2} - \dfrac{P_{ACO_2}}{0.8}$$

*From Murray JF: *The normal lung,* ed 2, Philadelphia, WB Saunders, 1986, pp. 173-174.
†P_{H_2O} varies according to humidity and has a proportionate effect on P_{O_2} and P_{N_2}.

III. Causes of arterial hypoxia (a reduction in Pa_{O_2}) and their effect on alveolar-arterial $P(A-a)_{O_2}$ differences ($[A-a]_{O_2}D$)

CAUSE	EFFECT ON ARTERIAL P_{O_2}	EFFECT ON $(A-a)_{O_2}D$
Hypoventilation	Decreased	No change
Diffusion abnormality	No change or decreased*	No change or decreased*
Ventilation perfusion imbalance	Decreased	Increased
Right-to-left shunt	Decreased	Increased
Reduction in inspired P_{O_2}	Decreased	No change

IV. Oxygenation

   A. Efficiency of oxygenation

      1. $P[A-a]_{O_2}D$

      2. Pa_{O_2}/PA_{O_2}

      3. Right-to-left shunt (when breathing 100% O_2)

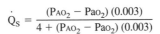

$$\dot{Q}_S = \frac{(PA_{O_2} - Pa_{O_2})\,(0.003)}{4 + (PA_{O_2} - Pa_{O_2})\,(0.003)}$$

   B. Adequacy of tissue oxygenation

      Pv_{O_2}

DELIVERY OF O_2 TO TISSUES

I. Dissolved

   A. Henry's law: Amount of O_2 dissolved is proportional to P_{O_2}. For each 1 mm Hg of P_{O_2}, there is 0.003 ml O_2/100 ml of plasma; content = solubility partial pressure

   B. Dissolved O_2 is not adequate to meet the animal's oxygen needs

II. Hemoglobin

   A. Conjugated protein of iron and porphyrin joined to the protein globin; globin has two alpha and two beta chains made of differing amino acid sequences

      1. Hemoglobin A: adult

      2. Hemoglobin F: fetal

---

*Effects of diffusion abnormalities are infrequently encountered at rest and are more likely to be evident during exercise.

    3. Hemoglobin S: sickle (valine-glutamic acid); poor oxygen carrying capability

B. Hemoglobin A is transferred from a ferrous to a ferric ion by oxidation (methemoglobin), which is not useful in O_2 carriage

    1. Nitrites

    2. Sulfonamides

    3. Benzocaine

O_2 DISSOCIATION CURVE (Fig. 16-1)

I. O_2 + Hb = HbO_2 (oxyhemoglobin); O_2 capacity is the amount of O_2 that can be combined with Hb

Example: 1 g Hb can combine with 1.39 ml of O_2. If there are 15 g Hb, then 1.39 × 15 = 20.8 ml O_2/100 ml at 100% saturation

II. O_2 saturation

$$\frac{O_2 \text{ combined with Hb X } 100}{O_2 \text{ capacity}}$$

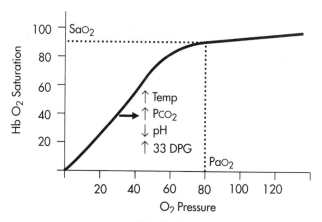

Fig. 16-1

The oxyhemoglobin dissociation curve. The effects of pH, P_{CO_2}, temperature, and 2,3-diphosphoglycerate on hemoglobin saturation with O_2 are noteworthy, as is the effect of anemia (low Hb) on O_2 content.

III. O_2 content is the amount of O_2 present as dissolved O_2 and combined with Hb

Example: $Po_2 = 100$ 12 g Hb

Sat $= 96\%$

$12 \times 1.39 \times 0.96 = 16$

$100 \times 0.003 = \underline{0.3}$

16.3 ml O_2/100 ml

IV. O_2 Dissociation curve shape (see Fig. 16-1)

A. Upper portion: Po_2 (partial pressure of oxygen) can fall slightly without affected O_2 loading of Hb

B. Lower portion: peripheral tissues can withdraw large amounts of O_2 with only small changes in Po_2; 5 g of reduced Hb can cause cyanosis (blue or purple discoloration)

V. Shifts in the O_2 dissociation curve are most commonly caused by changes in pH, Pco_2, and temperature

A. Increasing temperature and Pco_2 and decreasing pH shift the O_2 dissociation curve to the right; reverse changes have the opposite effect

B. 2,3-diphosphoglycerate (DPG) increases within red blood cells (RBC) occur in chronic hypoxia and shift the O_2 dissociation curve to the right

C. Rightward shifts mean more unloading of O_2 at a given Po_2 in a tissue capillary; the normal Po_2 at 50% O_2 saturation is approximately 26 mm Hg

D. Deoxygenated Hb can carry more CO_2

CARBON DIOXIDE

I. Transport

A. Dissolved in blood

1. In plasma as $[Hco_3^-]$

2. In RBCs as carbamino compounds

3. Carried in physical solution

B. The measurement of end-expired CO_2 ($Peco_2$) and Pao_2 permits the calculation of dead space ventilation (V_D)

$$V_D = \frac{Paco_2 - Peco_2}{Paco_2}$$

CARBON MONOXIDE

I. $Hb + CO \rightarrow COHb$ (carboxyhemoglobin)
II. Carbon monoxide has about 210 times the affinity for Hb than O_2
    A. Small amounts of CO can tie up large amounts of Hb, making it unavailable for O_2 carriage
    B. Results in a normal Po_2 but grossly reduced O_2 content
    C. Shifts the oxyhemoglobin curve to the left impair O_2 unloading in tissues

NORMAL PH AND BLOOD GAS VALUES

  I. pH = 7.40; range 7.35 to 7.45
  II. Pao_2 = 95 mm Hg; range 80 to 110 mm Hg
 III. Pvo_2 = 40 mm Hg; range 35 to 45 mm Hg
  IV. $Paco_2$ = 40 mm Hg; range 35 to 45 mm Hg
  V. $Pvco_2$ = 45 mm Hg; range 40 to 48 mm Hg
  VI. HCO_3^- = 24 mEq/L; range 22 to 27 mEq/L
 VII. The $Paco_2$/pH/HCO_3^- relationship

$Paco_2$ (mm Hg) (ACUTE CHANGE)	pH	HCO_3^- (mEq/L) (EFFECT)
80	7.2	28
60	7.3	26
40	7.4	24
30	7.5	22
20	7.6	20

VIII. Nomenclature
    A. Acidemia: pH 7.35 (acid blood)
       1. Metabolic acidosis: an abnormal physiologic process characterized by a primary gain of acid (H^+) or primary loss of base (HCO_3^-) from the extracellular fluid
       2. Respiratory acidosis: an abnormal process in which there is a primary reduction in alveolar ventilation relative to CO_2 production ($Paco_2$ increase)
    B. Alkalemia: pH 7.45 (alkaline blood)
       1. Metabolic alkalosis: an abnormal physiologic process characterized by a primary gain in base (HCO_3^-) or loss of acid (H^+) from the extracellular fluid

2. Respiratory alkalosis: an abnormal physiologic process in which there is a primary increase in alveolar ventilation relative to the rate of CO_2 production (Pa_{CO_2} decrease)

C. Compensation: an abnormal pH is returned toward normal by altering the component not primarily affected; for example, if the Pa_{CO_2} is elevated, the HCO_3^- should be elevated (retained) to compensate

1. If the P_{CO_2} or HCO_3^- values are outside normal limits, but the pH is within the normal range, then the patient is fully compensated

2. Because it takes time for the process of compensation to return the pH to within normal limits, a compensatory process implies a degree of chronicity

PRIMARY PH AND BLOOD GAS CLASSIFICATION

CLASSIFICATION	Pa_{CO_2}	pH	HCO_3^-	BE
Acute ventilatory failure	↑	↓	N	N
Chronic ventilatory failure	↑	N	↑	↑
Acute alveolar hyperventilation	↓	↑	N	N
Chronic alveolar hyperventilation	↓	N	↓	↓
Uncompensated metabolic acidosis	N	↓	↓	↓
Compensated metabolic acidosis·	↓	N	↓	↓
Uncompensated metabolic alkalosis	N	↑	↑	↑
Compensated metabolic alkalosis	↑	N	↑	↑

↓, Decreased; ↑, increased; N, normal.

I. Mixed respiratory and metabolic conditions can coexist. When this occurs, look at the individual values (pH, P_{CO_2}, HCO_3^-) to determine the severity

RAPID QUALITATIVE INTERPRETATION
OF pH AND BLOOD GASES

I. Determine pH: acidemia or alkalemia; the pH is the most important value in determining the animal's acid-base status; match subsequent values to it

II. Determine P_{CO_2}
   A. Respiratory alkalosis: <35 mm Hg
   B. Respiratory acidosis: >50 mm Hg

III. Determine BE or HCO_3^-
   A. Metabolic alkalosis: BE >+5 mEq/L (HCO_3^- >28 mEq/L)
   B. Metabolic acidosis: BE <−5 mEq/L (HCO_3^- <20 mEq/L)

IV. Determine primary problem by matching either the P_{CO_2} or BE or both with the pH; determine if compensation exists (pH near normal)

V. Next, look more closely at BE
   A. BE can be influenced by four things
      1. Free water (use $[Na^+]$ as the measure): Na, K and Cl are examples of strong ions
      2. $[Cl^-]$
      3. Protein concentration (A_{tot})
      4. Unidentified anion concentrations (lactic acid)
   B. Abnormalities in all four can exist simultaneously (Fig. 16-2); they can have opposite effects, and therefore can offset and hide each other; for example, a severe lactic acidosis from shock can be offset by a severe hyperchloremic

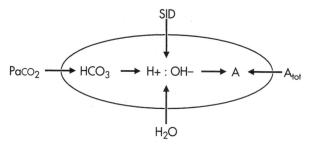

Fig. 16-2
Factors that effect acid-base balance.

alkalosis from sustained vomiting; the net (observed) BE could be zero

VI. Determine Pao_2
   A. If Pao_2 <80 mm Hg, suspect hypoxemia
   B. 5 g of reduced Hb results in cyanosis in patients with more than 5 g of Hb

RULES OF THUMB

I. The HCO_3^- concentration rises about 1 to 2 mEq/L for each acute 10-mm Hg increase in $Paco_2$ above 40; maximum change in HCO_3^- is about 4 mEq/L

II. The HCO_3^- concentration falls 1 to 2 mEq/L for each acute 10-mm Hg decrease in $Paco_2$ below 40; maximum change in HCO_3^- is about 6 mEq/L

III. Acute respiratory and nonrespiratory disorders can be distinguished by their $Paco_2$ and HCO_3^- values; HCO_3^- above 30 or below 15 mEq/L implies a nonrespiratory (metabolic) component

IV. During chronic elevation of the $Paco_2$ (hypercapnea), each 10-mm Hg increase in $Paco_2$ causes a 4-mEq/L increase in HCO_3^- concentration

V. An acute 10-mm Hg increase in $Paco_2$ results in a 0.05-unit decrease in pH; an acute 10-mm Hg decrease in $Paco_2$ results in a 0.10-unit increase in pH

VI. Rapid determination of the predicted respiratory pH
   A. Determine the difference between the measured $Paco_2$ and 40 mm Hg, then move decimal two places to left
   B. If the $Paco_2$ is greater than 40, subtract half the value from 7.40
   C. If the $Paco_2$ is less than 40, move decimal two places to left and add the value to 7.40
   D. Examples
      1. pH = 7.01; $Paco_2$ = 75 ($Paco_2$ > 40 mm Hg)
         $75 - 40 = 35$; $0.35 \times 0.5 > = 0.175$
         $7.40 - 0.18 = 7.22$
      2. pH = 7.43; $Paco_2$ = 23 ($Paco_2$ <40 mm Hg)
         $40 - 23 = 17$
         $7.40 + 0.17 = 7.57$

VII. Rapid determination of the metabolic component
   A. A 10-mEq/L change in HCO_3^- concentration changes pH

by 0.15 units; if the pH decimal is moved two places to the right, then a 10:15 or 2/3 relationship exists

   B. The absolute difference between the measured pH and the predicted respiratory pH is the metabolic component of the pH change; moving the decimal point two places to the right and multiplying by 23 yields an estimate of the mEq/L variation of the buffer baseline (usually assumed as HCO_3^- concentration change)

VIII. Rapid quantitative clinical determination of acid-base changes

   A. Determine predicted respiratory pH

   B. Estimate BE or deficit

   C. Examples

      1. pH = 7.02; $Paco_2$ = 75

         predicted respiratory pH:

            75 − 40 = 35; 0.35 × 0.5 = 0.175

            7.40 − 0.18 = 7.22

         metabolic component:

            7.22 − 7.02 = 20 × 2/3 = 13.3 mEq/L, or 13.3 mEq/L base deficit

      2. pH = 7.64; $Paco_2$ = 25

         predicted respiratory pH:

            40 − 25 = 0.15

            7.40 + 0.15 = 7.55

         metabolic component:

             7.64 − 7.55 = 9 × 2/3 = 6 mEq/L, or 6.0 mEq/L BE

IX. Quantitative analysis of nonrespiratory acid-base ratio state*

   A. Enter the observed BE at the bottom of a table (Table 16-1)

   B. Calculate and enter the expected contributions to BE of any free water abnormality, abnormality of the corrected $[Cl^-]$, and abnormal protein concentrations; be careful about sign (+ or −)

   C. Sum the values in "B"; be careful about sign (+ or −)

   D. Compare "A" and "C;" the observed BE should never be greater than the summed values in "C;" if the ob-

---

*Modified from Leith DE: Proceedings of the Ninth ACVIM Forum, New Orleans, May 1991.

TABLE 16-1

QUANTITATIVE ANALYSIS OF NONRESPIRATORY ACID-BASE RATIO STATE

Free water abnormalities:	$0.3 ([Na^+] - 140)$	=	___
Chloride abnormalities:	$102 - [Cl^-]corr$	=	___
Hypoproteinemia:	$3(6.5 - [P_{tot}])$	=	___
Unmeasured anions make up the balance:		=	___
Total, or the observed (reported) BE:		=	___

$[Cl^-]corr = [Cl^-]obs \times 140/[Na^+]$.
For [Alb] instead of $[P_{tot}]$, use $3.7 (4.5 - [Alb])$.

served BE is less, the presence of unmeasured anions (UA^-) equal in magnitude to the difference of the summed values in B and BE can be inferred

X. Example

If:

$$pH = 7.250, Na^+ = 135$$
$$Pco_2 = 75, Cl^- = 79$$
$$BE = 2; P_{tot} + 8.4$$

Then

Free water abnormality $= -1.5$
Chloride abnormality $= +20$
Hypoproteinemia $= -5.7$
Observed BE $= 2$

Therefore

$$UA^- = 16.3$$
$$[(14.3) + (2) = 16.3]$$

XI. Summary of acid-base disorders
  A. Acid-base state is determined by changes in $Paco_2$, SID (strong ion difference), and P_{tot}
  B. All acid-base disturbances are caused by changes in $Paco_2$, SID, and P_{tot}
  C. Since protein concentration is not manipulated clinically, all acid-base disturbances are corrected by changes in $Paco_2$ and SID

XII. Therapy
  A. Base deficits of less than 10 mEq/L are not routinely treated
  B. pH above 7.20 is not routinely treated unless there is evidence of shock

C. Since extracellular water is approximately 25% to 30% body weight, base deficits × body weight (kg) 25% = amount of HCO_3^- needed as replacement, or

$$\frac{\text{Base deficit} \times \text{wt (kg)}}{4} = \text{mEq } HCO_3^- \text{ required}$$

COMMON CAUSES OF ACID-BASE IMBALANCE

I. Respiratory acidosis
   A. Anesthesia or respiratory depressant drugs
   B. Obesity
   C. Pulmonary disease
   D. Rib or thoracic disease or trauma
   E. Brain damage
II. Respiratory alkalosis
   A. Anxiety, fear
   B. Fever
   C. Endotoxemia
   D. Pneumonia, pulmonary embolus
   E. Hypoxemia
   F. Left-to-right shunts
   G. Heart failure
III. Metabolic acidosis
   A. Renal disease (uremia)
   B. Chronic vomiting
   C. Diarrhea
   D. Severe exercise, hypoxia, ischemia, shock, trauma
   E. Diabetes
IV. Metabolic alkalosis
   A. Acute vomiting
   B. Hypokalemia
   C. Excessive use of diuretics

ACID-BASE AND ELECTROLYTE INTERRELATIONSHIPS

I. Most CO_2 entering the blood passes into RBCs, where the majority of CO_2 enters into a reversible formation with HCO_3^-

$$CO_2 + H_2O \overset{CA}{\leftrightarrow} H_2CO_3 \leftrightarrow H^+ + HCO_3^-$$

The HCO_3^- formed by this reaction diffuses out of RBCs; this movement sets up an electrostatic difference across the cell membrane, which is neutralized by the movement of Cl^- from plasma into the RBC (chloride shift)

II. The location and absolute numbers of positively and negatively charged ions (strong ions) and their difference in combination with CO_2 production, the resultant P_{CO_2} and the total protein determine pH ($[H^+]$) and $[HCO_3^-]$ changes in the body. The principal strong ions are Na^+, K^+, and Cl^-. SID $= [Na^+] + [K^+] - [Cl^-]$ (see Fig. 16-2)

III. Changes in strong ions in various body fluids result in changes in SID, which provide the major mechanism for acid-base interactions

IV. To maintain electrical neutrality, electrolyte shifts generally occur simultaneously with acid (H^+) or base (HCO_3^-) shifts. The most important electrolyte shift occurring with acid-base changes is K^+. For example, when HCO_3^- is added to the extracellular fluid, hydrogen ions (H^+) leave cells, causing K^+ to move intracellularly to maintain electrical equilibrium; therefore

  A. In metabolic alkalosis, suspect hypokalemia

  B. In metabolic acidosis, suspect hyperkalemia

CHAPTER SEVENTEEN

Pain

"Pleasure is nothing else but
the intermission of pain."

JOHN SELDEN

OVERVIEW

The definition, recognition, quantitation, and treatment of pain has become a central issue in veterinary practice. Once considered acceptable, physical restraint, sedation, hypnotics, and inhalation anesthesia are no longer appropriate unless pain is considered and treated. This is particularly true for pain in the perioperative period. Apprehension and stress produced by fear can initiate a variety of potentially deleterious neurohumoral reactions (stress response), in addition to sensitizing both the peripheral and central nervous systems to noxious stimuli. Improved understanding of pain pathways and the mechanism of action of analgesic therapies has evolved to the point of treating pain before it occurs, a method called preemptive analgesia. The optimal treatment of pain is to preempt the establishment of pain and pain hypersensitivity before, during, and after surgery.

GENERAL CONSIDERATIONS

I. Definitions

Allodynia: A change in the sensitivity to pain so that a stimuli that would never produce pain begins to do so

Analgesia: Absence of sensibility to pain

Analgesic, analgetic: Any method or drug that relieves pain

Analgia: Painlessness

Aseptic surgery: Surgery performed in ways and by means

sufficiently free from microorganisms so that appreciable infection or suppuration does not develop

Central sensitization: A change (prolonged response) in the excitability of neurons in the spinal cord to nociceptive afferent input

Deep pain: Originates in tendons, joints, viscera, muscles, and periosteum; it is not unusual for deep pain to cause a drop in blood pressure, a slowing of the pulse, nausea, vomiting, and sweating; can cause reflex cramping of nearby skeletal muscles

Distress: A state in which the animal is unable to adapt to an altered environment or altered stimuli

Field or production surgery: Any surgery performed on farm or free-ranging wild animals residing in their natural or production habitat

Hyperalgesia: An error in pain perception in which there is an excessive sensitivity to pain; secondary hyperalgesia is present when hypersensitivity to pain spreads to noninjured tissue

Institutional Animal Care and Use Committee: A committee whose existence is required by the United States Department of Agriculture and the Department of Health and Human Services at institutions conducting research on animals; consists of veterinarians, practicing scientists, nonscientists, and individuals not affiliated with the institution; responsible for evaluating the institutional animal care and use programs and making recommendations to the administration of the institution; ultimately responsible for approving or disapproving the use of animals in research at the institution on a case-by-case basis

Major surgery: Any surgical intervention that penetrates and exposes a body cavity; any procedure that has the potential for inducing permanent physical or physiologic impairment; and/or any procedure associated with orthopedics or extensive tissue dissection or transection

Minor surgery: Any surgical intervention that produces minimal impairment of physical or physiologic function (e.g., laparoscopy, superficial vascular cutdown, and percutaneous biopsy)

Neuralgia: Pain exhibiting periodic intensification, which extends along the course of one or more nerves

Nonsurvival/nonrecovery surgery: A surgical procedure performed under general anesthesia at the conclusion of which the animal is euthanized without regaining consciousness

Pain: Perception of an unpleasant sensory or emotional experience that results from potential or actual tissue damage

Perioperative: All events associated with a surgical procedure

Preemptive analgesia: The administration of an analgetic before pain develops

Projected pain: An error in the localization of pain; occurs with superficial pain, which is normally quite accurately located; injury to a nerve containing pain pathways causes a phantom pain to be projected into the uninjured area at the origin of the pain fibers

Referred pain: Pain originating in one part of the body but perceived as occurring in another; occurs as the result of the synapses in the spinal cord of visceral pain fibers with pain fibers from the skin

Stoic: Indifferent to pain or pleasure

Stress: The effect induced by external (e.g., physical or environmental) events or internal (e.g., physiologic or psychologic) factors, referred to as stressors, that induce alteration in an animal's biologic equilibrium

Superficial or cutaneous pain: Originating on an outer surface (skin) and well localized, it may be sharp or acute or it may be chronic, burning, or aching; may cause an increase in the pulse rate and blood pressure

Surgery: The act of incising living tissue; an operative procedure; and/or the room or facility where an operative procedure is done

Surgical facility: A group of interrelated rooms specifically designed for the conduct of surgery as well as for preoperative and postoperative functions associated with the conduct of surgery in animals

Survival/recovery surgery: A surgical procedure from which animals recover from the effects of general anesthesia and become conscious

The perception of pain: Only humans report and demand treatment of pain; pain in animals must be inferred by the observation of deviations from normal behavior; pain may be manifested as a limp or altered gait, withdrawal of an injured part, awkward, abnormal postures, a worried or distressed expression, looking at, licking, scratching, or kicking at the perceived pain; these and similar signs are the only ones a veterinarian can use to diagnose the presence and magnitude of pain; seems likely that the presence of pain in animals is underdiagnosed, and, when diagnosed, that its magnitude is underestimated

Visceral pain: Originating from internal organs, visceral pain is poorly localized; small injuries may not cause severe pain, whereas diffuse foci can produce extremely severe pain; pulling and twisting of viscera, mesenteries, and ligaments can cause pain in the body of an anesthetized patient; visceral pain can be perceived as a pain on the body surface; this error in pain localization is called *referred pain;* if the visceral involvement results in an inflammation that extends to an area of parietal peritoneum, pleura, or pericardium, pain fibers from these areas are also stimulated; pain fibers in the parietal peritoneum or pleura are innervated like the skin and are capable of sensing acute, highly localized pain referred to the corresponding area on the surface of the body; visceral pain can also reflexly produce skeletal muscle spasm of the abdominal wall over the affected area; usually involves the parietal peritoneum

II. Physiology of pain and pain pathways
   A. Peripheral pain receptors
      1. Mechanosensitive
         a. Stress, stretching
         b. Compression, crushing
      2. Thermosensitive; involves temperature change
         (1) Heat
         (2) Cold
      3. Chemosensitive
         a. Neurotransmitters (Ach)
         b. Prostaglandins (PGE_2)
         c. Autocoids
            (1) Bradykinin
            (2) 5-hydroxytryptamine (5HT)
            (3) Histamine

       (4) Potassium

       (5) Proteolytic enzymes

    d. Acids (e.g., lactic acid)

    e. Cytokines

       (1) Tumor necrosis factor

       (2) Interleukin-1,6,8

       (3) Calcitonin gene-related peptide

B. Peripheral nerves

  1. Myelinated A-δ nerve fibers transmit acute, accurately localized, (epicritic) sharp pain

  2. Nonmyelinated C nerve fibers transmit chronic, diffuse (protopathic), dull, burning, aching pain

C. Spinal cord pathways

  1. Peripheral nerves enter the spinal cord through the dorsal roots and then ascend or descend one or two segments in Lissauer's tract

  2. Peripheral nerves terminate in the dorsal horn gray matter (substantial gelatinosa)

  3. Peripheral nerves synapse with nerves of the spinothalamic tract and are carried centrally to the

    a. Thalamus: somatosensory cortex

    b. Reticular activating system, which is important in activating the autonomic nervous system and limbic system causing

       (1) Sleep arousal

       (2) Cardiopulmonary changes

       (3) Aversion reaction

       (4) Stress response

  4. Spinal cord pain receptors

    a. Facilitory

       (1) Substance P receptors (neurokin-1; NK-1 type)

       (2) Glutamate receptors (N-methyl-D-aspartate [NMDA type])

       (3) Prostaglandin receptors

    b. Inhibitory

       (1) Gamma amino butyric acid-B receptors

       (2) Opioid receptors (μ, κ, others)

       (3) α_2 Receptors (type unknown)

       (4) Adenosine receptors (A_1-type)

    5. Central perception

       a. Pain in animals is inferred by observation of deviations from normal behavior and physiologic responses

         (1) Altered gait

         (2) Increased locomotion

         (3) Reluctance to move

         (4) Abnormal posture

         (5) Licking, scratching

         (6) Self-mutilation

         (7) Aversion

         (8) Vocalization

         (9) Aggression

         (10) Tachycardia, tachypnea

       b. Pain in anesthetized animals is inferred by changes in response to manipulation, surgical or otherwise

         (1) Movement

         (2) Trembling

         (3) Increased heart or respiratory rate

         (4) Increased arterial blood pressure

       c. Pain or stress is inferred by increases in circulating "stress" substances

         (1) Adrenocorticotropic hormone

         (2) Glucose

         (3) Catecholamines (dopamine, epinephrine, norepinephrine)

         (4) Beta-endorphin

         (5) Leu-enkephalin

         (6) Lactic acid

         (7) Free fatty acids

III. Response to tissue injury

   A. Classification of pain

      1. Physiologic pain, which is experienced in everyday life in association with noxious stimuli (e.g., heat, cold, pressure)

         (1) Well localized

         (2) Transient

         (3) High threshold

         (4) Operates as a protective system

2. Clinical pain is composed of inflammatory pain and neuropathic pain
   a. Inflammatory pain is caused by peripheral tissue damage (crushing, burning, surgery)
      (1) Low threshold to pain (allodynia)
      (2) Exaggerated response to noxious stimuli (hyperalgesia)
      (3) Poorly localized (secondary hyperalgesia)
      (4) Initiates peripheral and central sensitization
   b. Neuropathic pain is caused by damage to the nervous system; characteristics are similar to those of inflammatory pain
3. Clinical pain differs from physiologic pain because of the presence of pathologic hypersensitivity

B. Peripheral and central hypersensitization
1. Peripheral sensitization causes decrease in pain threshold
   (1) At the site of injury
   (2) In surrounding tissue
2. Central sensitization
   a. Activity-dependent increase in the excitability of spinal neurons termed *spinal facilitation* or "windup"
      (1) Evokes progressively greater responses in dorsal-horn, wide dynamic-range neurons
      (2) Increases the size of peripheral receptive fields
      (3) Demonstrates continual changes (field plasticity) in spatial, temporal, and threshold qualities that parallel postinjury hyperalgesia
   b. Central sensitization includes "windup" and a prolonged phase of hyperalgesia; mediated by substance P (NK-1) and glutamate (NMDA) receptors
3. Differences between peripheral and central sensitization
   a. Peripheral sensitization is produced by low-intensity stimuli activating A-δ and C nociceptors
   b. Central sensitization is produced by normal, low-threshold A-β sensory fibers because of changes in central processing from neural inputs

C. Implications for pain therapy
1. Complete analgesia is required intraoperatively, whether or not the patient is conscious; intraoperative analgesia can be produced by general anesthesia, local anesthetics, and a variety of analgesic drugs (Table 17-1)
    a. Inhalation anesthetics (halothane, isoflurane)
    b. Hypnotics (barbiturates, etomidate, propofol)
    c. Dissociogenic drugs (ketamine, tiletamine)
    d. Local anesthetics (lidocaine, mepivacaine)
    e. Opioids (morphine, meperidine, oxymorphone, butorphanol)
    f. α_2 Agonists (xylazine, detomidine, medetomidine)
    g. Nonsteroidal antiinflammatory drugs (NSAIDs); flunixin megulamine, aspirin, phenylbutazone
2. Converting clinical pain to physiologic pain may be sufficient before and after surgery; best accomplished with behavior modifiers and antiinflammatory drugs
    a. Opioids
    b. α_2 agonists
    c. NSAIDs

TABLE **17-1**

INJECTABLE ANALGESIC DRUGS AND THEIR MECHANISM OF ACTION

DRUG	MECHANISM OF ACTION
Opioids (morphine, meperidine, oxymorphone)	Combine with opioid receptors to produce sedation, analgesia, and euphoria
α_2 agonists (xylazine, detomidine, medetomidine)	Combine with α_2 receptors to produce sedation, muscle relaxation, and analgesia
Nonsteroidal, antiinflammatory drugs;flunixin meglumine, phenylbutazone, aspirin	Act centrally (CNS) on the hypothalamus; antiinflammatory and analgesic activity mediated by peripheral inhibition of prostaglandins
Local anesthetics (lidocaine, bupivacaine)	Block nerve transmission of electrical impulses

CNS, central nervous system.

3. Prevent the establishment of pain and central sensitization (Table 17-2)
   a. Preemptive analgesia; drug combinations (opioids-tranquilizers) may be needed
   b. Dose and routes of drug administration can produce select effects; intravenous, intramuscular, subcutaneous, and oral versus epidural, intrathecal, and site-specific administration

TABLE 17-2

SOME DRUGS COMMONLY USED TO CONTROL PAIN

DRUG	GENERIC	DOSAGE (MG/KG)	ROUTE	DURATION (HOURS)	SPECIES APPROVED	COMMENT	SCHEDULE
Nonsteroidal antinflammatory drugs							
Aspirin	Aspirin	Dog: 10 Cat: 10	PO PO	12-24 48		Platelet dysfunction; GI hemorrhage	
Butazolidin	Phenylbutazone	Dog: 20	PO	24	Dog, Horse	Maximum daily dose = 800 mg; GI hemorrhage	
Banamine	Flunixin meglumine	Dog: 0.5-1	IV	24	Horse	GI hemorrhage	
Sedative							
Rompun Gemini Anased	Xylazine	Dog: 0.1-0.3 Cat: 0.05-0.2	IM, IV IM, IV	1-5 1-5	Dog, Cat, Horse	Cardiovascular and respiratory depression; cardiac dysrhythmias	
Opioid agonists							
Morphine	Morphine	0.2-0.5 0.1	IM Epidural	2-6 4-12		Bradycardia; respiratory depression	Schedule II
Oxymorphone/ PM	Oxymorphone	0.02-0.1	IM, IV	2-6	Dog, Cat	Bradycardia; respiratory depression	Schedule II

Trade name	Generic name	Dose	Route		Species	Comments	Schedule
Numorphan							Schedule II
Demerol	Meperidine	1-4	IM	0.5-1		Short duration	
Domosedan	Detomidine	0.01-0.05	IM, IV	1-5	Horse	Same as xylazine	
Opioid agonists-antagonists							
Talwin-V	Pentazocine	1-4	IM, IV	0.5-1	Dog, Horse	Short duration	Schedule IV
Torbugesic Torbutrol	Butorphanol	0.2-0.8	IM, IV	1-4	Horse		Noncontrolled
Nubain	Nalbuphine	0.5-1.5	IM, IV	1-5	Dog, Cat	Inconsistent activity	Noncontrolled
Buprenex	Buprenorphine	0.005-0.1	IM, IV	4-8		Long onset of action	Schedule V
Local anesthetics							
Lidocaine (2%)	Lidocaine		Selective nerve blocks	0.5-1		—	
Marcaine	Bupivacaine		Selective nerve blocks	4-6	Dog, Horse, Cat	—	

Schedule I: Substances in this schedule have no accepted medical use in the United States and have a high abuse potention (e.g., heroin, marijuana, LSD, methaqualone).

Schedule II: Substances in this schedule have high abuse potential with severe psychic or physical dependence liability (e.g., morphine, oxymorphone, meperidine, fentanyl, amphetamine, pentobarbital, phencyclidane, Innovar-Vet); records for Schedule II drugs must be maintained separately from those in Schedules III and IV

Schedule III: Less abuse potential than Schedule II: no examples in veterinary medicine

Schedule IV: Less abuse potential than Schedule III (e.g., chloral hydrate, diazepam, pentazocine)

Schedule V: Limited abuse potential (e.g., some drugs for antitussive and antidiarrheal use)

PO, by month; IM, intramuscular; GI, gastrointestinal.

CHAPTER EIGHTEEN

Anesthetic Procedures and Techniques in Small Animals

"Come now let us reason together."
LYNDON BAINES JOHNSON

OVERVIEW

Anesthetic procedures and techniques developed for small animals are designed to produce the desired result safely, effectively, and economically. The single drug technique in chemical restraint and anesthesia causes specific side effects. An experienced anesthetist knows the shortcomings of the various drugs and is prepared for likely adverse responses. The technique of combining drugs in reduced dosages to provide chemical restraint and anesthesia reduces unwanted side effects and toxicity. The advantage of combination drug therapy over single-drug therapy is a more ideal anesthetic state, which includes hypnosis, analgesia, and muscle relaxation. Combination drug therapy requires a comprehensive knowledge of the pharmacology of anesthetic drugs, their interactions, and potential side effects.

GENERAL CONSIDERATIONS

I. A variety of anesthetic procedures and techniques can be used to safely produce chemical restraint and anesthesia in dogs and cats
II. The choice of anesthetic regimen is influenced by
    A. Breed
    B. Temperament
    C. Health and physical condition

    D. The purpose of chemical restraint and anesthesia
    E. The familiarity of personnel with the drugs being used
    F. Concurrent medication
    G. The amount of available assistance
 III. Whenever possible, drugs that are reversible should be used
 IV. Endotracheal intubation should always be performed to assure an airway
  V. Careful monitoring is mandatory to avoid adverse effects
 VI. Food and water should be withheld for approximately 6 hours before surgery, except in very small, very young, or diseased patients

PREANESTHETIC EVALUATION (see Chapter 2)

   I. Review patient history
  II. Perform physical examination
 III. Review available laboratory data
 IV. Formulate a specific anesthetic plan
    A. Decide about further preoperative tests
    B. Choose drugs appropriate to patient needs
   V. Gather appropriate equipment and supplies
    A. Endotracheal tube
      1. Select diameter by patient size
      2. If using a cuffed tube, check cuff for leaks by injecting air
      3. Use a stylet for small-diameter, flimsy tubes (Fig. 18-1)
      4. Use a Cole catheter in neonates, rodents, birds, and reptiles (Fig. 18-2)
    B. Laryngoscope
      1. Aids intubation by allowing visualization, illumination, and manipulation of tongue and laryngeal structures
      2. May be optional, depending upon species, anatomy, and the physical size of the patient
    C. Anesthetic machine and breathing system
      1. Size and type of system determined by patient size
        a. For patients less than approximately 400 pounds, use the small-animal anesthetic machine (adult human anesthetic system)
          (1) Use the circle system for patients ≥ 10 pounds

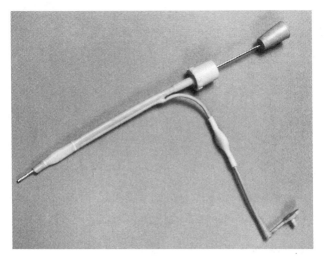

Fig. 18-1
A stylet can be used to stiffen small endotracheal tubes to facilitate tracheal intubation.

          (2) Use the nonrebreathing system for patient <10 pounds

  2. Rebreathing bag should be approximately five times the tidal volume

  3. Refill carbon dioxide–absorbent cannister if material is exhausted

  4. Evaluate anesthetic system for possible malfunctions (see Chapter 13)

    a. Fill vaporizer and check operation

    b. Turn on flowmeters and check for free movement of indicator balls or slides

    c. Close pop-off valve and pressurize the system to 40 cm water using oxygen flush valve; check for leaks

  5. Connect waste gas scavenging system to the anesthetic machine

D. Fresh gases

  1. Oxygen

    a. Use supply outside "house"

    b. Mate tanks to machine; change oxygen tank if pressure gauge reads <500 psi

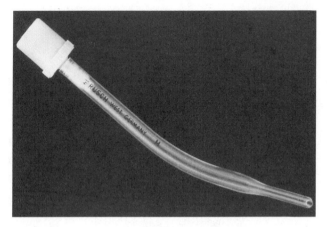

Fig. 18-2

A Cole catheter facilitates intubation of neonates, rodents, birds, and reptiles.

    2. Nitrous oxide
      a. Optional
      b. Change tank if pressure gauge reads <750 psi
  E. Intravenous administration supplies
    1. Intravenous catheter
    2. Appropriate intravenous fluids
    3. Solution administration set
  F. Drugs
    1. Calculate appropriate drug dosage and volume
    2. Withdraw drugs into labeled syringes
  G. Ancillary supplies
    1. 4 × 4–inch gauze sponges
    2. Adhesive tape
    3. Roll gauze
    4. Esophageal stethoscope catheter and earpiece

PREANESTHETIC MEDICATION

I. Choice of drug determined by the patient's preoperative condition and any other special considerations pertinent to the procedure

II. Drugs given intramuscularly (IM) or subcutaneously (SQ) should be administered 10 to 30 minutes before catheterization and induction

III. Drugs used as premedications
   A. Acepromazine 0.1 mg/lb IM, maximum total dose 4 mg
   B. Diazepam 0.1 mg/lb IV, maximum total dose 5 mg; use midazolam as an alternative, same dose
   C. Innovar-Vet 1 cc/20 to 40 lb IM, 1 cc/40 to 80 lb IV
   D. Anticholinergics
      1. Atropine 0.1 mg/lb IM or IV
      2. Glycopyrrolate 0.005 mg/lb IM or IV
   E. Narcotics
      1. Morphine 0.2 to 0.3 mg/lb IM (dogs), 0.1 mg/lb IM (cats)
      2. Oxymorphone 0.05 to 0.15 mg/lb IM
      3. Meperidine 0.5 to 3 mg/lb IM
      4. Innovar-Vet 1 ml/20 to 30 lb IM (dogs)
   F. Ketamine (cats) 3 to 5 mg/lb IM
   G. Xylazine 0.1 to 0.5 mg/lb IM
   H. Medetomidine 5 to 10 μg/lb IM
   I. Telazol 1 to 3 mg/lb IM

INDUCTION

I. Intravenous
   A. Catheterize vein(s)
   B. Start IV fluid administration to ensure catheter patency
   C. Lower fluid bag or bottle below patient's thorax, completely opening valve of fluid administration set valve to allow blood to siphon back into catheter; this confirms catheter placement within the vein
   D. Inject induction agent(s) at appropriate rate(s), allowing time for patient equilibration before administering further increments
   E. Specific IV induction drugs (see Chapter 8)
      1. Ultrashort–acting barbiturates
         a. Thiamylal 2% to 4%; 2 to 4 mg/lb
         b. Thiopental 2% to 4%; 3 to 5 mg/lb
         c. Methohexital 2%
      2. Pentobarbital

   3. Etomidate
   4. Propofol
   5. Combinations
      a. Innovar-Vet 1 cc/40 to 60 lb IV, followed by pentobarbital 2 to 3 mg/lb IV
      b. Diazepam 0.1 mg/lb IV, thiamylal 2 mg/lb IV, lidocaine 2 mg/lb IV
         (1) Useful in animals with CNS depression
         (2) Stabilizes myocardium
         (3) Reduces thiobarbiturate dosage
      c. Diazepam–ketamine: simultaneous administration of diazepam (0.125 mg/lb IV) and ketamine (2.5 mg/lb IV)
         (1) Mix equal parts of diazepam (5 mg/ml in stock vial) and ketamine (100 mg/ml in stock vial) to yield a mixture that is 2.5 mg/ml diazepam and 50 mg/ml ketamine
         (2) Use 1 cc of mixture per 20 pounds
      d. Diazepam, opioid, etomidate, or propofol; use etomidate at reduced dosage to produce hypnosis

II. Inhalant
   A. Face mask (Fig. 18-3)
      1. Be aware of potential for vomiting and possible resultant aspiration
      2. Ensure adequate restraint
      3. Environmental pollution is significant
   B. Induction box (Fig. 18-4)
      1. Cats, small dogs, rodents, birds, snakes
      2. Use high, fresh-gas flow rates
      3. Monitor patient closely for loss of righting reflex, then remove from box
      4. Atmospheric pollution with anesthetic gases is significant

ENDOTRACHEAL INTUBATION

I. Open patient's mouth and manipulate tongue to side with endotracheal tube; grasp tongue with a gauze sponge, and retract tongue firmly between lower canine teeth to hold mandible open (Fig. 18-5)

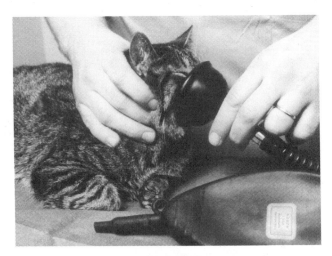

Fig. 18-3

A face mask is often used to induce cats and small dogs to anesthesia.

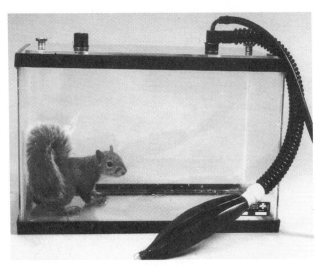

Fig. 18-4

An induction chamber is used to confine cats and small animals for induction to general anesthesia using an inhaled anesthetic.

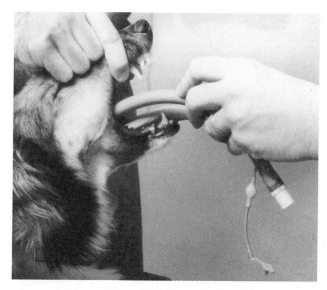

Fig. 18-5
Most dogs and cats are easily intubated without a laryngoscope.

II. Visualize larynx and insert endotracheal tube
   A. Direct visualization
   B. Use laryngoscope to facilitate visualization of the larynx
   C. Potential difficulties
      1. Laryngospasm (0.1 ml lidocaine sprayed into glottis reduces spasms)
         a. Patient too light
         b. Larynx sensitized
      2. Soft-palate displacement prevents rostroventral movement of epiglottis; push soft palate dorsally with endotracheal tube to release epiglottis
   D. Turn on oxygen
   E. Connect breathing system to endotracheal tube, and secure tube to patient (Fig. 18-6)
   F. Monitor respirations and pulse
      1. If pulses are present, turn on vaporizer and nitrous oxide if desired

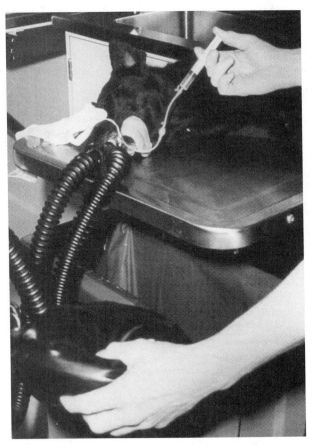

Fig. 18-6

Escape of gas from around the endotracheal tube can be eliminated by inflating the endotracheal tube cuff (right hand) until no gas escapes from the mouth during rebreathing bag compression (left hand) to 30 cm H_2O.

2. If pulses are absent, leave oxygen on and diagnose cause of absent or weak pulses; do not start inhalation drugs (see Chapter 26)
3. Spontaneous ventilation (assist ventilation if required)
4. Apnea, dyspnea
    a. Patient's ventilatory drive may be depressed by anesthetic induction drugs; begin mechanical ventilation using the breathing system
    b. Endotracheal tube may be obstructed or kinked
    c. For bronchial intubation, withdraw tube into trachea
    d. Pneumothorax or pneumomediastinum
        (1) Relieve intrathoracic pressure by percutaneous needle insertion
        (2) Evaluate hemodynamic status
G. Set vaporizer to a maintenance concentration determined by monitoring patient responses

MAINTENANCE OF ANESTHESIA

 I. Monitoring (see Chapter 15)
 II. Record concentrations, doses, and time administered for anesthetic drugs given; readjust dosages according to patient response, depth of anesthesia, and amount of analgesia needed
III. Frequently check patency of airway
    A. Blocked or kinked tube
    B. Overinflation of cuff
    C. Tube impinging at bifurcation of trachea
IV. Maintain endotracheal tube, head, and neck in a natural, slightly curved position to prevent kinking of the tube; position patient to avoid excessive flexion of neck, abduction of limbs, and pressure on thorax
 V. Calculate IV fluids needed and adjust fluid flow rate; record all fluids (total volumes), electrolytes, and other drugs administered
VI. Complete anesthetic record (Fig. 18-7)
    A. Note start and end of anesthetic period
    B. Note start and end of surgery period
    C. Note all major surgical events

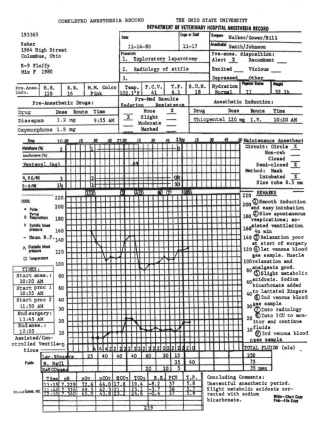

Fig. 18-7

Completed anesthesia record.

> D. Note all changes in patient status, cardiorespiratory variables, and anesthetic technique
>
> E. Note all laboratory results during anesthesia (e.g., blood gases)

VII. Nitrous oxide: turn off N_2O 5 to 10 minutes before the end of the surgical period; methoxyflurane: reduce concentration as surgery nears completion, and turn off 5 to 10 minutes before the end

VIII. Halothane; isoflurane: turn off at the end of surgery or before, depending on depth of anesthesia

IX. Oxygen: deliver a high flow rate (at least 3 L) into the recovery period; empty rebreathing bag several times to dump anesthetic gases

THE RECOVERY PERIOD

I. Deflate endotracheal tube cuff and extubate when animal is swallowing

II. Administer oxygen as necessary (endotracheal tube, mask, oxygen cage)

III. Position animal in sternal recumbency with head extended

IV. Observe animal until it can maintain sternal recumbency

V. Maintain airway free of secretions (use postural drainage, sponges, suction tubes)

VI. Check temperature; raise and maintain body temperature using towels, heating pads, and heat lamps

VII. Change animal's positions frequently, and stimulate by rubbing body and flexing and extending limbs

VIII. Tranquilizers and analgesics may be needed if the animal becomes excited or is in pain during recovery; observe for respiratory depression, especially if opioid analgesics are given

IX. Maintain IV fluids as needed

X. Monitor periodically until patient is able to stand unsupported

XI. Consider drug antagonists if necessary
- A. Opioids: naloxone
- B. a_2-Agonists: yohimbine, atipamazole
- C. Benzodiazepines: flumazenil
- D. Respiratory depression: doxapram
- E. Bradycardia: atropine, glycopyrrolate

CHAPTER NINETEEN

Anesthetic Procedures and Techniques in Horses

"The little neglect may breed mischief . . . for want
of a nail the shoe was lost; for want of a shoe
the horse was lost; and for want of a horse
the rider was lost."

BENJAMIN FRANKLIN

OVERVIEW

The ability to predict drug effects and drug actions is the single most important asset of a good equine anesthetist. Patient temperament varies and has considerable influence on the amount of drug required and anesthetic technique. Infusions of anesthetic drugs combined with physical restraint are frequently used to induce general anesthesia in horses to prevent injury to the patient and attending personnel. The majority of anesthetic techniques are designed to produce rapid and safe induction to and recovery from lateral recumbency and to maximize muscle relaxation and analgesia while maintaining normal cardiopulmonary status. Horses frequently benefit from assistance to regain and maintain a standing position following general anesthesia.

GENERAL CONSIDERATIONS

I. Preparation of the equine surgical patient
   A. Withhold food for approximately 6 to 12 hours before surgery
   B. Pull or pad all shoes to prevent injury; clip the surgical site before the induction to anesthesia (if possible)

    C. Groom the horse and wipe it with a moist cloth to remove dander; place an intravenous catheter before induction

    D. Perform a complete physical examination with emphasis on cardiorespiratory function

    E. Weigh each animal and enter in the anesthetic record

    F. Give each animal preanesthetic medication approximately 20 to 30 minutes before induction of anesthesia

    G. Rinse the mouth with water before induction

    H. Clean the feet before induction

  II. All horses develop acid-base disturbances under anesthesia, particularly respiratory acidosis

 III. Proper positioning and appropriate padding of the head, shoulder, and hip minimize cardiopulmonary compromise and the development of neuropathies and myopathies

 IV. Assisted or controlled ventilation is required to maintain normal arterial carbon dioxide concentrations during prolonged anesthesia in the horse

  V. Prevention of hypotension helps avoid postoperative complications, including myopathy

 VI. Observe all horses during the recovery period and, if needed, assist to a standing position

PREANESTHETIC EVALUATION

  I. Review patient history

 II. Conduct physical evaluation

    A. Determine age, weight, sex

    B. Judge the temperament of the horse

    C. Perform a physical examination; emphasize the cardiopulmonary system; check for subclinical respiratory disease

    D. Review the concurrent or previous drug history

    E. Assess the procedure to be performed

    F. Prepare anesthetic care plan

III. Conduct laboratory evaluation

    A. Routine evaluation

      1. Complete blood count (Hct, Hb)

      2. Total solids

      3. Fibrinogen

B. Suggested further evaluation
 1. Serum electrolytes
 2. Serum chemistry

PREANESTHETIC MEDICATIONS

I. Acepromazine (used to produce a calming effect)
 A. Dose: 10 to 40 mg/1000 lb intramuscularly (IM)
     5 to 20 mg/1000 lb intravenously (IV)
 B. Onset: within 10 to 20 minutes
 C. Duration: 2 to 3 hours
 D. Hypotensive effect may last for 12 hours
II. Promazine (like acepromazine); intravenous dose 0.1-0.5 mg/lb
III. Xylazine (used to produce sedation, analgesia, and muscle relaxation)
 A. Dose: 0.5-1 mg/lb IM
     0.2-0.5 mg/lb IV
 B. Onset of action: within 2 to 3 minutes of intravenous and within 10 to 15 minutes after intramuscular administration
 C. Duration: 30 minutes after intravenous and 60 minutes after intramuscular administration
 D. Sinus bradycardia, first- and second-degree heart block may occur
IV. Detomidine (like xylazine)
 A. Longer duration of action than xylazine
 B. Dose: 5 to 10 μg/lb IV
     10 to 20 μg/lb IM
V. Chloral hydrate (used to produce or enhance sedation); 10 to 50 mg/lb

ANESTHETIC EQUIPMENT

I. Collect the necessary equipment
 A. Endotracheal tubes
  1. Choose the largest tube possible (30, 26, 20, or 15 mm); most tube size designations are related to inside diameter
  2. Check the endotracheal tube cuff for leaks
  3. Use lubricating jelly for endotracheal tube
  4. Use 25- and 60-cc syringe to inflate the cuff

    5. Cotton mouth gag or speculum (2-inch polyvinylchloride plumber's pipe)

B. Intravenous catheter for intravenous anesthetic drug or fluid administration

    1. Commercially available 10-, 12-, and 14-gauge catheters

    2. Tubing for an adult patient 500 to 1000 pounds

       a. 240 polyethylene tubing or commercial catheter

       b. 10-gauge, 2-inch venapuncture needle

       c. 14-gauge disposable needle

       d. Three-way stopcock

       e. 12-ml syringe with heparinized saline solution

C. Pressure bag for administration of intravenous drugs (e.g., guiafenesin)

D. Chest rope for restraining front legs (Fig. 19-1)

E. Proper padding (see Fig. 19-1)

F. Monitoring equipment (see Chapter 15)

    1. EKG monitor

    2. Blood pressure recording device

    3. Stethoscope

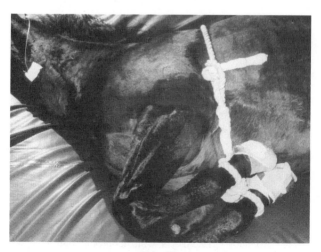

Fig. 19-1

During general anesthesia horses are usually positioned on large foam rubber pads or on air or water mattresses with their front legs restrained.

II. Before induction of general anesthesia

    A. The anesthetic machine should be examined to be sure the vaporizer has an adequate anesthetic level, and the circle system should be tested for leaks

        1. The anesthetic system can be checked for leaks by occluding the Y piece that connects to the endotracheal tube, closing the pop-off valve, and flushing oxygen through the system; if pressure is maintained, the system is not leaking

        2. The circle system should be capable of maintaining a pressure of approximately 40 cm of water

    B. Check gas pressures in the tanks

        1. Oxygen should be 2,500 psi

        2. Nitrous oxide should be 750 psi (used in foals)

    C. Fresh carbon dioxide absorbent should be placed in the cannister after approximately 6 hours of use

    D. Fresh gas flow rate

        1. Oxygen: 1 L/250 lb; minimum of 3 L/1000 lb; high flow rates, 1 L/100 lb, are used during induction and recovery to denitrogenate and remove anesthetic vapors, respectively

        2. Nitrous oxide, if used, is added to the oxygen flow (e.g., 3 L oxygen + 3 L nitrous oxide = 6 L total flow)

INDUCTION

  I. Thiopental sodium

    A. Dose: without guaifenesin 4 to 7 mg/lb
                 with guaifenesin 2 to 4 mg/lb

    B. Ultrashort-acting (5 to 10 minutes)

    C. Causes cardiovascular depression and may cause transient apnea (dose-dependent)

  II. Guaifenesin: centrally acting skeletal muscle relaxant

    A. Dose: 50 mg/lb to produce recumbency
              25 mg/lb to produce ataxia and relaxation

    B. 5% or 10% solution (50 or 100 mg/ml)

    C. Administered before or with thiopental sodium or ketamine

    D. Duration: 10 to 20 minutes

    E. Causes minimal analgesia and sedation by itself

    F. Toxic signs include

       1. Apneustic breathing pattern

       2. Muscle ridigity

       3. Hypotension

III. Diazepam (muscle relaxant)

    A. Dose: 0.02 to 0.05mg/lb

    B. Administered before thiamylal or ketamine

    C. Duration: 5 to 15 minutes

    D. No analgesia, minimal sedation

IV. Ketamine

    A. Dose: 0.7 to 1 mg/lb IV after xylazine, detomidine, or guaifenesin

    B. 10% contains 100 mg/ml

    C. Administered in combination with, but after, diazepam, xylazine, detomidine, or guaifenesin relaxation

    D. Short-acting (10 to 15 minutes)

    E. Causes apneustic breathing pattern

V. Telazol (tiletamine/zolazepam)

    A. Dose: 0.3 to 0.5 mg/lb

    B. Like ketamine and used the same way

    C. Longer duration of action

    D. Greater respiratory depression

    E. Greater muscle relaxation

VI. Halothane, isoflurane; 3% to 5% concentration and high oxygen flow can be used for induction in foals using a nasotracheal tube or mask

ENDOTRACHEAL INTUBATION

I. Endotracheal intubation (Fig. 19-2)

    A. Intubation is performed blindly

       1. Extend the head

       2. Advance the tube over the base of the tongue into the pharynx

       3. Rotate the tube as it is advanced into the trachea

       4. Repeat if unsuccessful

    B. If tube appears too small, choose a larger one

    C. Do not advance the tip past the thoracic inlet

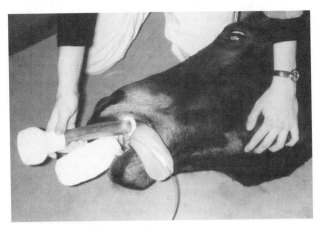

Fig. 19-2
Endotracheal intubation is performed blindly in the horse and foals.

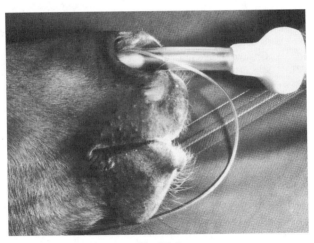

Fig. 19-3
Nasal intubation is easily performed in the adult horse and foal.

D. Secure the tube with gauze, if necessary

E. Nasal intubation can be performed in adult horses and foals (Fig. 19-3)

F. Two clean endotracheal tubes and a speculum or mouth gag should be available for induction

G. Connect the endotracheal tube to the anesthetic system; in the circle system for large animals, the rebreathing bag size should be at least five times the tidal volume; 30-L or 15-L bags are standard

H. Inflate the endotracheal tube cuff, and check to see that it does not leak by squeezing the rebreathing bag, thereby expanding the animal's lungs

   1. 15 to 20 cm water or 10 to 15 mm Hg pressure is sufficient

   2. Do not overinflate the cuff; generally, 50 to 75 ml is adequate in a 1000 pound patient (Fig. 19-4)

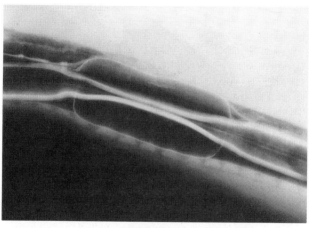

Fig. 19-4

Accidental overinflation of the endotracheal tube cuff can result in tube occlusion.

MAINTENANCE OF ANESTHESIA

I. Inhalation anesthesia
   A. Halothane: 1% to 3%
   B. Isoflurane: 1% to 3%
II. Intravenous anesthesia: a mixture of 500 ml of 5% guaifenesin, followed by 500 mg ketamine and 500 mg of xylazine until effective
III. Monitoring (see Chapter 15)
   A. Body temperature
      1. Generally increases in large animals during anesthesia
      2. May decrease in foals and during prolonged procedures
   B. Chart all anesthetic and surgical events and the animal's response
   C. Use sample anesthesia record (see Fig. 18-7)
   D. Monitor all vital signs (i.e., cardiovascular, respiratory) and the depth of anesthesia (i.e., unconsciousness, eye signs)
   E. Maintain arterial blood pressure (especially important)
IV. Administration of fluids (see Chapter 24)

THE RECOVERY PERIOD

I. Turn off the vaporizer and nitrous oxide before the oxygen
II. Administer oxygen until the patient is swallowing, if possible; then extubate
III. Oxygen is routinely administered by
   A. O_2 humidifier
   B. O_2 demand valve
IV. Keep tranquilizer, ropes, and emergency drugs available in case of rough recoveries
   A. Make sure the cuff on endotracheal tube is deflated
   B. Keep head and muzzle down to allow drainage
   C. Assist recovery to a standing position, if necessary
   D. Administer sedative (50 mg xylazine) to adult horses if necessary

CHAPTER TWENTY

Anesthetic Procedures and Techniques in Ruminants

"You've got to stop and eat the roses along the way."
ANONYMOUS BOVINE PHILOSOPHER

OVERVIEW

Physical restraint and local anesthetic techniques are frequently used in ruminants to provide immobility and analgesia. General anesthesia techniques are similar to those for dogs, cats, or horses. Regurgitation of rumen contents and bloat (distention of the rumen) are potential hazards not encountered in dogs, cats, or horses. Close observation and monitoring of palpebral and ocular reflexes, eyeball position, and pupil size can be used to monitor the depth of anesthesia in ruminants. Recovery from anesthesia is generally quiet and uneventful and does not routinely require assistance.

GENERAL CONSIDERATIONS

I. Preparation of the ruminant for anesthesia and surgery
   A. The most important factor in decreasing the risk of regurgitation is to decrease rumen pressure before anesthesia
      1. Withhold food for 24 to 36 hours in large ruminants
      2. Withhold water for 8 to 12 hours in large ruminants
      3. Withhold food for 12 to 24 hours in sheep and goats; there is no need to withhold water
      4. Withhold food for 2 to 4 hours in calves, lambs, and young kids; when these animals are less than 1 month

of age, they are essentially monogastric and are less
prone to regurgitation during anesthesia
  B. The side effects of withholding food are minimal
    1. Mild metabolic alkalosis is observed in healthy
       animals
    2. Bradycardia in adult cattle is due to increased vagal
       tone
  C. Endotracheal and rumen tubes can be placed, when
     appropriate, to avoid bloat and aspiration of rumen
     contents
 II. Most surgical techniques in cattle can be performed using
     local or regional anesthesia (see Chapter 5)
III. General anesthesia is required if local or regional anesthetic
     techniques are inadequate; light stages of anesthesia may
     predispose to stress
  A. Death may occur if painful procedures such as
     dehorning are attempted without adequate anesthesia or
     analgesia
  B. Cardiac arrest may be caused by catecholamine-induced
     ventricular fibrillation or vagally induced asystole

PREANESTHETIC EVALUATION

  I. Preanesthetic evaluation is very similar to that in horses
  A. Physical examination
  B. Basic laboratory tests
    1. PCV or Hb
    2. Plasma total protein
 II. The most frequently encountered problems associated with se-
     dation and general anesthesia
  A. Regurgitation
  B. Bloat
  C. Inadequate oxygenation
  D. Injury
  E. Respiratory depression and apnea
  F. Pulmonary aspiration
III. Regurgitation is caused by a vagal effect on reticular contrac-
     tions and parasympathetic effects on pharyngoesophageal and
     gastroesophageal sphincters

A. Anesthetic drugs increase the risk of regurgitation in the following ways
   1. By relaxing the pharyngoesophageal sphincter
   2. By relaxing the gastroesophageal sphincter
   3. By depressing the swallow reflex
B. Recumbency also increases the risk of regurgitation

PREANESTHETIC MEDICATION

I. Preanesthetic drugs are used to calm or sedate ruminants or to decrease the dose of a more potent intravenous or inhalation anesthetic
II. Tranquilizers are not approved for use in food animals; milk and meat drug residues must be taken into consideration
III. Popular preanesthetic medications include
   A. Acepromazine (to produce a calming effect)
      1. Dose: 20 to 40 mg/1000 lb intramuscularly (IM)
              25 to 10 mg/1000 lb intravenously (IV)
      2. Onset of tranquilization is within 10 to 20 minutes
      3. Duration of tranquilization is 2 to 4 hours
   B. Xylazine
      1. One tenth the intravenous dose used in horses: 0.05 mg/lb or less IV; 0-0.3 mg/lb IM
      2. Only low-concentration xylazine is recommended (20 mg/ml)
      3. Moderate dose of 0.01 to 0.05 mg/lb IV generally induces recumbency and depresses or abolishes pharyngeal and laryngeal reflexes, thus allowing easy intubation and inhalation anesthesia without barbiturates
      4. Side effects
         a. Cardiovascular depression
         b. Respiratory depression
         c. Rumen atony with bloat
         d. Hyperglycemia from decreased plasma insulin
         e. Diuresis
         f. Decreased hematocrit
         g. Abortion in late pregnancy
   C. Ketamine or Telazol

1. Dose: ketamine, up to 1 mg/lb IV or 1 to 3 mg/lb IM; Telazol, 0.5 mg/lb IV or 2 mg/lb IM
2. Prior administration of xylazine (0.1 mg/lb IM) decreases ketamine or Telazol dosage by one half
3. Ocular pharyngeal and laryngeal reflexes are depressed
4. Compatible with inhalation anesthetics
5. Side effects
   a. Respiratory depression
   b. Hypotension

D. Atropine, glycopyrrolate
1. Saliva flow is best controlled by having the head pointed downward and an endotracheal tube with an inflatable cuff in place
2. The use of anticholinergic drugs (atropine, glycopyrrolate) before surgery in ruminants is controversial
3. Atropine sulfate, 2 mg/100 lb IM or subcutaneously, may be useful in preventing bradycardia and hypotension during manipulation of viscera
4. The duration of action of atropine in ruminants is short
5. Anticholinergics increase the incidence of bloat because of a decrease in intestinal motility and an accumulation of gas from bacterial fermentation
6. Anticholinergics increase the viscosity of the saliva (without decreasing the volume of saliva significantly)

INDUCTION

I. Barbiturates
A. Thiopental sodium (Pentothal) and thiamylal sodium (Surital) are ultrashort-acting (10 to 15 minutes) barbiturates with predictable effects
1. Doses of 3 to 5 mg/ml thiamylal or 5 to 7 mg/lb thiopental will achieve light surgical anesthesia within 12 to 15 seconds
2. Less barbiturate is needed if the animal is premedicated or induced with guaifenesin
3. Barbiturates should be used with caution in animals less than 3 months of age

    4. Barbiturates rapidly cross the placental barrier and depress fetal respiration

II. Guaifenesin

    A. Dose: 50 mg/lb IV if used alone for recumbency

        25 mg/lb IV in small increments until effective

    B. 5% Solution (50 mg/ml) with 5% dextrose; more concentrated solutions (>7%) may cause hemolysis

    C. Can be used in combination with xylazine, thiamylal, ketamine or Telazol

III. Xylazine-ketamine combination

    A. Dose: 0.02 mg/lb xylazine and 1 mg/lb ketamine IV

        1. Both drugs can be administered in the same syringe

        2. When given IV, immobilization occurs in less than 1 minute, supplying anesthesia of 1-hour duration; recovery occurs standing, 2 hours or more after injection

        3. When given IM, induction time is 3 to 10 minutes; anesthesia and recovery time are increased

        4. Decreases heart rate, respiratory rate, and temperature; an apneustic respiratory pattern and salivation are seen in ruminants

IV. Xylazine-ketamine-guaifenesin combination

    A. Dose: 50 mg xylazine + 500 mg ketamine in 500 ml of 5% guaifenesin given in small increments until effective approximately 0.5 to 1 ml IV; anesthesia can be continued at a rate of 1 ml/lb/hr

        1. All three drugs are soluble in water

        2. Induction is gradual and generally uneventful but may require some physical restraint

        3. Anesthesia is adequate for periods of 30 to 90 minutes; respiration may need to be assisted

        4. Drug overdose causes apnea and hypotension

V. Telazol

    A. 0.025 to 0.5 mg/lb IV; 1 to 3 mg/lb IM

        1. Produces excellent, short-term (20 to 30-minute) surgical anesthesia

        2. May produce respiratory depression

VI. Masking down with an inhalation anesthetic: animals under 150 pounds can be induced using a mask induction technique with 3% to 4% halothane or 3% isoflurane, intubated and maintained at 1% to 2%

ENDOTRACHEAL INTUBATION

I. Intubation should immediately follow the induction of anesthesia

II. Several techniques are useful

    A. A dental speculum or mouth gag can be placed in the mouth

    B. Method 1: insert an arm into the oral cavity of the adult cow, reflect the epiglottis forward manually, and guide the endotracheal tube into the larynx

    C. Method 2: extend the patient's head and neck, and gently advance the tube into the trachea during inspiration

    D. Intubation may be facilitated by a laryngoscope and endoscopic light (Fig. 20-1)

    E. In small ruminants, a long, small-diameter wood, steel, or plastic dowel may be placed into the trachea first and the endotracheal tube passed over it (Fig. 20-2)

    F. Intubation should be done quickly to avoid regurgitation and aspiration of fluid

    G. A tracheostomy may be performed, if required

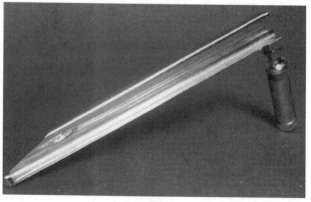

Fig. 20-1

Endotracheal intubation in cattle, sheep, and goats can be facilitated with a long-blade laryngoscope.

MAINTENANCE OF ANESTHESIA

I. Inhalation anesthetic drugs are an excellent means of producing general anesthesia, particularly for prolonged surgical procedures

II. Induction is completed with 3% to 5% halothane or 2% to 4% isoflurane

III. A surgical plane of anesthesia may be maintained at 0.5 to 2% halothane or 1% to 2% isoflurane

IV. A 50:50 mixture of nitrous oxide/oxygen may be used in small ruminants (preruminant); the use of N_2O in large ruminants may produce bloat

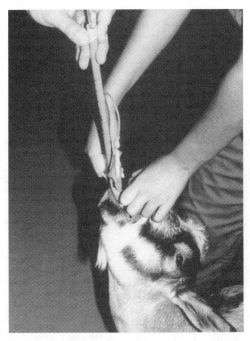

Fig. 20-2

To facilitate intubation in small ruminants, a steel dowel can be placed in the trachea and the endotracheal tube slid over it.

V. Ventilate ruminants to minimize respiratory acidosis, if surgical procedures last longer than 1 hour or blood carbon dioxide concentrations are greater than 70 mm Hg

MONITORING

I. The position of the eyeball provides a useful guide to anesthetic depth
   A. Ocular reflexes are good indicators of anesthetic depth; the corneal reflex should be present throughout anesthesia, and the palpebral reflex depressed by inhalation anesthesia
   B. The eyeball often rotates medioventrally when the patient is in a light surgical plane of anesthesia (Fig. 20-3)
   C. The iris and pupil are centered when the patient is in a deep surgical plane of anesthesia or awake; dilated pupils are a sign of anesthetic overdose when using inhalation anesthesia

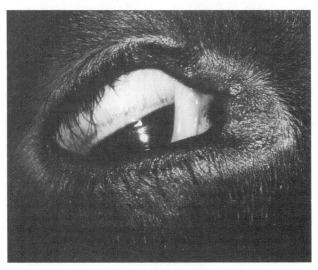

Fig. 20-3
The bovine eye rotates ventrally and medially during light planes of anesthesia.

    D. The auricular artery, located on the dorsal surface of the ear, can be cannulated to monitor arterial blood pressure

II. See Chapter 15

III. Administration of fluids (see Chapter 24)

THE RECOVERY PERIOD

I. Ruminants are allowed to breathe 100% oxygen for several minutes before being disconnected from the anesthetic machine

II. Leave the endotracheal tube in place until the laryngeal reflex returns

III. Position the head to allow drainage before pulling the endotracheal tube

IV. Leave the cuff inflated while the endotracheal tube is removed

V. Pass a stomach tube before removing the endotracheal tube to decompress the rumen if the animal has bloated

VI. Position ruminants on their right side or in sternal recumbency once the tube is pulled to avoid regurgitation

VII. Cattle generally need little assistance during recovery following inhalation anesthesia

CHAPTER TWENTY-ONE

Anesthetic Procedures and Techniques in Swine

"It is a bad plan that admits of no modification."
PUBLILIUS SYRUS

OVERVIEW

Swine anesthesia is a unique challenge. Swine have few superficial veins that are easily accessible, other than those on the dorsal surface of the ear. Ear veins may be difficult to use because of previous identification and tagging procedures; therefore most chemical restraining drugs are administered intramuscularly (IM). Pigs are difficult to intubate because of their small oral cavity, large tongue, and the presence of a pharyngeal diverticulum. Respiratory depression and elevations of body temperature are frequently associated with chemical restraint and general anesthesia. Respiratory depression may be caused by the combined respiratory-depressant effects of chemical restraining drugs and the limited expansion of the chest wall because of abnormal body positioning and body fat. Elevation in body temperature occurs because of the low body surface area to body mass ratio, the relative absence of sweat glands, and inefficient thermoregulatory mechanisms. Hyperpyrexia and malignant hyperthermia have been reported in genetically predisposed pigs and can be triggered by a variety of intravenous and inhalation anesthetics. Physical restraint combined with sedatives, tranquilizers, and local anesthetic techniques are the usual methods for simple surgical procedures in pigs. General anesthesia using inhalation anesthetics provides excellent, stable anesthesia for prolonged or complicated surgical procedures.

GENERAL CONSIDERATIONS

I. Surgical preparation of the pig
   A. Obtain a complete history, and do a complete physical examination, paying particular attention to the respiratory system
   B. Withhold food for 8 to 12 hours in adults, 1 to 3 hours in neonates
   C. Do not withhold water
   D. Use drugs that are potentially reversible, such as xylazine and opioids
   E. Avoid stress by leaving the pig with other pigs until tranquilized

II. Respiratory depression is a frequent sequela to the administration of depressant drugs in pigs
   A. Use low doses of drugs that are potentially reversible, such as xylazine and opioids
   B. Obtain an estimate of the size of the trachea before drug administration; a pig's trachea may be very narrow
   C. Be prepared for respiratory emergencies
      1. Have a variety of endotracheal tube sizes available
      2. Be prepared to do a tracheotomy
         a. No. 10 blade and scalpel
         b. Hemostat
         c. Cuffed tracheostomy tube
         d. Respiratory stimulants, such as doxapram, may be necessary

III. Increases in body temperature are frequently associated with inhalation anesthesia in pigs
   A. The pig has a low body surface area relative to body mass
   B. The pig has relatively poor thermoregulatory mechanisms and relatively few sweat glands
   C. Depolarizing neuromuscular blocking agents and inhalation anesthetics can trigger malignant hyperthermia
      1. Several strains of pigs (e.g., Landrace, Poland China) are genetically predisposed to malignant hyperthermia
      2. Dantrolene (1 mg/lb intravenously [IV]) is the only known truly effective therapy for malignant hyperthermia

IV. The preanesthetic evaluation
   A. Physical examination
   B. Basic laboratory tests, including a complete blood count
V. The most frequently encountered problems associated with sedation and general anesthesia
   A. Respiratory depression and apnea
   B. Increased body temperature

ANESTHETIC PROCEDURES

I. Lumbosacral epidural anesthesia is a commonly used local anesthetic technique in pigs (see Chapter 5)
   A. The major advantages are minor systemic effects and the minimal effect on the fetuses during cesarean section
   B. Disadvantages include lack of unconsciousness, necessitating physical restraint of the forelimbs
   C. A 3- to 5-inch, 18-gauge spinal needle is used to facilitate administration of 2% lidocaine hydrochloride
   D. The dose varies from 0.2 to 0.5 ml/10 lb, with the higher dosage providing anesthesia cranially to the paralumbar fossa

II. Intratesticular injection
   A. Large boars can be castrated by using physical restraint and the injection of 15 to 30 mg/kg of sodium pentobarbital into each testicle
   B. Anesthesia occurs in approximately 5 minutes
   C. As soon as the testicles are removed, the source of anesthetic is removed

III. Azaperone
   A. Butyrophenone tranquilizer is approved for use as an aid to mixing and sorting pigs
   B. Dose: 0.5 to 1 mg/lb IM
   C. Prevents porcine stress syndrome
   D. Used before mask induction of anesthesia or the administration of ketamine
   E. Produces a calm pig that does not squeal
   F. Does not produce analgesia

IV. Azaperone/ketamine
   A. Administer azaperone (0.5 mg/lb IM) before ketamine (3 to 5 mg/lb IM)

    B. Produces a light plane of anesthesia with good peripheral analgesia

    C. Compatible with inhalation anesthesia

    D. Pigs may be hypersensitive

V. Fentanyl-droperidol (Innovar-Vet) and ketamine combination

    A. Intramuscular dosages

       1. < 200 pounds body weight

          Innovar-Vet: 1 ml/60 to 80 lb

          Ketamine: 3 to 5 mg/kg

       2. > 200 pounds body weight

          Innovar-Vet: 1 ml/100 lb

          Ketamine: 3 to 5 mg/lb

    B. Onset of analgesia is within 5 to 10 minutes and lasts for 30 to 45 minutes

    C. Supplemental doses of Telazol or ketamine (1 to 3 mg/lb IM) or sodium pentobarbital (1 to 3 mg/lb IM) may be given to prolong anesthesia

    D. Advantages

       1. Ease of administration

       2. Useful for longer procedures in which some movement is allowable

       3. Reversibility of the depressant effects of fentanyl

    E. Disadvantages

       1. Pigs may develop muscle tremors and hyperpyrexia following ketamine administration

       2. Hyperthermia is occasionally observed

       3. Excitability, salivation, and respiratory depression can occur

       4. Atropine (0.02 mg/lb IM) or glycopyrrolate (0.005 mg/lb IM) may be necessary to prevent bradycardia caused by fentanyl

VI. Atropine-acepromazine-ketamine combination

    A. Dosage: 0.02 mg/lb atropine and 0.05 to 0.2 mg/lb acepromazine IM, followed in 20 minutes by 5 mg/lb IM ketamine

    B. Azaperone can be used as an alternative to acepromazine at dosages ranging from 0.2 to 1 mg/lb IM

C. Useful for minor surgical or medical procedures, such as detusking or castration of large boars

D. Advantages
   1. Ease of administration
   2. Some analgesia and muscle relaxation within 5 minutes and lasting 10 to 15 minutes

E. Disadvantages
   1. Additional analgesia is required using a local anesthetic
   2. 20-minute waiting period between administration of drugs
   3. Hypotension

VII. Atropine-xylazine-ketamine combination

A. Dosage: 0.02 mg/lb atropine and 0.1 to 0.3 mg/lb xylazine IM, followed in 10 minutes with 5 mg/lb IM ketamine

B. Advantages
   1. Ease of administration
   2. Some analgesia and muscle relaxation within 5 minutes and lasting 10 to 15 minutes

C. Disadvantages
   1. Xylazine has a short duration of action because it is rapidly metabolized
   2. Muscle movement is involuntary during the anesthetic period

VIII. Xylazine-ketamine-guaifenesin combination

A. Dosage: 500 mg xylazine + 500 mg ketamine mixed in 500 ml 5% guaifenesin given in small increments until effective, approximately 1 to 2 ml/lb IV

B. Advantages: gradual induction, stable hemodynamics, and good muscle relaxation

C. Disadvantages: respiratory depression may require assisted ventilation

IX. Xylazine-Telazol or Azaperone-Telazol

A. Dosage: xylazine 0.1 to 0.5 mg/lb IM or azaperone 0.5 mg/lb IM followed in 5 minutes by Telazol 1 to 3 mg/lb IM

B. Advantages
   1. Ease of administration

       2. Good analgesia and muscle relaxation

       3. Minimal cardiovascular depression

    C. Disadvantages

       1. Occasional respiratory depression

       2. Light plane of anesthesia

       3. Short duration of action; may need to be supplemented

       4. Pigs may remain drowsy for 24 hours

       5. Increased salivation

X. Atropine-acepromazine-thiopental combination

    A. Dosage: 0.02 mg/lb atropine and 0.2 mg/lb acepromazine IM, followed in 10 minutes by 5 mg/lb thiopental sodium (3% to 5% solution) administered into an ear vein

    B. Advantages

       1. Anesthesia immediate and lasts for 15 to 30 minutes

       2. Thiopental can be redosed but produces respiratory-depressant effect and prolongs recovery time

    C. Disadvantages

       1. Difficulty of venapuncture

       2. Respiratory and cardiovascular depression

XI. Inhalation anesthesia

    A. The inhalation anesthetics, halothane, isoflurane, or methoxyflurane, are administered

       1. For induction (by mask) to anesthesia

       2. For maintenance of anesthesia after the pig is induced with other drugs

    B. Inhalation drugs (Fig. 21-1) can be administered in the following ways

       1. Through a face mask

       2. Through nasal tubes, which are made from human nasal tube adapters and small-animal endotracheal tubes (6 to 8 mm)

       3. Through endotracheal intubation, which is preferred; laryngoscope or long, rigid dowel rods can be used to pass the endotracheal tube

    C. Advantages

       1. Good control of anesthesia

       2. Excellent muscle relaxation

       3. Ease of administration

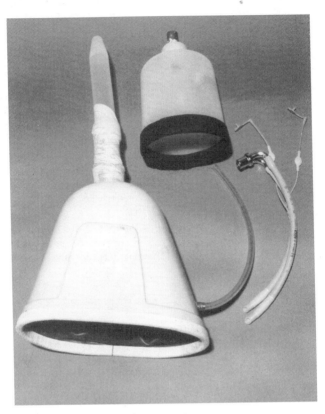

Fig. 21-1
Face masks and nasal endotracheal tubes can be used as an alternative to endotracheal intubation in pigs.

    D. Disadvantages
        1. Expensive equipment required
        2. Not generally suited for field conditions
        3. Halothane can induce hyperthermia in pigs

MONITORING

I. Monitoring anesthesia in pigs is similar to that for other species (see Chapter 15); the auricular artery, located on the dorsal surface of the ear, can be cannulated to monitor arterial blood pressure

II. Signs of malignant hyperthermia
   A. Extreme muscle rigidity
   B. Increased temperature ($>107°$ F); hot to the touch
   C. Tachycardia
   D. Tachypnea
   E. Metabolic acidosis
III. Treatment of hyperthermia in pigs
   A. Dantrolene: 1 to 3 mg/lb IV; 10 mg/lb per os
   B. Supportive treatment
      1. Fluids
      2. Bicarbonate
      3. Steroids
      4. Oxygen
      5. Body cooling

THE RECOVERY PERIOD

I. Administer oxygen and/or assist ventilation if necessary
II. Position in sternal recumbency
III. Place in a well-ventilated, cool, quiet environment
IV. Assess vital signs periodically

CHAPTER TWENTY-TWO

Anesthesia for Cesarean Section

"The hand that rocks the cradle is the hand that rules the world."

WILLIAM ROSS WALLACE

OVERVIEW

Anesthetic drugs used in pregnant animals affect the fetus. Generally, the effects of anesthetic drugs are more pronounced and longer-lasting in the fetus than in the mother. Drugs that cross the placental barrier slowly, or not at all, are preferred because they have minimal fetal effects. Anesthetic drugs may induce or inhibit parturition by altering uterine function. This chapter describes the changes that occur in maternal physiology during advanced pregnancy and the effects of anesthetic drugs in pregnant animals.

GENERAL CONSIDERATIONS

I. Pregnancy, especially the immediate preparturient period, causes significant alterations in maternal physiology
   A. Altered pharmacokinetics and pharmacodynamics
   B. Changes in hemodynamics
      1. Increased heart rate
      2. Increased cardiac output
      3. Increased blood volume
   C. Changes in respiration
      1. Increased breathing rate
      2. Decreased functional residual capacity (FRC)

II. Anesthetic drug and technique considerations
   A. Providing optimal analgesia for surgery
   B. Preventing maternal hypoxemia or hypotension
   C. Minimizing fetal depression
   D. Minimizing postoperative maternal depression
   E. Neither inducing nor preventing uterine contractions

CHANGES IN MATERNAL PHYSIOLOGY IN ADVANCED PREGNANCY

I. Central nervous system (CNS)
   A. Increased progesterone concentration decreases inhalation anesthetic requirement; there is minimum alveolar concentration
   B. Vascular engorgement decreases the size of the epidural space; decreased volume of local anesthetic is required for epidural anesthesia

II. Respiratory system
   A. Alveolar ventilation is increased because of increased respiratory center sensitivity to CO_2, which is progesterone–induced; increased alveolar ventilation and decreased FRC result in a more rapid alveolar rate of rise in inhalation anesthetics·
   B. FRC is decreased because of anterior displacement of diaphragm
      1. Relative anemia refers to the pregnant patient not tolerating blood loss as well as the nonpregnant patient
      2. Patients with a history of heart disease may decompensate
   C. Small airways constrict at higher lung volumes; airway closure and decreased FRC cause greater ventilation perfusion mismatches, which may result in decreased oxygenation

III. Cardiovascular system
   A. Maternal blood volume is increased by approximately 30%
   B. Packed cell volume and plasma-protein concentration are decreased
   C. Cardiac output is increased 30% to 50% because of increases in stroke volume and heart rate

    D. The weight of the gravid uterus causes aortocaval compression during dorsal recumbency; cardiac reserve is decreased because of increased cardiac output and aortocaval compression

    E. Central venous pressure and systemic blood pressure remain relatively unchanged but may increase during labor

IV. Gastrointestinal system

    A. Placental gastrin secretion increases gastric acidity

        1. Increasing the chance of regurgitation and aspiration pneumonia

        2. Increasing the need for a properly fitting cuffed endotracheal tube

    B. The stomach is displaced cranially and the tone to the lower esophageal sphincter is altered

V. Other changes: decreased plasma cholinesterase (pseudocholinesterase)

    A. Prolonged duration of action of succinylcholine

    B. Prolonged duration of action of ester local anesthetics

DRUG TRANSFER ACROSS THE PLACENTA

I. Factors influencing drug transfer

    A. Surface area and diffusion characteristics of the placenta; the surface area of placenta is large, and diffusion distance is small in all species

    B. Diffusion properties of drugs

        1. High lipid solubility, which increases diffusibility

        2. Lower molecular weight, which increases diffusibility

        3. Decreased degree of ionization and protein binding, which increases diffusibility

    C. Relative maternal and fetal drug concentrations

        1. Discrete bolus doses of drugs result in rapid transfer of drug to the fetus initially and rapidly declining maternal concentrations

        2. Continuous-infusion, repeated bolus administration and the administration of inhalation anesthetics result in continuously high maternal drug concentration and continual drug transfer to the fetus

UTEROPLACENTAL CIRCULATION
AND FETAL VIABILITY

I. Conditions that decrease circulating maternal blood volume can decrease placental perfusion, resulting in fetal hypoxia and acidosis; this includes maternal dehydration, hemorrhage (shock), and drug-induced hypotension
  A. Dehydration
     1. Prolonged labor
     2. Concurrent disease
  B. Hemorrhage and shock
     1. Prolonged labor
     2. Positioning: decreases venous return
     3. Anesthetic drugs
     4. Surgically related hemorrhage
     5. Hemorrhagic or endotoxic shock
  C. Drugs: anesthetic drugs cause peripheral vasodilation and hypotension

MATERNAL AND FETAL EFFECTS
FROM ANESTHETIC DRUGS
USED FOR CESAREAN SECTION

I. Anticholinergics—drug effects
  A. Both atropine and scopolamine pass placental barriers rapidly
       a. Fetal tachycardia noted within 10 to 15 minutes
       b. Fetal disorientation or excitement may be caused by central action of atropine of scopolamine
       c. Fetal effects may vary, depending on the amount of drug absorbed
  B. Glycopyrrolate does not cross the placenta in significant quantities because of its large molecular size and charge
  C. Anticholinergics can reduce placental activity
II. Local anesthetic drugs
  A. Drug effects
     1. Local anesthetic drugs administered by any route cross the placental barrier
       a. Drug effects depend on total dose, interval between

final dose and delivery, and whether or not epinephrine is used

   b. Doses of local anesthetics used clinically usually do not produce significant depression in the fetus

B. Lidocaine

   1. The preferred local anesthetic for cesarean section because of clinical experience and relatively low toxicity

   2. Appears in umbilical venous blood of the fetus within 2 to 3 minutes

   3. No correlation has been found between degree of neonatal depression and umbilical venous concentration of lidocaine

C. Procaine

   1. Low doses do not produce significant drug concentrations in fetuses

   2. Procaine metabolism is slow because of low concentrations of pseudocholinesterase in the fetus

III. Preanesthetic (sedatives, tranquilizers, opioid) drug effects

A. Drug effects: preanesthetic drugs reduce the amount of potentially more dangerous anesthetic drugs

   1. Phenothiazines (acepromazine, promazine)

      a. Rapidly appear in fetal blood

      b. Produce little to no apparent effect on the newborn when used in clinical dosages

      c. α-Adrenergic blockade may produce hypotension in stressed mother, resulting in decreased uterine blood flow and fetal hypoxia

      d. Decrease uterine tone

   2. Benzodiazepines (diazepam, midazolam)

      a. Concentrations higher in fetal blood than in maternal blood

      b. Produce minimal respiratory and cardiovascular depression

      c. Duration of action depends on redistribution away from the CNS

   3. α_2-Agonists (xylazine, detomidine, medetomidine)

      a. Respiratory depression may be severe in both mother and fetus

      b. Use in low doses and be prepared to administer an antagonist (yohimbine, atipamazole)

      c. Increases uterine pressure in cattle; may be an abortifacient; effect in other species is unknown

  4. Opioids

      a. Frequently used as preanesthetic medication for sedation and analgesia or administered epidurally

      b. Readily cross the placenta

      c. Concentrations may be higher in the fetus than in the mother because of a lower fetal pH

      d. Moderate maternal doses do not produce serious CNS depression in neonates; the effect can be reversed by opioid antagonists (naloxone)

      e. Since naloxone has a shorter duration of action than most opioids; neonates should be observed for several hours and redosed as needed

      f. Specific opioid drugs

        (1) Meperidine (Demerol)

          (a) Reaches the fetal circulation rapidly

          (b) No significant depression is apparent if birth is within the first hour

        (2) Morphine

          (a) Causes observable clinical CNS depression in the newborn

          (b) Has direct vasoconstrictor effect on placental vessels

        (3) Oxymorphone (Numorphan)

          (a) Better analgesia and sedation than meperidine

          (b) Can produce neonatal depression

        (4) Fentanyl (Sublimaze); 100 times more potent as an analgesic than morphine, with respiratory depression of shorter duration

IV. Injectable anesthetic drugs

  A. Barbiturates

    1. Readily cross the placenta into fetal circulation

    2. Barbiturates that depend on metabolism for their duration of action should be avoided because of prolonged fetal CNS depression and reduced fetal ability to metabolize drugs

    3. Dose of barbiturates that does not produce anesthesia in the mother can completely inhibit fetal respiratory movements

B. Short-acting barbiturates (pentobarbital)
1. Should not be used because of prolonged fetal respiratory depression, which is the biggest problem in the newborn and results in high mortality
2. Prolongs anesthetic recovery, preventing newborn from nursing

C. Ultrashort-acting barbiturates (thiamylal, thiopental)
1. Thiobarbiturates cross placenta readily and achieve equilibrium within 5 minutes
2. A single dose of 4 mg/lb at induction produces only modest placental transfer and does not endanger the normal fetus
   (a) Because of their dependence on redistribution for their duration of action, the use of small doses of ultrashort-acting barbiturates has not been associated with a significant degree of fetal CNS depression
   (b) Redosing is discouraged
   (c) Peak drug concentrations occur in the fetus within 10 minutes

D. Dissociogenic Agents (ketamine, tiletamine)
1. Used to produce restraint and analgesia
2. Produce poor muscle relaxation
3. Rapidly cross the placenta producing fetal depression within 5 to 10 minutes
4. Specific dissociogenic drugs
   a. Ketamine
      (1) Good restraint in queens with minimal fetal depression when used intravenously (IV) or intramuscularly (IM) in low dosages (1 mg/lb IV; 5 mg/lb IM)
      (2) Poor muscle relaxation and questionable ability to block deep pain
      (3) May increase uterine tone and decrease uterine blood flow, leading to fetal hypoxia
      (4) Fetal blood levels reach 70% of those found in the mother
      (5) Little clinical CNS depression is evident in the neonate

b. Telazol (tiletamine-zolazepam)
    (1) Similar to ketamine but better muscle relaxation
    (2) Greater respiratory depression
c. Propofol
    (1) Crosses the placenta readily but with minimal effects on the fetus
    (2) Single bolus useful for induction
    (3) Shows promise but further evaluation is needed

V. Peripheral muscle relaxants; neuromuscular blocking drugs include succinylcholine, pancuronium, atracurium, vecuronium

  A. These drugs are highly ionized with a high molecular weight, resulting in poor if any placental transfer

  B. There is no demonstrable effect on the newborn

  C. Succinylcholine metabolism is reduced because of a decrease in pseudocholinesterase

VI. Inhalation anesthetic drugs

  A. All inhalation anesthetic drugs readily cross the placenta because of their low molecular weight and lipid solubility

  B. The degree of fetal CNS depression depends on the depth and duration of maternal anesthesia

  C. Specific inhalation drugs

    1. Nitrous oxide
      a. Rapidly crosses the placenta
      b. Administration exceeding 15 minutes may result in fetal CNS depression
      c. Diffusion hypoxia, which may occur in the fetus, can be minimized with oxygen therapy
      d. When used in the mother with adequate amounts of oxygen, there is minimal effect on the neonate

    2. Halothane
      a. Quickly appears in the fetal circulation
      b. A rapid and potent uterine relaxant
        (1) Inhibits uterine involution
        (2) Increases the risk of uterine hemorrhage
      c. If used for cesarean section, the procedure should be performed as quickly as possible; neonatal CNS depression should resolve rapidly if adequate ventilation is provided at birth

TABLE 22-1

ANESTHETIC TECHNIQUES BY SPECIES

SPECIES	DRUG/TECHNIQUE	DOSAGE	COMMENTS
Cow	**Local techniques**		
	1. Standing paravertebral analgesia, line block, inverted L block	2% lidocaine (see Chapter 5 for techniques)	Suitable for tractable animals without a sedative Suitable for animals in good physical condition
	2. Anterior epidural	2% lidocaine, 1 ml/lb at Cx_1-Cx_2 junction	Induces recumbency and sensory block anterior to umbilicus Watch for hypotension Intubate if possible
	General techniques		
	3. Guaifenesin-ketamine-xylazine	500 mg ketamine 25 mg xylazine 500 ml and 5% guaifenesin + 0.25-0.5 mg/lb until effective for maintenance	
Horse	1. Premed: acepromazine, xylazine, or detomidine	Acepromazine: 0.02 mg/lb IV Xylazine: 0.1-0.3 mg/lb IV Detomidine: 5-10 µg/lb	Adjust dosage for physical condition of mother; rely on guaifenesin to produce relaxation and to allow less thiobarbiturate or ketamine to be used
	Induction: guaifenesin plus thiobarbiturate (low dose) or ketamine	Guaifenesin: 25-50 mg/lb Thiobarbiturate: 1-2 mg/lb Ketamine: 0.7-1 mg/lb	

Maintenance: halothane, isoflurane

Sheep, goat	1. Guaifenesin-ketamine	500 ml 5% guaifenesin containing 500 mg ketamine 0.25-1 mg/lb induction maintenance until effective	Intubate; copious salivation Moderate to poor muscle relaxation Can add 25 mg xylazine to mixture, but fetal CNS depression is greater Use for induction to gas or as IV technique Guaifenesin allows small bolus doses of thiobarbiturate
	2. Guaifenesin-thiobarbiturate induction or guaifenesin-ketamine induction; halothane, isoflurane	25 mg/lb guaifenesin 1-2 mg/lb thiobarbiturate	Useful in sick, toxic animals and when fetal viability is of no concern
	3. Mask induction halothane or isoflurane	Until effective	
	Local techniques		
Dog, cat	1. Epidural with 2% lidocaine or morphine	1 ml/7.5 lb body weight lidocaine; 0.1 mg/lb body weight morphine	Requires assistant for physical restraint; use sedative/tranquilizer in all but extremely tractable patients *Continued*

TABLE 22-1-cont'd
ANESTHETIC TECHNIQUES BY SPECIES

SPECIES	DRUG/TECHNIQUE	DOSAGE	COMMENTS
	General techniques		
	2. Diazepam-ketamine induction	0.125 mg/lb diazepam plus 5 mg/lb ketamine combined	Single-bolus dose not depressant to fetus
	Telazol induction	1-3 mg/lb IM	Single administration causes minimal fetal CNS depression
	Thiobarbiturate induction	4-8 mg/lb	Diazepam-ketamine good in patients who are depressed, and in shock
	Maintenance		
	Halothane or isoflurane in 50% N_2O and oxygen followed by muscle relaxant (atracurium, pancuronium) if needed	See Chapters 8, 9, and 11	Administer inhalation agent as late into procedure as possible

Intractable animal

3. Pre-med
   Dogs: Innovar-Vet or aceptromazine-oxymorphone

   1 ml/30-40 lb IM
   0.5 mg/lb of each maximum
   4 mg of each

   Controlled ventilation necessary when using relaxants

   Cats: ketamine induction then-thiopental

   4 mg/lb IM
   1-3 mg/lb IV

   Sedative-hypnotics generally increase fetal CNS depression; therefore use sparingly

Maintenance

Isoflurane or halothane

Pig:
1. Epidural

   2% lidocaine (see Chapter 4 for technique)

   Restraint of sow's head and front legs necessary

2. Innovar-Vet plus ketamine

   1 ml/50-80 lb
   3-5 mg/lb

   Good chemical restraint; however, relatively more fetal CNS depression than with epidural
   Requires placement of IV catheter

3. 500 mg ketamine plus 500 mg xylazine in 500 ml 5% guaifenesin

   1 ml of mixture per lb until effective for maintenance

IV, intravenously; *IM*, intramuscularly.

3. Methoxyflurane
   a. Quickly appears in the fetal circulation
   b. Minimal depression in the newborn at analgesic levels
   c. Minimal uterine relaxation in analgesic dosages
   d. Neonatal depression may resolve slowly because of high blood gas partition coefficient
4. Isoflurane
   a. Quickly appears in fetal circulation
   b. Rapid and potent uterine relaxant
   c. If used for cesarean section, the procedure should be performed as quickly as possible
      (1) The degree of fetal CNS depression does not correlate with maternal blood concentration
      (2) Neonatal respiratory depression may be severe, requiring postparturient ventilation
   d. Rapid elimination of this agent with ventilation may be an advantage
5. Enflurane and desflurane are similar to isoflurane; desflurane's rapid onset and elimination minimize the duration of maternal and fetal CNS depression

ANESTHETIC TECHNIQUES

I. General principles
   A. The choice of a particular anesthetic technique should be influenced by familiarity with the technique or drug and avoidance of excessive fetal CNS depression
   B. Intubation is desirable in all patients when possible
   C. Presurgical preparation and oxygenation should be completed before the administration of anesthetic drugs
   D. Avoid excessive physical restraint; sedatives, tranquilizers, and other drugs that can be antagonized are preferred over excessive physical force and subsequent maternal-fetal distress
   E. Avoid dorsal recumbency if possible; left lateral recumbency may be safest
II. Anesthetic techniques by species (Table 22-1)

CHAPTER TWENTY-THREE

Anesthetic Procedures in Exotic Pets

" 'The time has come,' the walrus said, 'to talk
of many things.' "

LEWIS CARROLL

OVERVIEW

The number of exotic animals being maintained as pets and for
profit is increasing. Anesthesia of nontraditional species is accomplished by applying techniques and drugs used in domestic animals. Because exotic species demonstrate idiosyncracies and
widely varying sensitivities to drugs, it is frequently necessary to
make modifications. This chapter is an overview of the basic information needed to successfully immobilize the exotic animals
that are likely to be encountered by general practitioners. Consult
current literature for more detailed descriptions of the anatomy,
physiology, recognition and treatment of disease, and response to
chemotherapeutics of specific species.

GENERAL CONSIDERATIONS

I. Preanesthetic considerations
  A. Discussions with owners
    1. Ensure that client has realistic expectations
    2. Detail prognosis and risks; owners may not understand
       that exotic animals respond differently to immobiliza-
       tion than do domestic animals
    3. Discuss who will be the aftercare provider; owners
       may not be able to administer treatments to exotic pets

       4. Discuss costs

  B. Reduce animal's stress; exotic animals have high sympathetic drive; excessive stress can induce complications that include arrhythmias, hypertension, and hyperthermia and that can result in death

  C. Presurgical evaluation and patient selection

     1. Physical examination: contraindications to anesthesia

       a. Abnormally high respirations; a respiratory recovery rate > 3 to 5 minutes is the amount of time an animal needs to return to normal respirations after 2 minutes of physical restraint or pursuit; normal is less than 3 to 5 minutes

       b. Shock/septicemia/acidosis

       c. Anemia or cyanosis

       d. Prolonged clotting

       e. Cachexia/obesity

       f. Unfasted, if regurgitation likely

       g. Severe weakness and CNS depression

       h. Dehydration

       i. Ascites

     2. Laboratory evaluation: contraindications to anesthesia

       a. If packed cell volume (PCV) is low, a blood transfusion may be needed

GENUS	PCV (%)
Avian	<25
Reptile	<17-20
Amphibian	<20
Rodent/lagomorph	<20
Mustelid	<25
Felid	<15
Swine	<20
Camelid	<20

       b. If PCV is high, fluids may be needed

GENUS	PCV (%)
Avian	>50-60
Reptile	>50-60
Amphibian	>60
Rodent/lagomorph	>55-60
Mustelid	>60
Felid	>50
Swine	>50
Camelid	>50

c. If total protein is <3 g/dl, amino acid or plasma supplementation may be needed; refractometers and colorimetric tests frequently used at diagnostic laboratories for mammalian blood often register falsely low proteins in nonmammalian species; the biuret method is the most accurate in avian species

d. If glucose is low, administer 5% dextrose or delay anesthesia

GENUS	GLUCOSE (mg/dl)
Avian	<150
Reptile	<50-80
Amphibian	<50
Rodent/lagomorph	<80-100
Mustelid	<80-100
Felid	<80
Swine	<60
Camelid	<60

e. If calcium is <8 mg/dl, correct level

f. If potassium is <3.5 mg/dl, correct level

3. Further evaluation

a. Oral/fecal gram stains in nonmammalians

b. Culture and sensitivity

c. Fecal/urinalysis

d. Complete hemogram/serum profile

e. Radiographs/ultrasound

f. Clotting profile

g. Electrocardiogram (EKG)/echocardiography

II. Preanesthetic fasting

	TIME (HOURS)
Avian <100 g	0
Large psittacine	1-2
Raptor, ratite, fowl, waterfowl	12-24
Carnivorous reptile ingesting whole prey	>5 days
Reptile <200 g	2-4
Reptile 200-500 g	12
Reptile >500 g	24+
Amphibian	24
Fish	24
Rodent <200 g	2
Rodent >200 g/lagomorph	>6
Mustelid	12

continued.

	TIME (HOURS)—con't
Felid	24
Swine	24
Camelid	24-48

III. Maintenance of homeothermy

    A. Hypothermia depresses the respiratory control system

        1. Small animals are predisposed to hypothermia; they lose heat rapidly and have secondary-to-high surface area–to-volume ratios

        2. Ectotherms (reptiles, fish, amphibians) do not generate their own heat; they require external heat sources to maintain their body temperature; hypothermia depresses the immune system and slows healing

        3. Hypothermia can result in brain damage, shock, electrolyte imbalances, and disseminated intravascular coagulation

            a. Well-insulated small animals such as rabbits, chinchillas, water birds, and birds in winter plumage are susceptible to hyperthermia

            b. Ungulates are prone to malignant hyperthermia; stress, high ambient temperature, and high relative humidity during immobilization increase the likelihood of hyperthermia

    B. Methods of monitoring core body temperature (skin temperature is not reliable)

        1. Esophageal thermometer

        2. Rectal/cloacal thermometer

    C. Heat sources

        1. To avoid iatrogenic burns and hyperthermia, *always* monitor heat sources

            a. Skin temperature

            b. Temperature of surfaces the patient's body contacts

            c. Ambient temperature in incubators

        2. Water circulating heating pad

            a. Very safe

            b. High maintenance cost if punctured

        3. Electric heating pads

            a. Likely to cause iatrogenic burns

            b. Inexpensive

            c. Should *never* be set on high

4. Incubators
   a. Must be preheated
   b. Useful before and after anesthesia
   c. Must be escape proof
5. Hot water bottles
   a. Very safe
   b. Act as heat sink after they are cool

IV. Fluids
   A. Preheat to 80° to 95° F for animals <1kg and for all ectotherms
      1. Incubator
         a. Even, reliable temperature must be maintained
         b. Microbial growth may occur
      2. Warm water bath
         a. Even, reliable temperature must be maintained
         b. Water must be kept warm
      3. Microwave fluids
         a. Frequently have hot spots
         b. Should be well mixed
      4. Placing intravenous tubing in warm water bath
         a. Quick method to warm fluids in emergency
         b. Effluent temperature must be carefully monitored
   B. Administration (route)
         a. Intravenous or intraosseous administration is best; the humerus in all birds and the femur in many birds are pneumatic bones; placing intraosseous catheters in these bones causes iatrogenic drowning
         b. Subcutaneous fluids (usually 5% to 10% of body weight) are given before induction of anesthesia to allow absorption and volume expansion
         c. Intraperitoneal fluids
            (1) More rapidly absorbed than subcutaneous
            (2) Could cause peritonitis
            (3) Must be warmed to body temperature
            (4) Not in birds
            (5) Not in gravid animals
            (6) Bladder should be expressed before administration
   C. Fluid rates
      1. Standard maintenance: 40 to 100 ml/kg/24 hr; the

higher end of the range is used for neonates, birds, and animals with high metabolisms

2. Intraoperative: 10 to 20 ml/kg/hr
3. Shock: 30 to 80 ml/kg in 20 minutes

D. Fluid rate control
   1. Rates <10 ml/hr require an intravenous fluid infusion pump to ensure accuracy
   2. Rates of 10 to 50 ml/hr are accurately measured with in-line flow controls or burette fluid chambers
   3. Rates >50 ml/hr are accurately measured off of most fluid containers

E. Fluid choice (see Chapter 24)

F. Blood transfusion
   1. See Chapter 24
   2. Ethylenediamine tetraacetic acid should not be used in small patients to avoid hypocalcemia
   3. Heparin is the anticoagulant of choice for birds
   4. Birds can receive *one* interspecies or genera transfusion if a donor of the same species is not available
      a. Pigeons are the most common donors
      b. Transfusion should not be repeated before 3 weeks

V. Premedication

A. If needed, administer antibiotics to achieve adequate serum levels before induction of anesthesia

B. Avian
   1. Atropine is *not* indicated in the presence of respiratory secretions because it makes them more viscous
   2. Preanesthetics are rarely indicated if the bird is small enough to be manually restrained
      a. Most are overridden
      b. They may delay recovery
      c. They may depress respirations
      d. Diazepam/midazolam overall is the most efficacious and safe—0.5-1 mg/kg intramuscularly (IM)
   3. Because their long legs are susceptible to trauma, ratites, storks, and long-legged wading birds >30 lbs

may benefit from sedation before capture and/or restraint

    a. Xylazine: 0.2 to 0.4 mg/kg IM

    b. Tiletamine-zolazepam (Telazol): 2 to 5 mg/kg IM

C. Reptile

  1. Atropine is not indicated in the presence of respiratory secretions, because it makes them more viscous

  2. Preanesthetics are rarely indicated, except for large, aggressive and/or venomous reptiles

D. Amphibian: preanesthetics are not routinely used

E. Fish: preanesthetics are not routinely used

F. Rodent

  1. Atropine is useful to decrease airway secretions

    a. 0.04 mg/kg IM, subcutaneously (SQ) (rat, mouse, hamster, gerbil)

    b. 0.2 mg/kg IM, SQ (guinea pig, chinchilla)

    c. 0.2 to 1 mg/kg IM, SQ (rabbit)

  2. One third of rabbits possess atropinase

  3. Acepromazine and diazepam are effective preanesthetics

    a. Acepromazine: 1 to 2 mg/kg IM

    b. Diazepam: 3 to 5 mg/kg IM; 0.4-3 mg/kg IM for guinea pigs

  4. Acepromazine is not recommended in gerbils because it may cause seizures

G. Mustelid (ferrrets)

  1. Preanesthetics are usually not necessary

  2. Atropine: 0.04 mg/kg IM, SQ

  3. Acepromazine and diazepam are effective preanesthetics

    a. Acepromazine: 0.1 to 0.5 mg/kg IM

    b. Diazepam: 1 to 2 mg/kg IM

H. Felid

  1. Preanesthetics not routinely used

  2. Atropine can be used at standard domestic cat doses

    a. Atropine: 0.045 mg/kg SQ, IM, IV

    b. Glycopyrrolate: 0.01 mg/kg SQ, IM, IV

I. Swine; preanesthetics are not generally used

J. Camelid; preanesthetics are not generally used

VI. Monitoring plane of anesthesia

  A. Generalities

    1. Pulse rate and character: a decrease in the heart rate to <80% of stabilized rate after induction is a sign to lighten anesthesia

    2. Respiratory rate and character

      a. A decreasing pulse rate or apneustic/erratic patterns are signs to lighten anesthesia

      b. Ectotherms normally develop apnea at surgical planes of anesthesia; plan to administer positive pressure ventilation at least 4 to 6 times per minute

  B. Equipment

    1. EKG modifications

      (1) Attach clips to steel sutures or metal hubbed needles placed through skin at lead sites to protect delicate skin or penetrate thick skin

      (2) Attach clips to alcohol-soaked pads placed at the usual lead sites

      (3) Wings are used for forelimb lead sites in birds

      (4) Place one clip cranial and one caudal to the heart in legless animals

    2. Doppler placement

      (1) Over the heart in small animals

      (2) Over the peripheral artery

        (a) Avian: medial metatarsal, brachial

        (b) Reptile: tail artery

        (c) Rodent/lagomorph: ear, femoral, saphenous, footpad

        (d) Mustelid: tail, footpad, saphenous

    3. Pulse oximeter

      a. Measures oxygenation in addition to heart rate

      b. Placement

        (1) Measures across any nonpigmented capillary bed

        (2) Mucous membranes are excellent sampling sites: oral or nasal mucosa, cloaca, vulva

        (3) Measures through nonpigmented skin: ear, wing web, thin skin of flank or abdomen

4. Respiratory monitor must be sensitive enough to detect small tidal volumes

AVIAN ANESTHESIA (<30 pounds)

I. Attainment of surgical anesthesia
   A. Toe, tail, cloacal pinches should induce slow withdrawal
   B. Most birds have a slow third-eyelid response; loss of this response in a bird that previously had a reflex is an indication to lighten anesthesia
   C. See Table 23-1
II. Anesthetic agent recommendations
   A. Inhalation anesthesia is preferred over injectable anesthesia
      1. The safety and efficacy of injectable anesthetics vary by species and individual animal
      2. It is extremely difficult to titrate the dose of injectable anesthetics

TABLE 23-1
AVIAN ANESTHESIA

SPECIES	DRUG	DOSAGE
Birds >250 g	Ketamine	10 mg/kg
Birds <250 g	Ketamine	30 mg/kg
Parakeet	Ketamine	30 mg/kg
	Xylazine	6.5 mg/kg
Cockatiel	Ketamine	25 mg/kg
	Xylazine	2.5 mg/kg
Amazon	Ketamine	10-20 mg/kg
	Xylazine	1-2 mg/kg
African Grey	Ketamine	15-20 mg/kg
	Xylazine	1.5 mg/kg
Cockatoo	Ketamine	20-30 mg/kg
	Xylazine	2.5-3.5 mg/kg
Macaw	Ketamine	15 mg/kg
	Xylazine	1.5-2 mg/kg
Hawks, falcons	Ketamine	25-30 mg/kg
	Xylazine	2 mg/kg
Owls	Ketamine	10-15 mg/kg
	Xylazine	2 mg/kg

B. Oxygen flow rates
1. 500 ml/min in small birds
2. 0.5 to 2 L/min/kg; maximum dosage is 3 to 4 L
C. Use nonrebreathing system for all birds <15 pounds
1. Hand-hold or use toweling to restrain bird
2. Place bird's head inside a clear plastic bag taped to the end of the Y or T piece while oxygen and anesthetic gas are flowing
3. Hold bird until relaxed and then maintain anesthesia with mask or intubation
D. Intubate all birds >100 g
1. Birds <100 g should be intubated for procedures >30 minutes or for procedures involving the coelomic cavity; small face masks are commercially available or can be fashioned from 35- to 60-cc syringe cases and rubber gloves
2. The glottis is easily visualized at the base of the tongue
   a. The trachea is composed of nonexpansible, complete tracheal rings; cuffs are not recommended
   b. Tissue swelling secondary to tube-induced tracheitis can occlude the trachea in birds <100 g
   c. Small endotracheal tubes can be fashioned from catheters, the hub end of butterfly catheters, or red rubber feeding tubes; the hubs of these items fit into adapters made for commercially available 3.5 to 4.5 mm endotracheal tubes
   d. Dead space can be minimized by making the tubes just long enough to ensure secure placement
   e. Tubes should be taped securely to beak to avoid the sensitive cere
   f. Tubes should be monitored for occlusion; mucous plugs and kinking are common; always have a replacement tube immediately available
3. If the trachea is occluded, the caudal thoracic air sacs can be cannulated at the site usually used for surgical sexing with a red rubber feeding tube cut to 2 to 5 cm in length; suture the tube in place; use the tube in the same fashion as an endotracheal tube; use aseptic technique to prevent life-threatening air sacculitis

4. Birds do not tolerate apnea
   a. Positive pressure ventilation is required at least 2 times per minute to assist self-ventilating bird; ventilate 10 to 15 times per minute in apneic bird; tidal volume is approximately 15 ml/kg
   b. Birds have no pulmonary reserve; air is stored in the air sacs, which have no gas exchange capability
E. Isoflurane is the anesthetic agent of choice in birds
   1. Induce at 3% to 4%
   2. Maintain at 0.5% to 2.5%
   3. Induction usually takes <5 minutes
      a. Induction is more rapid in birds than in mammals because of the cross-current system of the blood and air capillaries in addition to the greater proportional surface area of the lung; this makes the gas exchange in birds more efficient than in mammals
      b. Small changes in the vaporizer setting can cause rapid and dramatic changes in the plane of anesthesia; monitoring the level of anesthesia is critical
      c. Recovery is rapid, usually <5 minutes for a <45-minute procedure; hand-hold bird in toweling until it is able to walk
      d. Apnea is an important sign, usually a signal to lighten anesthesia immediately; cardiac arrest often follows within 2 to 5 minutes of onset of apnea; the endotracheal tube should always be checked for occlusion
F. Halothane is an acceptable anesthetic in birds
   1. Induce at 2.5% to 3.5%
   2. Maintain at 1% to 2%
   3. Induction usually takes 5 to 10 minutes
   4. *Peracute cardiac arrest with no prior warning* is a recognized risk of using halothane as an anesthetic in birds
   5. Recovery usually requires 5 to 15 minutes for a 45-minute procedure
G. Methoxyflurane has been used successfully in birds, but is associated with higher mortality rates than isoflurane or halothane

H. Injectable anesthetics
   1. Accurate body weight in grams is critical
   2. Effects of injectable anesthetics vary markedly by species and individual birds
   3. The dosages given are guidelines only
   4. Administer intramuscular injections in the pectoral muscles only
   5. Use of ketamine alone produces poor relaxation and turbulent recoveries; ketamine does not produce acceptable anesthesia in most fowl
   6. Xylazine causes excellent muscle relaxation and produces calm recoveries, but is a marked respiratory depressant; avoid using in ill birds
   7. Benzodiazepines have markedly variable effects; when they are not overridden, they produce safe sedation and muscle relaxation
   8. The combination of ketamine with xylazine or a benzodiazepine given IM usually produces adequate anesthesia for minor procedures
      a. Diazepam: 0.5 to 1 mg/kg; ketamine: 10 to 50 mg/kg IM; use higher doses for smaller birds
      b. Xylazine and ketamine: see Table 23-1
      c. Tiletamine/zolazepam: 4 to 25 mg/kg IM
         (1) Parakeet: 15 to 20 mg/kg IM
         (2) Duck: 5 to 10 mg/kg IM
      d. If a deeper plane of anesthesia is needed, after waiting 10 minutes readminister one fourth to one half of the ketamine dose only
      e. If the plane of anesthesia is still inadequate, it is advisable to postpone the procedure for 24 hours before attempting anesthesia again
   9. Recovery from injectable anesthetics is variable, but it usually takes >45 minutes after a 45-minute procedure
      a. Wrap bird in towel to control wings
      b. Place in warm, dark, quiet recovery area
      c. If the bird panics, hand-hold until it completely recovers
   10. Use one fourth to one half of the intramuscular dose if administering intravenously (IV)

I. Anesthetic emergencies
  1. Apnea
     a. Positive-pressure ventilation; if no endotracheal tube is available, lift and compress sternum
     b. Flush system free of anesthetic gas, administer 100% O_2
     c. Doxapram: IV, intraosseously (IO), or IM 5 mg/kg
     d. To reverse xylazine: yohimbine 1 mg/kg IV, IO
  2. Cardiac arrest
     a. Epinephrine 5 to 10 μg/kg IV, IO, intratracheally (IT)
     b. Lift and compress sternum
     c. Perform laparotomy and use fingertips or cotton-tipped applicators to perform internal cardiac massage
     d. See Chapters 25 and 26 for additional information on treatment of anesthetic emergencies
J. Recovery
  1. It is important to continue to monitor patient until recovered
  2. Provide warmth
  3. Monitor hydration and energy needs
  4. Reduce incidence and severity of self-induced trauma

AVIAN ANESTHESIA (>30 POUNDS, LONG LEGGED)

I. The same general principles apply as for smaller birds
II. Unless very weak, these birds are large enough to require chemical sedation before induction of inhalant anesthesia
  A. Large ratites (ostriches) are extremely dangerous; they should never be approached from the front; a forward kick can disembowel a person
  B. Using large sheets of wood as shields, herd large ratites from the sides and rear head first into a corner or chute
  C. Long-billed birds such as storks and herons strike swiftly with their beaks; it is *imperative* that eye protection be worn; first restrain these birds from over the back by their wings and neck; then a seond person should grasp and protect the legs; if the likelihood of hyperthermia is

low, the beak may be taped shut and padding placed on its tip

D. If the head can be reached safely, hood it with soft material to aid in calming and restraining the bird; ensure that the mouth and nares are open to the air to decrease the likelihood of hyperthermia

E. Capture myopathy, compartmentalization syndrome, hyperthermia, and leg fractures secondary to violent recoveries are complications associated with anesthesia in large long-legged birds

　1. Adequate padding, maintenance of blood pressure and oxygenation during procedures is critical; see Chapter 19

　2. Reduce handling needed to administer sedatives to a minimum; keep the induction and recovery areas as quiet and dark as possible

　3. Well-padded induction and recovery areas are desirable; a recovery stall slightly larger than the bird when recumbent often makes it feel secure; after the bird is completely recovered, the hood can be removed and the crate opened to release the bird; give it time to stand on its own; if a bird becomes agitated before it is fully recovered, injecting 0.1 to 0.2 mg/kg of diazepam has a calming effect

F. If the bird has not been fasted, it is wise to inflate the cuff on the endotracheal tube to prevent aspiration; regurgitation is common in unfasted birds

III. Injectable anesthetics are useful for short procedures and for induction of inhalant anesthesia

A. Intravenous injections can be administered in the brachial veins in standing animals such as ostriches and emus; some calm birds tolerate jugular injections; rheas have poor brachial veins, but are small enough to be manually restrained for inhalant anesthesia after a sedative is administered IM

B. Brachial, jugular, and medial metatarsal veins are excellent sites for indwelling intravenous catheters

C. Ratites

　1. Xylazine: 0.5 to 1 mg/kg IM, followed by ketamine: 2 to 4 mg/kg IV after 15 minutes

2. Xylazine: 0.25 mg/kg, and ketamine: 2.2 mg/kg IV
3. Tiletamine/zolazepam: 4 to 10 mg/kg IM
4. Tiletamine/zolazepam: 2 to 6 mg/kg IV
5. Diazepam 0.2-0.3 mg/kg, and ketamine 2.2 mg/kg IV

REPTILE ANESTHESIA

I. Never use hypothermia
   A. It depresses bodily functions, including the immune system and delays healing
   B. It does not provide analgesia
   C. It delays recovery from anesthesia
II. Induction of anesthesia
   A. Excitement is followed by loss of motor control; loss of the righting reflex is followed by muscle relaxation, which signifies attainment of surgical anesthesia when toe, tail, and cloaca pinches do not elicit a withdrawal
   B. Most reptiles with third eyelids retain this reflex; a decrease in heart rate to <80% of the stabilized rate is a sign to lighten anesthesia; often heart rate is the only reliable indicator of a reptile's level of anesthesia and needs to be carefully monitored
   C. Most reptiles can be induced by mask or chamber at 2% to 4% isoflurane; avoiding injectable anesthetics shortens recovery
      1. Watch for apnea
      2. Chelonians, aquatic squamates, and crocodilians can hold their breath for long periods of time; it can be difficult to extract a chelonian head from its shell and open the beak; injectable sedatives are often required to allow intubation and positive-pressure respiration to maintain inhalant anesthesia; venomous or large aggressive reptiles may require injectable anesthetics for safe restraint
         a. Ketamine: 20 to 60 mg/kg IM
         b. Ketamine: 5 to 15 mg/kg IV, IO
         c. Tiletamine/zolazepam: 10 to 40 mg/kg IM (squamates), 5 to 15 mg/kg IM (chelonians, crocodilians)

    d. Succinylcholine: *for intubation only*
      (1) No analgesia
      (2) Paralyzes muscles, including muscles of respiration
      (3) Intubate and assist respiration for approximately 1 hour after injection, sometimes longer
      (4) Do not repeat within 24 hours
      (5) 0.25 to 1.5 mg/kg IM (chelonans, crocodilians) in front half of animal

D. Intubation (similar to birds)
   1. Glottis is located at the base of tongue
   2. Glottis harder to see in chelonians
   3. Crocodilians possess a pharyngeal membrane that allows them to breathe with a mouth full of food or water; this membrane must be pushed aside to visualize the glottis
   4. In some crocodilians the trachea is bent in on itself; therefore the endotracheal tube does not advance as far as expected
   5. The tracheal rings are complete in chelonians and crocodilians
   6. All reptiles attaining surgical levels of anesthesia must be intubated; exceptional care is needed in individual reptiles <100 g to prevent tube-induced tracheitis

E. Maintenance
   1. Isoflurane is the anesthetic of choice at 1% to 2%
   2. Oxygen flow rates: 1 L/0.3 to 1 kg, 1 L/5 to 10 kg for larger reptiles
   3. Ventilate a minimum of 3 to 6 times per minute
   4. Halothane has been used successfully
   5. Methoxyflurane is associated with death in snakes
   6. Maintaining body temperature is essential

F. Recovery
   1. Usually <20 minutes with isoflurane for procedures <1 hour
   2. Hours to days with injectable anesthetics
   3. Positive-pressure ventilations must be continued until animal is breathing regularly on its own
     a. Some reptiles breathe when stimulated, but not on their own

       b. During recovery, reduce ventilations to 2 per minute; room air or exhaled air may be used to increase the carbon dioxide concentration to stimulate respirations; be careful not to induce anoxia

    4. Heat and fluids speed recovery times

  G. Emergencies

    1. Respiratory arrest

      a. Apnea is frequent; if the animal is stable administer positive-pressure ventilation

      b. In turtles extending and retracting the front legs can temporarily support respirations while an endotracheal tube is being placed

      c. To reverse xylazine: yohimbine 1 mg/kg IV

      d. Doxapram: 5 mg/kg IV, IO, IM

    2. Cardiac arrest

      a. Administer 100% oxygen

      b. Use chest compressions in nonshelled reptiles

      c. Perform laparotomy and manually compress heart

      d. Epinephrine: 5 to 10 mg/kg IV, IO, IC, IT

      e. See Chapters 25 and 26 for further information

AMPHIBIAN ANESTHESIA

  I. Indications

    A. Any painful procedure

    B. Diagnostic imaging

 II. Preanesthetic considerations

    A. See general considerations

    B. Withhold food from the animal 24 hours before anesthesia

    C. Significant respiration occurs across moist skin

      1. Do not allow skin to completely dry out

      2. Handle with wet latex gloves or wet hands

    D. Preanesthetic medications are not commonly used

    E. Ectotherm

      1. Maintain adequate body temperature with external heat sources

      2. Hypothermia prolongs recovery and depresses immune system

F. Animals greater than 100 g bodyweight should be intubated (see avian anesthesia earlier in chapter)

III. Stages of anesthesia

A. Similar to mammals

B. Erythema of ventral abdomen during induction

C. Abdominal respirations cease with heavy sedation but pharyngeal (gular) respirations continue

D. Corneal reflex is lost before loss of withdrawal reflex

IV. Anesthetic agents

A. Tricaine methane sulfonate (3-aminobenzoic acid ethyl ester; ethyl m-aminobenzoate, MS222; Finquel)

1. Routes

a. Immersion bath; keep tank of untreated water for recovery tank

b. Parenteral—IM or SQ; use sterile solution

2. Dose is species dependent

a. Immersion bath: 50 to 100 mg/L

b. 100 mg/kg SQ or IM (0.1 ml/10 g body weight with a 1% solution)

3. Induction takes 5 to 20 minutes

4. Recovery takes 10 to 30 minutes; keep skin moist with untreated water, maintain normal temperature

5. Wide margin of safety

6. Suppliers

a. Argent Chemical Laboratories
8702 152nd Ave NE
Redmond, WA 98052
1-800-426-6258

b. Crescent Research Chemicals
5301 N 37th Place
Paradise Valley, AZ 85253

B. Isoflurane

1. Intubate and ventilate after masking down

2. Induce at 3% to 4% for 5 to 15 minutes

3. Maintain at 1% to 2.5%

4. Keep skin moist and maintain normal temperature

5. Isoflurane is irritating to amphibian skin

6. Isoflurane is a respiratory depressant; use intermittent positive-pressure ventilation

7. Recovery takes 10 to 30 minutes; keep warm and moist

   C. Ketamine
     1. Good for diagnostics but not surgery
     2. 100 to 200 mg/kg SQ or IM
     3. Reflexes remain intact
     4. Induction takes 10 to 20 minutes
     5. Recovery takes 20 to 60 minutes

FISH ANESTHESIA

I. Indications
   A. Any painful procedure
   B. Sedation during shipping
   C. Diagnostic imaging
   D. Stripping milt or eggs
II. Preanesthetic considerations
   A. See previous general considerations
   B. Obligate water breathers
     1. Require oxygenated water moving over gills to oxygenate blood
     2. Normal water flow pattern is through the mouth, over gills, and out the operculum
     3. Provide water flow during anesthesia using frequent immersion or a small recirculating pump and airstone; a pump tube should be placed in the mouth of the fish so that water flow is maintained across the gills
   C. Exterior mucus layer is an important part of the integument
     1. Use the minimum restraint possible
     2. Use wet latex gloves when handling to minimize disruption to mucus layer
   D. Withhold food 24 hours before anesthesia
   E. Have recovery tank ready with water identical to the fish's preanesthetic conditions
   F. Preanesthetic medications are not commonly used
   G. Ectotherm
     1. Maintain adequate body temperature with external heat sources
     2. Hypothermia prolongs recovery and depresses immune system

III. Stages of Anesthesia

STAGE	PLANE	CATEGORY	FISH RESPONSES
0		Normal	Normal
I	1	Light sedation	Decreased response to visual stimuli
I	2	Deep sedation	Voluntary swimming stopped, normal posture, no response to external stimuli
II	1	Light narcosis	Excitement, loss of balance
II	2	Deep narcosis	Equilibrium lost, normal respiratory rate responds to pain
III	1	Light anesthesia	Decreased respiratory rate, deep pain present
III	2	Surgical anesthesia	Low respiratory rate, low heart rate, no deep pain
IV		Medullary collapse	Cardiac and respiratory arrest

IV. Anesthetic Agents
   A. Tricaine methane sulfonate (3-aminobenzoic acid ethyl ester; ethyl m-aminobenzoate, MS222; Finquel)
      1. The only anesthetic licensed for use in fish
      2. Commonly used as an immersion bath; keep tank of untreated water for recovery bath
      3. Dose is species dependent; generally sedation is 20 to 50 mg/L, anesthesia 50 to 100 mg/L; depth of anesthesia is controlled by switching from water bath containing anesthetic to untreated water bath
      4. Acidic solution: buffer with imidazole, or sodium hydroxide to normal tank pH
      5. Rapid induction takes 1 to 5 minutes
      6. Rapid recovery takes 10 to 15 minutes; keep water moving over gills to prevent hypoxia
      7. Wide margin of safety
      8. Suppliers
         a. Argent Chemical Laboratories
            8702 152nd Ave NE
            Redmond, WA 98052
            1-800-426-6258
         b. Crescent Research Chemicals
            5301 N 37th Place
            Paradise Valley, AZ 85253

B. Halothane
1. 0.5 to 40 mg/L of water; liquid halothane added to water
2. Narrow margin of safety
3. Not a preferred anesthetic agent
C. Isoflurane
1. Not a preferred anesthetic agent
2. Liquid isoflurane can be added to water
V. Treatment of anesthetic overdose
A. Move to untreated, oxygenated water
B. Increase gentle water flow over gills
C. If spontaneous respirations do not occur in 2 minutes, assist respirations
1. Move fish gently through the water
2. Slowly pump oxygenated water into mouth and across gills

POCKET PETS

I. Generalities
A. Rabbits, guinea pigs, and chinchillas frequently hold their breath and then take deep rapid breaths when being masked down or induced in a chamber; this behavior can result in death if the concentration of anesthetic gases is high; to reduce risk
a. Use preanesthetics
b. Use nitrous oxide followed by anesthetic agent
c. Use a low induction setting
B. Levels of anesthesia
1. Excitement phase
2. Loss of coordination
3. Muscle relaxation
4. Surgical anesthesia is attained when toe, ear, and tail pinches do not generate a withdrawal
5. Loss of corneal reflexes varies markedly between individual animals and anesthetic agents; loss in an animal that previously had them is a sign to lighten anesthesia
6. A decreasing respiratory or heart rate or abnormal breathing patterns are signs to lighten anesthesia

II. Intubation

    A. It is difficult to intubate rodents and lagomorphs because of their small size and long, thin oral cavities

    B. Masks are effective for short procedures

    C. Intubation techniques and considerations

        1. Small endotracheal tubes clog and kink easily

           a. Check tube patency with positive pressure ventilation at least every 2 minutes

           b. Have a replacement tube handy

           c. If a tube is clogged, try to reposition or suction; if the tube does not become patent, maintain anesthesia by mask or injectables or place a new tube

        2. Be careful not to create iatrogenic tracheitis

        3. Prolonged, oral, or thoracic procedures require intubation

        4. Oxygen flow

           a. 500 ml/min minimum

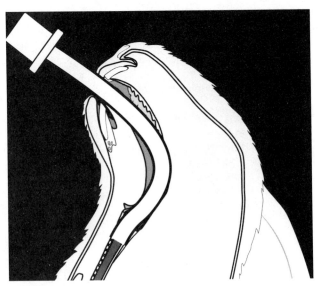

Fig. 23-1
Rodent/lagomorph endotracheal intubation. Extend head and neck. Bounce endotracheal tube off the roof of the mouth and into the larynx.

b. 0.5 to 2 L/min/kg, 3 to 4 L/min maximum
c. 1 L every 5 to 10 kg

D. Oral intubation: requires practice and luck (Fig. 23-1)
   1. Dorsal, lateral, or ventral recumbency
   2. Extend head and neck
   3. Keep straight
   4. Grasp tongue and pull forward
   5. Stylet or tube is bounced off the roof of the mouth and into the larynx
   6. A laryngoscope is helpful in larger individuals (Fig. 23-2)

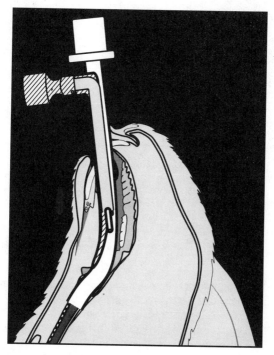

Fig. 23-2

Rodent/lagomorph endotracheal intubation with laryngoscope. Extend head and neck. Depress tongue with laryngoscope. Bounce endotracheal tube off of the roof of the mouth and into the larynx.

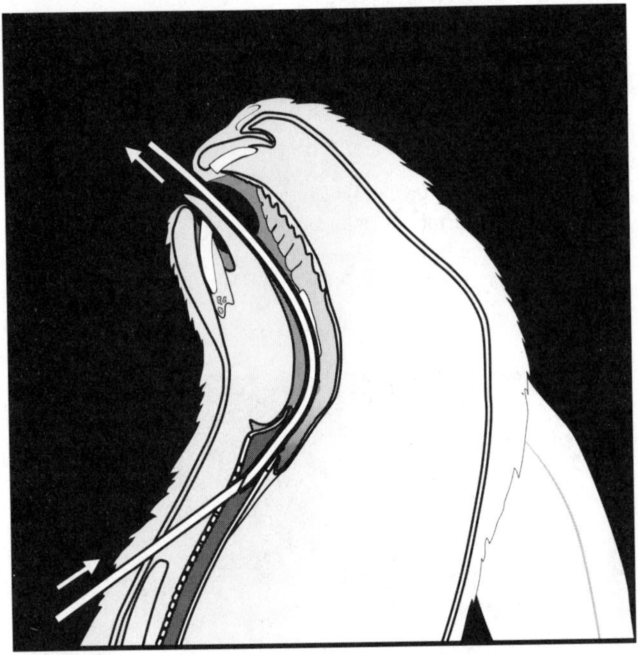

Fig. 23-3

A, Rodent/lagomorph endotracheal intubation, retrograde technique. Aseptically prepare ventral neck. Locate trachea (may require a cut down). Insert a through-the-needle catheter into the trachea as if performing a tracheal wash, *except* direct the catheter proximally.

7. Use of topical lidocaine can suppress laryngospasm
8. Repeated attempts at intubation can cause life-threatening hemorrhage and swelling
E. Retrograde technique (Figs. 23-3, *A* and *B*)
   1. Aseptically prepare ventral neck
   2. Pass an over-the-needle catheter into the trachea
   3. Retrograde it through the larynx
   4. Use the catheter as a stylet for the endotracheal tube
   5. Remove catheter

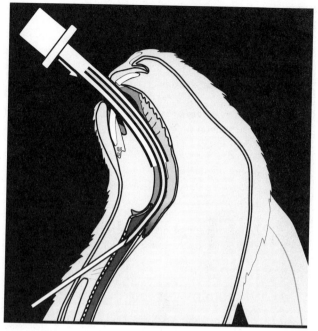

Fig. 23-3—cont'd

B, Use the catheter as a stylet to direct the endotracheal tube into the larynx. Once the endotracheal tube is correctly positioned, remove the catheter.

    6. In animals with fat necks, a "cut down" to the trachea is required

F. Induction
    1. Isoflurane: 2% to 3%
    2. Halothane: 2% to 4%

G. Maintenance
    1. Isoflurane: 0.25% to 2%
    2. Halothane: 0.25% to 2%
    3. Methoxyflurane: not recommended
    4. Use of nitrous oxide is similar to use in other domestic mammals

H. Recovery
1. Isoflurane takes 5 to 15 minutes for surgeries <1 hour
2. Halothane takes 10 to 20 minutes for surgeries <1 hour
3. Keep animal warm
4. Watch animal's hydration and energy needs

I. Injectables
1. Results vary markedly between individuals
2. Most frequent problem is poor muscle relaxation and poor analgesia
3. Injectable anesthetics are most useful for diagnostics or minor procedures
4. Dosages listed are only guidelines (Table 23-2)
5. Barbiturates produce excellent analgesia and muscle relaxation
   a. Their margin of safety is very low
   b. They are not recommended for use in pets

TABLE 23-2
POCKET PET ANESTHESIA

SPECIES	DRUG	DOSAGE
Rat, mouse, hamster, chinchilla, gerbil	Diazepam	Sedation only 3-5 mg/kg IM
Guinea Pig	Diazepam	Sedation only 0.5-3 mg/kg IM
Rabbit	Diazepam	Sedation only 1-4 mg/kg IM
All but gerbils	Acepromazine	Sedation only 1-2 mg/kg IM
Rat, mouse	Ketamine Xylazine	60-80 mg/kg IM 7-15 mg/kg IM
Rabbit, guinea pig, chinchilla	Ketamine Xylazine	30-40 mg/kg IM 5-8 mg/kg IM
Hamster, gerbil	Ketamine Xylazine	50 mg/kg IP 2-5 mg/kg IP
Rabbit, guinea pig	Ketamine Xylazine	35-40 mg/kg IM 4-6 mg/kg IM
Rat, mouse, guinea pig	Ketamine Acepromazine Xylazine	20-40 mg/kg IM 0.75 mg/kg IM 2-5 mg/kg IM

IM, intramuscularly; *IP*, intraperitoneally.

    c. Barbiturates are useful for euthanasia

    d. Pentobarbital: dilute to <10 mg/ml

Rat	25-40 mg/kg IP, IV
Mouse	40-80 mg/kg IP, IV
Guinea Pig	30-40 mg/kg IP, IV
Chinchilla	35-40 mg/kg IP
Rabbit	25-40 mg/kg IV
Hamster	50-90 mg/kg IP
Gerbil	40-60 mg/kg IP

J. Emergencies (see Chapters 25 and 26)

MUSTELIDS

I. Information in Chapters 7 and 18 is applicable to ferrets

II. Introduction

    A. Ferrets are easier to hold in a towel and mask down with isoflurane than cats, because they lack substantial claws

    B. Mask induction is used for very ill ferrets to eliminate the side effects associated with many injectable anesthetics and for short procedures such as diagnostics so that the ferret can be returned to the owner quickly

    C. Monitoring of depth of anesthesia is similar to cats

    D. Ferrets are small enough to require a nonrebreathing system

    E. Ferrets are easily intubated

        a. 2.5 to 3 mm endotracheal tubes

        b. A laryngoscope is helpful

III. Isoflurane

    A. Induce at 2.5% to 4%

    B. Maintain at 1% to 2.5%

    C. Recovery time is similar to cats

IV. Halothane

    A. Do not use for mask induction

    B. Maintain at 0.5% to 1.5%

    C. Recovery time is similar to cats

V. Injectables

    A. Tiletamine/zolazepam

        a. Light sedation: 3 to 5 mg/kg IM

        b. Anesthesia: 8 to 12 mg/kg IM

    B. Ketamine: 20 to 25 mg/kg IM

    Diazepam: 2 to 3 mg/kg IM

    C. Ketamine: 25 to 35 mg/kg IM
       Acepromazine: 0.2 to 0.3 mg/kg IM
    D. Ketamine: 10 to 20 mg/kg IM
       Xylazine: 2.2 mg/kg IM
VI. Emergencies (see Chapters 25 and 26)

EXOTIC CAT ANESTHESIA

  I. Preanesthetic considerations
    A. See general considerations at the beginning of this chapter
    B. Withhold food from animal for 24 hours; withhold water for 12 hours
    C. Respect animal's strength
    D. Remote delivery (pole syringe, darting equipment) is often needed to ensure human safety
    E. Premedication is similar to that used in the domestic cat but often is not needed
    F. Higher drug doses are needed for excited animals; make environment calm and quiet for induction to anesthesia
  II. Stages of anesthesia
    A. Similar to other mammals
    B. Sudden arousal of animals sedated with xylazine alone is possible
  III. Anesthetic agents
    A. Xylazine
      1. Rarely used alone because of possible sudden arousal
      2. Significant respiratory depressant
    B. Ketamine
      1. Used alone for short procedures in small cats 5 to 20 mg/kg IM
      2. Seizures have been reported in some species of exotic cats recovering from ketamine or ketamine combination anesthesia; control with diazepam
    C. Ketamine/xylazine combination IV
      1. Ketamine: 8 mg/kg
      2. Xylazine: 0.6 mg/kg
      3. Intubate and place on isoflurane inhalation anesthesia if procedure takes longer than 20 minutes
    D. Ketamine/diazepam combination IV
      1. Ketamine: 5 to 8 mg/kg
      2. Diazepam: 0.1 mg/kg

      3. Intubate and place on isoflurane inhalation anesthesia if procedure takes longer than 20 minutes

  E. Tiletamine/zolazepam (Telazol)

      1. Can reconstitute 500 mg vial to final concentration of 100 to 500 mg/ml depending on volume of diluent added for use in darting equipment

      2. Dose: 1.5 to 4 mg/kg IM for most species

         a. Sufficient for intubation

         b. Intubate and place on isoflurane inhalation anesthesia if procedure takes longer than 20 minutes

         c. Snow leopards require higher dose

         d. Excessive salivation seen in some species

         e. Recoveries from anesthesia smooth but prolonged compared to ketamine alone or ketamine combinations

         f. Delayed (3 to 10 days after immobilization) adverse drug reaction seen in some Siberian and white tigers

  F. Isoflurane is the inhalation anesthetic of choice; halothane can be used

      1. Small cats can be anesthetized in a chamber

      2. Face mask delivery can be used to supplement other anesthetics

      3. Dose

         a. Induce at 3% to 4%

         b. Maintain at 1% to 2%

         c. Oxygen flow rate is 1 to 6 L/min

      4. Intubate if procedure takes longer than 20 minutes

IV. Treatment of anesthetic overdose

  A. Treat as anesthetic emergency in domestic cat but be prepared for arousal of animal

  B. Xylazine can be reversed with yohimbine, although results are not as dramatic as other species

  C. Adverse tiletamine/zolazepam reaction in tigers has been treated with diazepam and dexamethasone

CAMELID ANESTHESIA (llamas, camels, alpacas)

I. Preanesthetic considerations

  A. See general considerations at beginning of chapter

  B. Withhold food from animal for 24 to 48 hours; withhold water for 24 hours weather permitting

    C. Patient positioning is important to reduce regurgitation
       1. Keep head elevated above rumen
       2. Do not roll anesthetized animal dorsally
       3. If regurgitation occurs, position head with muzzle below level of poll and ensure an open airway
    D. Intubate animals if procedure takes longer than 20 minutes
    E. Place jugular catheter
II. Stages of anesthesia are similar to other mammals
III. Anesthetic agents
    A. Neonates: mask with isoflurane; intubate if procedure takes longer than 20 minutes
    B. Juveniles and adults
       1. Sedation: xylazine 0.1 to 0.2 mg/kg SQ or IM
       2. Anesthesia
         a. Xylazine: 0.4 to 0.7 mg/kg SQ or IM
         b. Tiletamine/zolazepam: 0.75 to 1.5 mg/kg IM
IV. Treatment of anesthetic overdose
    A. Treat as anesthetic emergency in other mammals
    B. Xylazine can be reversed with yohimbine 0.125 mg/kg IV

POT-BELLIED PIG ANESTHESIA

I. Preanesthetic considerations
    A. See general considerations at beginning of chapter
    B. Withhold food from animal for 24 hours
    C. Warn owner and hospital staff that pig may squeal upon restraint
    D. Premedication is not generally needed
    E. Endotracheal intubation can be challenging (see Chapter 21)
    F. Watch for hyperthermia, although it is less of a problem in pot-bellied pigs than in food pigs
II. Stages of anesthesia are similar to other mammals
III. Anesthetic agents
    A. Isoflurane
       1. Can be used as the sole anesthetic agent in small animals which can be masked down
       2. Agent of choice for inhalation anesthesia

    3. Deliver from a precision vaporizer with face mask or
       endotracheal tube
       a. Induction: 3% to 4%
       b. Maintenance: 1% to 2%
       c. Oxygen flow rate: 2 to 3 L/min
  B. Tiletamine/zolazepam/ketamine/xylazine injectable com-
     bination
     1. Reconstitute a 500 mg vial of telazol with 2.5 ml of
        10% ketamine and 2.5 ml of 10% xylazine
     2. Each ml of resultant mixture contains
        a. 50 mg tiletamine
        b. 50 mg ketamine
        c. 50 mg zolazepam
        d. 50 mg xylazine
     3. Dose
        a. Sedation: 0.006 to 0.012 ml/kg body weight IM
        b. Surgical anesthesia and intubation: 0.018 to 0.024
           ml/kg body weight IM
        c. Requires 20 to 40 minutes to take effect
        d. Can supplement with 0.1 to 0.5 ml bolus in the au-
           ricular vein
IV. Treatment of anesthetic overdose
  A. If using isoflurane, turn vaporizer off and flush system
  B. Administer oxygen
  C. If xylazine has been given, reverse with yohimbine 0.125
     mg/kg IV
  D. Perform cardiopulmonary resuscitation as for other mam-
     mals

CHAPTER TWENTY-FOUR

Fluid Administration During Anesthesia

"One can drink too much, but one never drinks enough."

GOTTHOLD EPHRAIM LESSING

OVERVIEW

Fluid and blood replacement therapy are vital adjuncts to any anesthetic plan. Their use is extremely important during prolonged surgical and anesthetic procedures when hemorrhage is excessive or when the patient is dehydrated, debilitated, or in shock. Almost all drugs used to produce chemical restraint and anesthesia decrease the force of cardiac contraction and relax blood vessels, increasing vascular volume. The net effect of these actions is a decrease in cardiac output (blood flow) and arterial blood pressure. The routine administration of fluids during anesthesia is indicated to maintain an adequate and effective circulating blood volume and near-normal cardiac output. Blood loss must be replaced with at least two to three times as much isotonic fluid, since this fluid does not contain protein and will distribute throughout the extracellular fluid space (approximately three times the vascular volume). When blood loss is excessive, it should be replaced with blood on a one-to-one basis.

GENERAL CONSIDERATIONS

I. Anesthesia, surgery, and many of the diseases for which surgical intervention is required interfere with water and acid-base balance and decrease the effective circulating blood volume

A. Diseases producing changes in fluid, electrolyte, and acid-base balance (Table 24-1)

B. Imbalances caused by anesthesia
1. Most inhalation and intravenous (IV) anesthetic agents
a. Depress myocardial contractility and thus decrease cardiac output; metabolic acidosis may ensue
b. Induce generalized vasodilation; relative hypovolemia and hypotension may result
c. Depress minute ventilation; respiratory acidosis may occur
d. Decrease urine formation and renal concentrating ability
2. General anesthesia usually depresses the sympathoadrenal response to hypercapnia and decreases effective circulating blood volume

C. Imbalances caused by surgery
1. Blood loss
2. Drying of exposed tissues
3. Removal of effusions
4. Insensible losses

II. Fluid losses leading to a decrease in effective circulating blood volume usually cause metabolic acidosis

III. Blood loss can be replaced with crystalloid fluids, providing the hematocrit remains above 20% and total protein above 3.5 mg/dl

IV. Fluid administration to young or small patients should be supplemented with a source of calories (dextrose) and monitored very closely to prevent overhydration

V. The administration of large quantities of room-temperature fluids can produce hypothermia and hemodilution; packed cell volume (PVC) and total protein should be monitored

VI. Fluid administration
A. Most fluid administration sets deliver 10 drops/ml (regular drip) or 60 drops/ml (minidrip)
B. Larger-diameter needles or IV catheters offer less resistance to fluid flow and increase the rate of fluid administration

TABLE 24-1

COMMON DISEASES AND ASSOCIATED ELECTROLYTE ABNORMALITIES

DISEASE SYNDROME	WATER	NA⁺	K⁺	CA⁺⁺	MG⁺⁺	HPO₄⁻	CL⁻	HCO₃⁻
Gastric loss, vomiting	Loss	↓↓	↓↓		↓↓		↓↓	↑—↓
Pancreatic or intestinal fluid loss	Loss	↓	↓↓		↓↓		↓	↓
Diarrhea	Loss		↓↓				↓	
Starvation	Loss	—↓	↓	↓			↓	
Acute hemorrhagic pancreatitis	Loss	↓—		↓↓			↑	
Malabsorption syndrome	Loss		↑	↓↓	↓↓	↓↑		↓
Acute renal failure (oliguric)	Excess	—↑	↑	↓—	↓	↑↑	↓	↓↓
Renal tubular dysfunction	Loss	↓↓	—↓	—↓		—↑	—↓	
Chronic renal disease	Loss	—↓	—↓			—↑		↓↓
Diabetes insipidus	Loss	↑						

Burns	Loss	→	←→	→	→		→	←→
Primary aldosteronism	Excess	←–	←					→
Stress, surgery, including ADH	Excess	→	→					
Hypoadrenocorticalism (Addison's disease)	Loss	→	←	–↑		–↑	→	←
Hypopituitarism	Excess		→	→	→			
Hyperadrenocorticalism (Cushing's disease)	Excess	–↑	→	→←–→	→→	→		
Excess citrated blood								
Hyperparathyroidism								
Excess lactation (milk fever)								
Acidosis (metabolic)			←→				–→	→←
Alkalosis (metabolic)								

↑, Increased serum concentration; ↓, decreased serum concentration; –, normal serum concentration.

    C. Occasionally, fluids are administered at extremely rapid rates using electrical fluid pumps

    D. Infusion pumps and syringe infusion pumps facilitate delivery of accurate volumes of fluid (Figs. 24-1 and 24-2)

NORMAL BODY WATER DISTRIBUTION

    I. Total body water represents 55% to 75% of body weight (use 60%), primarily depending on age and body fat

    II. Extracellular water constitutes 23% to 33% of body weight (use 30%); percentage is greater in very young animals

    III. Intracellular water constitutes 35% to 45% body weight

    IV. Plasma water constitutes approximately 5% body weight

    V. Blood volume constitutes 8% to 10% of body weight (approximately 40 ml/lb), depending on the hematocrit; blood volume equals plasma water plus red blood cell (RBC) volume

    VI. Interstitial water constitutes 15% to 25% of body weight

    VII. Extracellular water equals plasma plus interstitial water

ELECTROLYTE DISTRIBUTION

    I. Extracellular water contains large quantities of sodium and chloride ions

    II. Intracellular water contains large quantities of potassium ions

    III. Table 24-2 shows the normal electrolyte composition of serum

PRINCIPLES OF FLUID ADMINISTRATION

    I. Correct dehydration and electrolyte and acid-base imbalances before anesthesia

    II. Do not attempt to replace chronic fluid losses acutely; severe dilution of plasma proteins, blood cells, and electrolytes may be produced

    III. Monitor pulmonary, renal, and cardiac function when administering fluids rapidly (e.g., for shock)

        A. Pulmonary function; overhydration can lead to pulmonary edema

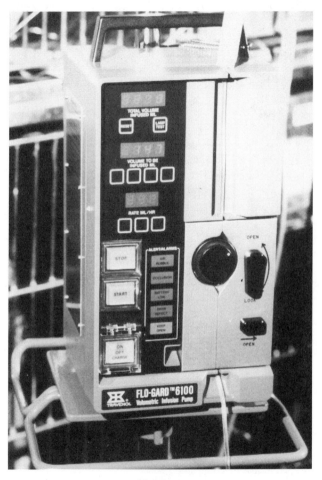

Fig. 24-1
Volumetric infusion pump.

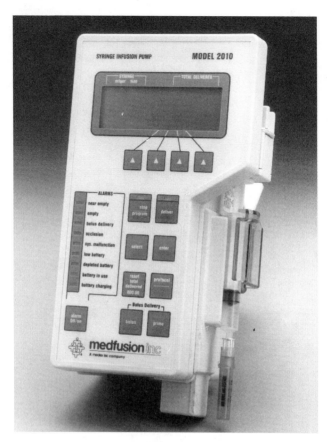

Fig. 24-2
Syringe infusion pump.

B. Renal function
1. Improve or reestablish glomerular perfusion rate (renal perfusion) before anesthesia
2. Administer mannitol at 0.5 to 1 g/lb over 30 minutes after hydration has been restored
3. Monitor urine output

TABLE 24-2
NORMAL ELECTROLYTE COMPOSITION OF SERUM

	NA⁺	K⁺	CA⁺⁺	MG⁺⁺	HPO₄⁻	CL⁻	HCO₃⁻
Dog	145-155	4.0-5.4	9.8-12.8	1.8-2.4	2.5-7.3	104-117	18-25
Cat	150-170	3.7-6	9.1-12.3	—	2.8-8.7	111-128	18-22
Horse	137-143	3.2-4.5	11.6-13.4	2.2-2.8	1.5-5.1	98-105	23-31
Cow	137-148	3.1-5.1	8.9-11.6	2.2-3.4	4.5-8.2	84-102	23-31

C. Cardiac function
   1. Monitor central venous pressure (CVP) if heart failure is right-sided or biventricular heart failure is suspected (see Chapter 15)
   2. Monitor pulmonary capillary wedge pressures, if possible, in cases of left-sided heart failure
   3. Auscult the chest; if the total protein drops below 3 and 4 mg/dl from fluid administration, pulmonary edema may occur

FLUID ADMINISTRATION DURING ANESTHESIA

I. Fluids administered during anesthesia are usually polyionic isotonic crystalloid solutions (Table 24-3)
II. Rate of fluid administration depends on fluid loss during surgery

| Small animals | 5-10 ml/lb/hr |
| Large animals | 3-5 ml/lb/hr |

A. Increase this rate if significant hypotension develops
B. Monitor for hemodilution or pulmonary edema
III. Estimate blood loss and administer 3 ml of crystalloid solution for each milliliter of blood loss (unless blood transfusion is indicated) over and above the basic fluid rate provided during anesthesia
IV. Maximum rate of fluids that can be administered safely during shock therapy varies considerably; the rule of thumb is 40 ml/lb/hr

POSTOPERATIVE FLUID THERAPY

I. When continued IV fluid therapy is necessary before or after surgery, the normal daily fluid maintenance rates are
   A. 20 to 30 ml/lb/24 hr (mature animal)
   B. 30 to 45 ml/lb/24 hr (young animal)
II. Calculation of replacement fluid volume in dehydrated animals
   A. Body weight (kg) × % dehydration (figured as a decimal) = fluid deficit (L) (e.g., 20 kg [dog] 10% = 2 L fluid deficit); periodic reassessment is indicated to determine response to volumes administered

TABLE 24-3
COMPOSITION OF COMMONLY USED FLUIDS

	TONICITY	pH	CALORIFIC VALUE	Na⁺	K⁺	Ca⁺⁺	MG⁺⁺	Cl⁻	LACTATE	HCO₃
Normal saline (0.9% NaCl)	Isotonic	5	0	155	0	0	0	155	0	0
2.5% dextrose (0.45% NaCl)	Isotonic	4.5	85	77	0	0	0	77	0	0
5% dextrose	Isotonic	4	170	0	0	0	0	0	0	0
Ringer's	Isotonic		0	147	4	5	0	156	0	0
Lactated Ringer's	Isotonic	6.5	9	130	4	3	0	109	28	0
Eltrad	Hypertonic		0	140	10	5	3	103	55	23
Whole blood	Isotonic	6.5	150	144	5.3	10	0	103	0	300
THAM*	Hypertonic		0	0	0	0	0	0	0	

*Contraindicated in anuria or uremia.
Potassium chloride: 20 or 40 mEq/ampule; 50 g/1 gal = isotonic
Sodium bicarbonate: 84 g = 1000 mEq; 50 g/1 gal = isotonic

B. Replacement fluids can be administered over a 4- to 6-hour period or added to the maintenance fluid volume and administered over a 24-hour period

CLINICAL ASSESSMENT OF HYDRATION

	MINIMAL (4%)	MODERATE (6% TO 8%)	SEVERE (10%-12%)
Skin resiliency	Pliable	Leathery	Absolutely no pliability
Skin tenting	Twist disappears immediately and tent persists up to 2 seconds	Twist disappears immediately and tent persists 3 seconds or more	Twist and tent persists indefinitely
Eye	Bright Slightly sunken	Duller than normal Obviously sunken	Cornea dry Deeply sunken, 2- to 4-mm space between eyeball and bony orbit
Mouth	Moist, warm	Sticky to dry, warm	Dry, cyanotic, warm to cold

BLOOD TRANSFUSION— MAJOR BLOOD GROUPS

I. Dog
   A. At least eight specific antigens have been identified on the dog erythrocyte
      1. Dog erythrocyte antigen (DEA)$_1$ DEA$_2$, and DEA$_7$ have the greatest potential to induce hemolytic antibody production in recipients; dogs negative for these RBC antigens are desirable as donors
      2. Transfusion reactions related to the remaining blood-group antigens are usually clinically insignificant
      3. Dogs should test negative for heartworm
II. Cat
   A. Three major antigens have been identified on the cat erythrocyte

      1. Transfusion reactions are rare in the cat; blood typing is rarely performed
      2. RBC survival time may decrease after multiple transfusions

III. Horse
    A. At least nine specific blood group antigens have been identified in the horse
      1. Compatibility testing should be done in horses before transfusion
        a. Blood typing
        b. Major and minor antigen agglutination
        c. Lysis cross-matching test
      2. A healthy male horse that has never had a transfusion is the most suitable donor in situations on which compatibility cannot be tested

IV. Cow: 11 antigenic blood groups are recognized
V. Swine: 15 antigenic blood groups are recognized
VI. Sheep: eight antigenic blood groups are recognized

INDICATIONS FOR BLOOD TRANSFUSION

  I. Restoration of oxygen-carrying capacity
    A. Anemia
      1. PCV is <20%, Hb is <5 g/dl in a normally hydrated patient that is being prepared for surgery
      2. Nonsurgical chronically anemic patients may not require transfusion unless PCV is <15 in dogs or PCV is <10 in cats
    B. Hemorrhage
      1. Crystalloid infusion may be adequate to treat 30% to 40% total blood volume loss
      2. Whole blood is necessary for replacement of more than 50% total blood volume loss
  II. Restoration of blood volume
  III. Coagulation factor replacement
    A. Poor viability of platelets and coagulation factors in stored blood
    B. Choose fresh blood (stored for <12 hours) when treating coagulopathies

COLLECTING AND STORING BLOOD
FOR TRANSFUSION

I. Obtain blood from jugular vein or cardiac puncture
II. Anticoagulant solutions used
   A. Acid citrate dextrose (ACD)
   B. Citrate phosphate dextrose (CPD) maintains higher pH, adenosine triphosphate (ATP), and 2,3-diphosphoglycerate (DPG) content during storage
   C. Heparin
      1. Heparin activates platelet aggregation and inhibits thrombin formation by inhibiting factor IX activation
      2. Do not use blood collected with heparin as the anticoagulant if it has been stored longer than 48 hours
III. Plastic containers are recommended for blood collection; they are less likely to activate platelet and coagulation factors
IV. Suggested guidelines for blood storage
   A. Maintain temperature between 1° and 6° C for the following storage times
      1. ACD anticoagulant: 21 days
      2. CPD anticoagulant: 28 days
      3. Feline blood: 30 days
   B. 70% to 75% RBCs are viable at the end of the storage times listed above

MODIFICATIONS OF STORED BLOOD

I. RBCs undergo less deformability as the fluidity of cytosol decreases because of the following conditions
   A. Hypertonicity of anticoagulant solution
   B. Decreasing erythrocyte ATP content
II. Erythrocyte 2,3-DPG content is decreased
   A. The oxygen dissociation curve shifts to the left; decreased oxygen is released at the tissue level
   B. 2,3-DPG content in RBCs is restored within hours of transfusion
III. pH decreases (pH <6.5 after 3 weeks of storage); citrate anticoagulants are converted to bicarbonate within minutes by the liver; bicarbonate therapy with blood transfusion is not necessary unless inadequate liver blood flow or altered liver metabolism is suspected

IV. Platelet numbers decrease; functional platelets are nonexistent after 2 to 3 days of storage

V. Ammonia content increases; may be detrimental in patient with impaired hepatic function

VI. Plasma potassium concentration increases because of progressive hemolysis during storage

VII. Metabolic transformations in stored blood are largely reversed during the first 24 hours following transfusion

BLOOD ADMINISTRATION

I. Blood administration sets
  A. Use set with a filter to remove aggregated debris
    1. Micropore filter with pore size 20 to 40 μm
    2. Cloth filter of administration set with pore size 170 μm
  B. Flush tubing before introducing blood
    1. This reduces resistance to blood flow
    2. Isotonic saline is fluid of choice
    3. Lactated Ringer's or other calcium-containing solutions may recalcify blood and trigger coagulation
    4. Dextrose solutions may cause agglutination and/or hemolysis

II. Sites of blood administration
  A. A peripheral or jugular vein
  B. Intraperitoneal administration
    1. Administer slowly
    2. RBCs are poorly recovered into system; approximately 40% blood is absorbed in 24 hours
  C. Medullary cavity of femur, tibia, or humerus
    1. Adequate for neonatal small animals
    2. Use 20-gauge needle or bone-marrow aspiration needle
    3. 95% of the blood is absorbed within 5 minutes

III. Rewarm stored blood to decrease viscosity and prevent hypothermia in recipient; immerse transfusion tubing in water bath maintained at a temperature below 40° C; autoagglutination occurs at higher temperatures

IV. Volume of blood to be administered
  A. General rule: 1 ml whole blood per pound raises the PCV by 1% (assuming a donor PCV of 40%)
  B. Blood volume needed to obtain target PCV

$$\text{Amount of donor blood needed} = \frac{\text{Desired PCV} - \text{Actual patient PCV}}{\text{PCV of anticoagulated donor blood}} \times \text{Recipient blood volume}$$

Estimate total blood volume at 40 ml/lb (30 ml/lb in the cat)

C. The amount of blood lost in aspirated fluids

$$\text{Volume of blood in suction fluid} = \frac{\text{PCV of fluid} \times \text{volume of fluid}}{\text{PCV of animal}}$$

D. Plasma volume needed to attain a target total protein (TP)

$$\text{Amount of donor plasma needed (ml)} = \frac{\text{Desired TP} - \text{Acutal TP}}{\text{Donor Plasma TP}} \times \text{Recipient plasma volume (ml)}$$

V. Blood administration rate depends on clinical circumstance
   A. Administer rapidly following massive hemorrhage
   B. In other cases
      1. Transfuse slowly at 0.1 ml/lb during the first 30 minutes, and observe for adverse reactions
      2. Afterward the rule of thumb is 5 ml/lb/hr, until the desired PCV is achieved
      3. Monitor for signs of fluid overload (CVP, thoracic auscultation)

ADVERSE, IMMUNE-MEDIATED EFFECTS OF TRANSFUSION

I. Hypersensitivity nonhemolytic reactions
   A. Activation of kallikrein-kinin system or immunoglobulin E
   B. Release of biogenic amines
   C. Clinical signs are muscle tremor, pyrexia, hypotension, tachycardia, and urticaria
II. Hemolytic reactions
   A. Hemolysis results from
      1. Recipient antibodies interacting with incompatible antigen of donor
      2. Antibodies of a previously sensitized donor interacting with recipient antigen
   B. Immediate transfusion reactions are unlikely during a first transfusion

C. Clinical signs usually develop within an hour posttransfusion and include hypotension, pyrexia, muscle tremor, emesis, convulsions, hemoglobinemia/uria, bilirubinemia/uria

D. Shock, renal failure, and disseminated intravascular coagulation may ensue

E. Delayed transfusion reactions for up to 2 weeks posttransfusion
   1. The recipient mounts an immune response to incompatible erythrocytes
   2. Clinical signs include pyrexia, anorexia, jaundice, and bilirubinuria

F. Hemolysis in the newborn resulting from previous sensitization of the mother (neonatal isoerythrolysis) can be avoided by preventing colostrum absorption; withhold mother's milk from neonate for first 48 hours of life

NONIMMUNOLOGIC ADVERSE TRANSFUSION REACTIONS

I. Sepsis; improper collection, storage, or handling may result in bacterial contamination and overgrowth

II. Transmission of infectious or parasitic diseases

III. Circulatory overload

IV. Citrate toxicity
   A. Rarely seen because of rapid metabolism of citrate by the liver; more likely in animal with liver dysfunction or excessively rapid blood administration
   B. Excessive circulating citrate causes chelation of serum ionized calcium

PLASMA TRANSFUSION

I. Indications
   A. Hypoproteinemia: total protein 4 g/dl; albumin 1.5 g/dl
   B. Failure of passive transfer; inadequate colostral antibody absorption
   C. Thrombocytopenia: use fresh plasma
   D. Coagulopathies: use fresh plasma

II. Plasma can be stored in a conventional freezer for up to 1 year

CHAPTER TWENTY-FIVE

Respiratory Emergencies

"Each person is born to one possession which
outvalues all his others—his last breath."

MARK TWAIN

OVERVIEW

Respiratory depression occurs during almost all chemical restraint
and anesthesia. Frequently respiratory depression causes apnea and
hypoxemia, leading to respiratory emergencies. Hypoventilation
cannot always be determined by visual inspection but can be as-
sessed by arterial blood gases. Although potentially devastating,
respiratory depression, if recognized early, is easily treated by establishing a patent airway and providing adequate inflation of the
lungs to ensure appropriate gas exchange.

GENERAL CONSIDERATIONS

I. Definition: A respiratory emergency is the inability to
    maintain adequate ventilation and normal blood gas
    values
II. Common causes
    A. The causes are diverse and may vary among animal
       species
    B. Major causes
       1. Hypoventilation caused by drug-induced respiratory
          depression
       2. Airway obstruction
       3. Parenchymal pulmonary disease
       4. Pleural cavity disease

      5. Iatrogenic causes

        a. Laryngeal spasm with intubation of cats

        b. Small or plugged endotracheal tube

III. When considering assisted or controlled ventilation, patient age and size determine respiratory frequency, rate of lung inflation, inflation pressure, and tidal volume delivered; large adult patients generally require slower inflation rates, lower frequencies of inflation, and larger inflation pressures and volumes

    A. Pneumothoraces should be corrected immediately to ensure adequate lung expansion

    B. Intrathoracic air or fluid should be removed

IV. A patient's total lack of respiratory effort or increased respiratory frequency using the accessory muscles of respiration, particularly the abdomen, are signs of a respiratory difficulty or emergency

V. Support of ventilation should be continued until the patient can maintain consciousness, normal mucous membrane color, and normal blood gases

CLINICAL SIGNS

  I. Apnea or dyspnea

 II. Respiratory rate, depth, and effort are generally increased in animals with respiratory disease

III. Stridor or sonorous breathing are sounds associated with airway obstruction

IV. Cyanosis may be absent in severely anemic animals (Hb <5 g/dl)

 V. Abnormal upper airway and lung sounds (wheezes, crackles)

VI. Deformities of head, neck, and thorax

VII. Abnormal positions

    A. Extension of the head and neck

    B. Abduction of the forelimbs

HYPOVENTILATION

  I. Treat primary cause

 II. Control or assist breathing when necessary

III. Use respiratory stimulants when necessary: doxapram 0.05 to 0.2 mg/lb intravenously (IV), repeat if necessary, or, 5- to 10-μg/kg/min-intravenous infusion

AIRWAY OBSTRUCTION

I. Partial airway obstruction is frequently associated with respiratory disease and endotracheal intubation

II. Anatomic conformations that predispose animals to airway collapse
  A. Stenotic nares in brachycephalic breeds
  B. Edema of the nasal turbinates in horses
  C. Elongated or displaced soft palate
    1. Brachycephalic breeds
    2. Beagle and cocker spaniel
    3. Horses
  D. Collapsing arytenoid cartilages
    1. Congenital in Bouvier, bull terrier, Siberian husky
    2. Acquired in giant-breed dogs (e.g., St. Bernard)
  E. Everting laryngeal ventricles
    1. Brachycephalic breeds
    2. English bulldog
    3. May be associated with hypothyroidism
  F. Collapsing trachea
    1. Middle-aged to older obese toy-breed dogs, especially miniature poodle, Yorkshire terrier, Chihuahua
    2. Calves
  G. Laryngeal paralysis
    1. Congenital, especially in Bouvier, bull terrier, Siberian husky
    2. Acquired in giant-breed dogs, especially St. Bernard
    3. Hemiplegia or postsurgical paralysis in horses
  H. Hypoplasia of the trachea
    1. Congenital in brachycephalic breeds
    2. English bulldog

III. Other causes of airway obstruction
  A. Endotracheal or tracheotomy tubes
  B. Nasal disease (e.g., tumor, fungal)
  C. Chronic obstructive pulmonary disease
  D. Other species

1. Cat: asthma
   a. Stage I (asymptomatic)
   b. Stage V (severe distress)
2. Horse: gutteral pouch infections, ethmoidal hematoma, tumors
3. Sheep : nasal parasites
4. Pig: atrophic rhinitis

IV. Clinical signs
- A. Noisy, stridorous, or labored breathing
  1. Loudest at larynx and pharynx during upper airway obstruction
  2. Low-pitched honking sound during tracheal collapse
- B. History of exercise intolerance, cyanosis, and/or collapse
- C. Choking, retching, and vomiting
- D. Severely distressed animals may paw or claw at the face and throat
- E. Abnormal body positions

V. Diagnosis (consider establishing a patent airway before attempting a diagnosis)
- A. History of facial injuries, epistaxis, or wounds to the neck
- B. The presence of stenotic nares, foreign bodies or tumors, and soft tissue swelling
- C. Radiography
  1. Survey
  2. Contrast
  3. Fluoroscopy
- D. Bronchoscopy to confirm presence or absence of lower airway obstruction
- E. Electromyography to confirm denervation of laryngeal muscles

VI. Treatment
- A. Provide oxygen
- B. Avoid stress
- C. Establish patent airway
  1. Intubate
  2. Remove oral, nasal, or tracheal foreign material or blood using forceps, suction, and postural drainage
  3. Perform tracheotomy if necessary to bypass obstruction (Fig. 25-1)
  4. Apply local anesthetic creams (5%) to prevent laryngospasm

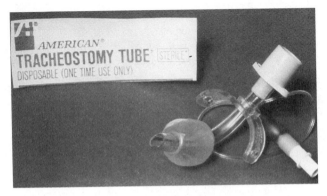

Fig. 25-1
Tracheotomy tubes are available in different sizes and are cuffed or un-cuffed. Cuffed tubes are preferred.

    D. If apneic, institute artificial ventilation with air or, prefer-ably, oxygen
        1. Mouth-to-mouth
        2. Mouth-to-nose
        3. Nasal intubation with oxygen administration
        4. Face mask and oxygen
        5. Deliver oxygen to endotracheal or tracheotomy tube
    E. Control breathing rate if apneic; assist ventilation if breathing
        1. Rate: 6 to 15 breaths per minute
        2. Inspiratory time: 1 to 3 seconds, depending on size of patient
        3. Maintain proper inspiratory/expiratory ratio of 1:2, 1:3, or 1:4
        4. Inflate lungs to 15 to 20 cm H_2O if chest is closed (up to 30 to 50 cm H_2O in large animals)
        5. Inflate lungs to 20 to 30 cm H_2O if chest is open or atelectasis of lungs has occurred (up to 50 cm H_2O in large animals)
        6. Tidal volume
            a. approximately 5 to 7 ml/lb
            b. 7 to 10 ml/lb if mechanical ventilator is used
    F. Discontinue all anesthetic agents, including nitrous oxide

G. Supportive care
1. Intravenous fluid therapy
2. Bronchodilators
3. Respiratory stimulants if necessary
4. Sedation
5. Antibiotics
6. Corticosteroids
7. Maintain normal body temperature

H. Treat coexisting problems; prepare for surgery
   a. Remove foreign bodies or tumors
   b. Repair fractures and wounds of the respiratory system
   c. Drain chest
   d. Correct anatomic defects when necessary

I. Care of tracheotomy tube
1. Apply suction every 2 hours using aseptic technique
2. Nebulize with saline or acetylcysteine diluted with saline
3. Maintain normal hydration
4. Monitor body temperature
5. Take periodic chest radiographs

PARENCHYMAL EXCHANGE DISEASES

I. Classification
A. Life-threatening pneumonias
1. Acute, fulminating bronchopneumonia
2. Smoke inhalation
3. Aspiration pneumonia
B. Pulmonary contusion
C. Pulmonary edema
D. Cat asthma

II. Diagnosis
A. Physical signs, including lethargy
B. Radiographs of the chest
C. Laboratory tests
1. Complete blood count
2. Transtracheal aspirate
3. Bronchoscopy
4. Blood gas determination

III. Treatment
  A. Remove aspirated material
  B. Maintain the patency and function of the airways
  C. Apply positive end-expiratory pressure
  D. Treat infection
  E. Enhance removal of secretions (acetylcysteine, guaifenesin)
  F. Supportive care
    1. Administer oxygen (≥40%) by
       a. Face mask
       b. Nasal catheter
       c. Pediatric incubator
       d. Oxygen cage
       e. Tracheotomy and positive-pressure ventilation, if laryngeal spasm or airway obstruction with secretions persist
    2. Humidify the air by nebulization with normal saline to improve removal of secretions
    3. Maintain normal body hydration with fluids intravenously or subcutaneously (SQ) to prevent drying and thickening of secretions
    4. Perform periodic coupage (percussion of the chest)
    5. Provide physiotherapy with deep breathing aids removal of secretions, increases lymphatic drainage of the lungs, and activates surfactant
    6. The use of diuretics, corticosteroids, and antiprostaglandins in pneumonia is controversial
    7. Bronchodilators are helpful in reversing bronchial spasm and constriction (e.g., aminophylline)
    8. Pneumonias with viscous secretions may require expectorants (e.g., guaifenesin)
    9. Antibiotic use should be based on culture and sensitivity results
    10. Analgesics may be used for extreme pain and apprehension in selected patients
    11. Medical therapy of pulmonary edema
        a. Decrease the workload of the heart by cage rest; administer oxygen, sedation, and digitalization
        b. Improve ventilation by endotracheal suctioning

      c. Nebulize with 40% alcohol

      d. Eliminate excessive fluids with diuretics and vaso-
dilators

PLEURAL CAVITY DISEASE

I. Definition: Pleural cavity disease includes problems that decrease the functional capacity of the lungs because of occu-
pation of space in the pleural cavity and damage to the integrity of the thoracic wall

II. Classification

    A. Pneumothorax

      1. Open

      2. Closed

      3. Spontaneous

      4. Tension

    B. Pleural effusion

      1. Chylothorax

      2. Pyothorax

      3. Hydrothorax

      4. Hemothorax

      5. Neoplastic effusion

      6. Infectious, inflammatory effusion

    C. Diaphragmatic hernia

    D. Flail chest

III. Causes

    A. Pneumothorax: accumulation of free air in the pleural cav-
ity

      1. Spontaneous pneumothorax—most common in Afghan
hounds

      2. Tension pneumothorax: air accumulates in pleural
space during inspiration and is not expelled during expiration; intrapleural pressure increases, collapsing the
lungs and great vessels

      3. Trauma resulting in pleural or parenchymal lacerations
or tracheobronchial ruptures is the most common cause
of pneumothorax

      4. Other causes

        a. Penetrating injuries from bite wounds and projec-
tiles

      b. Rupture of congenital bullous emphysematous or granulomatous lung lesions (blebs or bullae)

      c. Rupture of parasitic cysts (Paragonimus); neoplasia

      d. Hardware disease in cattle

      e. Pleuritis

      f. Iatrogenic causes

          (1) Intrathoracic surgical procedures

          (2) Cardiopulmonary resuscitation

          (3) Overzealous intermittent positive-pressure ventilation

      g. Following pneumomediastinum from trauma to trachea or esophagus (rare)

B. Pleural effusion: abnormal fluid accumulation within the pleural cavity

  1. Hemothorax

      a. Rupture of cardiac and intrathoracic blood vessels from trauma

      b. Clotting disorders

      c. Bleeding neoplasms (e.g., hemangiosarcoma)

      d. Lung-lobe torsion

      e. Pleuritis

  2. Chylothorax

      a. Rupture of the thoracic duct

      b. Idiopathic lymphatic obstruction

  3. Hydrothorax

      a. Hypoproteinemia

      b. Heart failure and cardiomyopathy

  4. Pyothorax

      a. Penetrating wounds of thorax or esophagus

      b. Migrating foreign bodies

      c. Spread of pulmonary infection and pleuritis

      d. Organisms: Escherichia coli, Staphylococcus, β-streptococcus, Pasteurella, Nocardia

C. Chest wall abnormalities

      a. Diaphragmatic hernias displace the lungs with abdominal viscera

      b. Flail chest caused by proximal and distal fractures of several consecutive ribs

          (1) Chest wall is drawn inward with inspiration and blown outward with inspiration (paradoxic movement)

(2) Lung contusion and hemopneumothorax may be present, precipitating acute respiratory distress

IV. Diagnosis
- A. Auscultation and percussion
- B. Thoracic radiography
- C. Ultrasound examination
- D. Thoracentesis

V. Treatment
- A. Establish a patent airway
- B. Oxygen therapy
- C. Shock therapy
- D. Bandage penetrating wounds, flail segments
- E. Assess status of animal
- F. Remove the cause
  1. Needle aspiration (air or liquid)
  2. Tube thoracostomy
     a. Indications
        (1) Acute severe pneumothorax
        (2) Tension pneumothorax
        (3) Pneumothorax associated with rib fractures, emphysema, or hemothorax
        (4) In situations where repeated needle evacuations are necessary
        (5) Postthoracotomy
     b. Methods of drainage
        (1) Intermittent aspiration using a syringe and three-way stopcock
        (2) Unidirectional flutter (Heimlich) valves (Fig. 25-2)
        (3) Intermittent connection of the chest tube to a suction pump (10 to 15 cm H_2O negative pressure)
        (4) Connection of chest tube to underwater seal units
           (a) One-bottle system
           (b) Two-bottle system
           (c) Three-bottle system
  3. Complications
     a. Chest tube attaches to underwater seal and requires

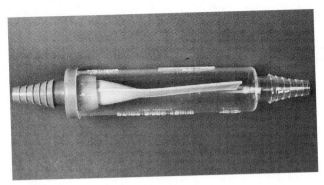

Fig. 25-2

A unidirectional valve (Heimlich valve) is used to evacuate air from the chest.

      constant monitoring (disconnection causes pneumo-thorax)
  b. Accumulation of fibrin and blood
  c. Displacement of tube
  d. Kinking of tube
  e. Subcutaneous emphysema
  f. Lung tissue entrapment and infarction after vigor-ous suction
  g. Infection

IATROGENIC CAUSES OF RESPIRATORY EMERGENCIES

  I. Inadequate patient evaluation
 II. Faulty anesthetic techniques
    A. Anesthetic overdose (e.g., barbiturates)
    B. Excessive dead space in anesthetic equipment
    C. Lack of oxygen delivery
      1. Nitrous oxide on; oxygen off
      2. Excessive use of N_2O (>70%)
      3. Oxygen supply depleted
      4. Anesthetic system not connected properly
      5. Endotracheal tube too small

   6. Overdistended endotracheal tube cuff
      a. Stenosis of trachea in horses
      b. Postsurgical stenosis of trachea
   7. Inappropriately placed endotracheal tube
      a. In esophagus
      b. In pharynx
      c. At or caudal to bifurcation of trachea
  D. Kinked or obstructed anesthetic delivery hoses and tubes
  E. Overdistention of lungs during mechanical ventilation
  F. Neuromuscular paralysis of diaphragm and intercostal muscles without ventilatory support
III. Restrictive bandages
IV. Inadequate monitoring of the patient
  A. Patterns of respiration
    1. Eupnea: normal rate and rhythm

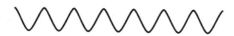

    2. Tachypnea: increased respiratory rate; causes: fever, hypoxia, hypercapnia, pneumonia, lesions of central nervous system (CNS) respiratory centers

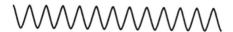

    3. Bradypnea: slow but regular respirations; causes: sleep, anesthesia, opiate narcotics, hypothermia, neoplasia, respiratory decompensation

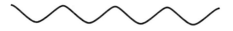

    4. Apnea: absence of respiration; may be periodic; causes: drug depression, muscle paralysis, overventilation, obstruction, shock, increased cerebral blood pressure (BP), surgical manipulation of vagus and splanchnic nerves

5. Hyperpnea: large respirations (increased tidal volume); rate normal; causes: excitement, pain, surgical stimulation, hypoxia, hypercarbia, heat, cold

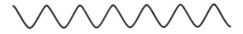

6. Cheyne-Stokes asthma: respirations become faster and larger, then slower, followed by apneic pause; causes: increased intracranial pressure from head trauma or neoplasia, meningitis, renal failure, severe hypoxia, drug overdose, high altitude

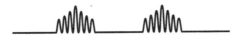

7. Biot's respirations: respirations that are faster and deeper than normal, with abrupt pauses between them; each breath has approximately the same tidal volume; causes: anesthesia in normal athletic horses and greyhounds, spinal meningitis, drugs that cause generalized CNS depression

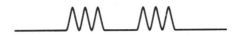

8. Kussmaul's respirations: regular and deeper respirations without pauses; patient's breathing usually sounds labored, with breaths that resemble sighs; causes: renal failure or metabolic acidosis, diabetic ketoacidosis

9. Apneustic: prolonged gasping inspiration, followed by extremely short, inefficient expirations; causes: high doses of drugs (e.g., ketamine in cats and horses,

guaifenesin in horses), lesions in the pons and thalamus

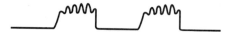

OTHER CAUSES OF PULMONARY INSUFFICIENCY

I. Ventilation-perfusion inequalities
   A. Decreased cardiac output
   B. Atelectasis
   C. Gravitational effects
   D. Severe abdominal distention (e.g., obesity, neoplasia)
   E. Airway obstruction
   F. Hypoventilation
II. Increased venous admixture (shunts)
   A. Pulmonary arterial-venous shunts
   B. Bronchial vessel shunts
   C. Atelectasis (physiologic shunt)
   D. Pulmonary neoplasia

RESPIRATORY ARREST

I. Cessation of breathing from any of the previously discussed causes
II. Correct immediately (within 3 to 5 minutes)
III. Treatment
   A. Establish a patent airway
      1. Remove obstruction, foreign material
      2. Intubate
      3. Consider tracheostomy if unable to orotracheally intubate
   B. Provide artificial ventilation
      1. Room air delivered through Ambu bag
      2. 100% delivered through anesthetic system
      3. Transtracheal insufflation of O_2, 3 to 6 L/min in dogs
      4. Refer to Chapter 14

C. Proceed with cardiopulmonary resuscitation (see Chapter 26)

D. Interestingly an acupuncture resuscitative technique has been used successfully in an emergency situation
   1. Use 25 to 28-gauge hypodermic needle, 25 to 50 mm long
   2. Insert 10 to 20 mm into the nasal septum at point GV 26, along the midline of the nasolabial cleft at the left of the lower canthi of the nostril
   3. Twirl the needle strongly and move it up and down
   4. Use this technique as an adjunct to but not a replacement for conventional techniques

PREVENTION OF RESPIRATORY EMERGENCIES

I. Proper preanesthetic evaluation
   A. Clinical signs
   B. Auscultation
   C. Radiography
   D. Blood gas analysis
II. Use of proper anesthetic and monitoring equipment (Figs. 25-3 and 25-4)
III. Adequate inspection of anesthetic equipment
IV. Proper administration of preanesthetic and anesthetic agents
V. Careful and continuous monitoring during anesthesia
VI. Awareness of possible problem

USE OF ANALEPTICS, BICARBONATE, BRONCHODILATOR DRUGS; OTHER DRUGS

I. Doxapram hydrochloride (0.5 to 0.2 mg/lb in small animals; 0.1 to 0.3 mg/lb IV in large animals); doxapram can be administered by infusion (5 to 10 μg/kg/min) until effective; a centrally acting respiratory stimulant; increases tidal volume and, in larger doses, respiratory rate; causes small elevations in arterial BP and heart rate and may cause arousal from anesthetic depression

II. Sodium bicarbonate (0.5 to 2 mEq/lb); use to correct metabolic acidosis, which may occur in severe hypoxia, hypercapnea, or complete respiratory and cardiac arrest; excessive ad-

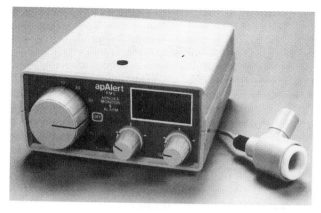

Fig. 25-3

Respiratory rate monitor, which uses a temperature device attached to the endotracheal tube.

ministration may produce hypokalemic metabolic alkalosis or paradoxic cerebrospinal fluid acidosis

III. Aminophylline: up to 2 mg/lb IV slowly over 30 minutes, 1 to 2 mg/lb intramuscularly (IM); dilates bronchial smooth muscle and may be useful in asthmatics and bronchospasm; has inotropic action on heart

IV. Narcotic antagonists (naloxone, nalorphine, levallorphan); Nalline (nalorphine): 1 mg/5 lb; acts by competitively displacing narcotic analgesics from opiate and nonopiate receptors

V. Other specific antagonists

    A. Neostigmine, edrophonium: reversal of nondepolarizing neuromuscular blocking drugs (see Chapter 11)

    B. α_2-Antagonists (yohimbine, tolazoline, atipamazole): reversal of xylazine, medetomidine, or detomidine (see Chapter 3)

TREATMENT OF PULMONARY EDEMA

I. Measures to improve ventilation-gas exchange

    A. Reduction of activity (cage rest): to decrease oxygen demand

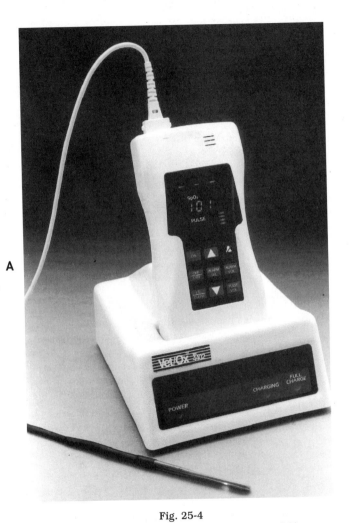

Fig. 25-4

A pulse oximeter (**A** and **B**) can be used to monitor hemoglobin saturation with oxygen.

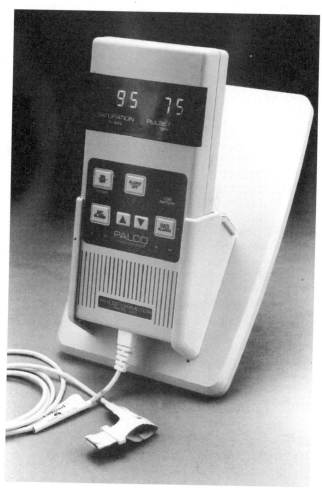

Fig. 25-4—cont'd

For legend, see facing page.

B. Sedation, relief of anxiety
   1. Morphine (dogs): 0.2 to 0.5 mg/kg SC, IM, IV
   2. Acepromazine (cats): 0.1 to 0.2 mg/kg SC, IM
C. Oxygen therapy (40% to 50%)
D. Endotracheal suctioning in severe cases to clear foam from airways
E. Bronchodilator (e.g., aminophylline 6 to 10 mg/kg by mouth [PO], SC, IV q6h)
F. Ethyl alcohol nebulization (40%) into O_2 (prevents foaming in airways)
G. Positive-pressure ventilation through endotracheal tube
   1. Manual or mechanical (PEEP, continuous positive airway pressure)
   2. Use only as a last resort when life-threatening respiratory failure persists despite other measures
   3. Criteria: Pao_2 <60 mm Hg, $Paco_2$ >50 mm Hg, persistent cyanosis, dyspnea, or tachypnea (all while breathing 60% O_2)

II. Measures to reduce capillary hydrostatic pressure
   A. Decrease circulating blood volume
      1. Diuretics: furosemide 2 to 4 mg/kg IV, IM, SC, PO q6 to 8h
      2. Phlebotomy: remove 6 to 10 ml/kg, rarely used
   B. Redistribute pulmonary blood flow to other circulatory beds
      1. Morphine; in addition to sedative effects, increases systemic venous capacitance
      2. Furosemide (Lasix); in addition to diuresis, redistributes pulmonary blood flow by increasing systemic venous capacitance
      3. Vasodilators
         a. Na nitroprusside, nitroglycerine, hydralazine, prazosin
         b. Peripheral vasodilation redistributes circulation away from pulmonary beds (noncardiogenic) and decreases resistance to outflow (afterload; cardiogenic)
   C. Improve cardiac function (cardiac output); mostly used in cardiogenic edema

     1. Positive inotropes: dopamine, dobutamine
     2. Antiarrhythmics to control arrhythmias, if present
III. Other therapy involves corticosteroids, e.g., prednisolone sodium succinate 10 to 15 mg/lb IV
IV. Monitoring of response to therapy
    A. Physical examination (including rate and depth of breathing, auscultation, mucous membrane color)
    B. Sequential arterial blood gas analyses
    C. Thoracic radiography
    D. Pulmonary capillary wedge pressure

CHAPTER TWENTY-SIX

Cardiac Emergency and Shock

"It is by presence of mind in untried emergencies that the native metal of a man is tested."

JAMES RUSSELL LOWELL

OVERVIEW

Bradycardia, hypotension, and decreased peripheral perfusion leading to shock can occur following the administration of chemical restraining drugs and anesthetics. The potential for these emergencies is increased in severely debilitated or traumatized patients. A variety of physical and pharmacologic approaches have been developed to prevent further deterioration of the circulation or return abnormal hemodynamics to normal. Since it is difficult to perform external/internal cardiac massage in animals in excess of 500 pounds, it is imperative that practitioners have a working knowledge of the various pharmacologic approaches to cardiopulmonary resuscitation. Generally most therapeutic responses to acute cardiovascular crises must be followed by continued care and close patient monitoring.

GENERAL CONSIDERATIONS

I. Definition: A cardiac emergency is any acute or chronic condition involving the heart that results in the inability to maintain adequate cardiac output

II. Common causes
   A. Respiratory failure (hypoxia)

      1. Hypoventilation

      2. Low inspired PO_2

      3. Ventilation-perfusion abnormalities

      4. Shunt

      5. Diffusion abnormality

B. Acid-base imbalance

      1. Respiratory acidosis

      2. Metabolic acidosis leading to myocardial depression

      3. Respiratory alkalosis

      4. Metabolic alkalosis leading to myocardial irritability

      5. Mixed metabolic and respiratory alkalosis or acidosis

C. Electrolyte imbalance

      1. Hyperkalemia (bradycardia; poor contractility, vasodilation)

      2. Hypokalemia (tachycardia)

      3. Hypocalcemia (hypocontractility, hypotension)

D. Autonomic imbalance

      1. Increased sympathetic tone; increased myocardial automaticity and irritability

      2. Increased parasympathetic tone; predisposition to bradycardia and various forms of heart block; predisposition to atrial arrhythmias, including atrial fibrillation

E. Hypothermia

F. Air embolism

G. Toxicity

      1. Myocardial depressant factors produced by ischemic organs (e.g., pancreas)

      2. Any hypersensitivity or drug overdose
         Hypotensive crisis secondary to phenothiazine administration

         (1) Most commonly observed after intravenous (IV) drug administration

         (2) Treatment includes fluids, steroids, and occasionally vasopressors

H. Excessive or inappropriate drug administration

      1. Administration of catecholamines during inhalation anesthesia with halothane (ventricular arrhythmias, tachycardia)

      2. Accidental intraarterial drug administration, for

example, accidental intracarotid administration of preanesthetic drugs (phenothiazines, xylazine) in horses and cattle; treatment should include adequate padding, anticonvulsants (diazepam), fluids, and steroids

I. Cardiac disease and/or arrhythmias (Table 26-1)
1. Bradycardia
a. Increased parasympathetic tone
b. Hypothermia
c. Hyperkalemia
d. Specific medications (opioids, α_2-agonists)
e. Conduction disease (sick sinus syndrome, atrioventricular block)
f. Drug overdose
2. Tachycardia
a. Increased sympathetic tone
(1) Pain
(2) Excitement, stress
(3) Hypotension
(4) Hypoxia
(5) Hypokalemia
b. Specific drug administration (catecholamines, atropine, ketamine)
3. Atrial or ventricular arrhythmias (atrial tachycardia, ventricular tachycardia); associated with conditions that include ischemia, hypoxia, hypotension, hypercarbia, metabolic acidosis or alkalosis, hypothermia, hypotension, surgical manipulation, anesthetic drugs, and cardiac catheterization
4. Atrial fibrillation
a. Variable-intensity heart sounds
b. Variable-strength pulses
c. Irregular heart rates
5. Ventricular fibrillation
a. Most likely to occur during induction and recovery from anesthesia because of the instability of autonomic reflexes and the endogenous release of catecholamines
b. May be associated with too rapid an infusion of thiobarbiturate or high initial concentrations of inhalation anesthetics

TABLE 26-1

DISTINGUISHING CHARACTERISTICS OF SEVERAL TYPES OF CARDIAC FAILURE OR ARREST

CAUSE	PERIPHERAL PULSE	AUSCULTATION OF HEART SOUNDS	ELECTROCARDIOGRAM	VISUAL OBSERVATIONS
Bradycardia	Slow; may be irregular	Slow	Infrequent or irregular PQRST complexes; junctional or ventricular escape complexes	Infrequent coordinated ventricular contractions
Ventricular tachycardia	Rapid, irregular Pulse deficit	Muffled; may be variable intensity	Wide QRST complexes; absence of PQRS relationship	Disorganized, rapidly beating heart
Ventricular fibrillation	None	None	Absence of QRST complexes; fibrillation waves	Fine-to-coarse rippling of the ventricular myocardium
Ventricular asystole	None	None	Absence of QRST complexes; straight-line EKG	No cardiac movement
Electromechanical dissociation*	None	None	Normal PQRST complexes	Feeble or absent cardiac contractions

EKG, Electrocardiogram.
*Results clinically in pulseless electrical activity.

     c. May follow severe hypercarbia, hypoxia, hypovolemia, or acidosis

  6. Ventricular asystole (lack of ventricular contraction)

     a. Usually associated with anesthetic overdose

     b. Seen during shock or in toxic animals that must be anesthetized

  7. Electromechanical dissociation (electrocardiogram [EKG] present, no myocardial contraction)

     a. Hypoxia and ischemia

     b. Drug overdose

  8. Cardiovascular collapse

     a. Cardiac failure that is unresponsive to therapy

     b. Occurs primarily in patients who have chronic heart disease or are extremely toxic

INDICATIONS OF POOR CARDIAC FUNCTION

    I. Cyanosis (not seen in anemic patients)
    II. Poor perfusion; prolonged refill time (>2 seconds)
  III. Irregular or absent pulse or heart sounds
   IV. Signs of shock (see later section on Shock)
    V. Cardiac arrhythmias
   VI. Abnormal breathing pattern or apnea
  VII. Dilated pupils
 VIII. Depression or loss of consciousness
   IX. No bleeding from cut surfaces

EQUIPMENT NEEDED FOR CARDIAC EMERGENCIES

I. Should be readily accessible in the event of cardiovascular collapse

  A. Cuffed endotracheal tubes

    1. Small

    2. Medium

    3. Large

  B. Lighted laryngoscope with blades

  C. Ambu bag, demand valve, or anesthetic machine (Fig. 26-1 and 26-2)

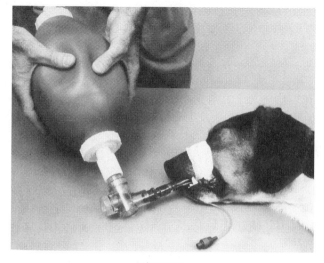

Fig. 26-1
A self-inflating Ambu bag can be used to assist or control breathing in small animals.

    D. Tongue depressors
    E. Syringes
        1. Five 3-ml
        2. Five 5-ml
        3. Five 12-ml
        4. Five 30-ml
    F. Three-way stopcock
    G. One roll 1-inch adhesive tape
    H. One roll 2-inch gauze
    I. One pack sterile 4 × 4-inch gauze pads
    J. One roll elastic bandage
    K. Blood administration set
    L. Needles
        1. Five 20-gauge
        2. Five 18-gauge
        3. Two 16-gauge

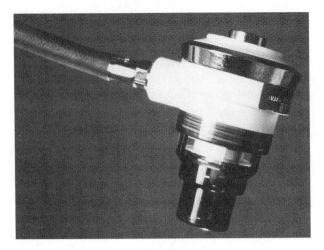

Fig. 26-2
A demand valve connected to an oxygen hose can be attached to an endotracheal tube for assisting or controlling breathing in small or large animals.

M. Butterfly administration needles
1. Two 21-gauge
2. Two 19-gauge
N. IV fluid administration set
O. Sterile emergency surgery pack
1. Scalpel handle
2. Blades: two No. 10, two No. 15
3. Two small hemostats
4. Thumb forceps
5. One pair Metzenbaum scissors
6. One pair curved forceps
7. Several packages suture of preference swaged to needles
8. Needle holders
9. One set medium-sized rib retractors
P. IV catheters: one 16-gauge, one 18-gauge
Q. Chest tube: Heimlich valve
R. Defibrillator/EKG

TREATMENT (TABLES 26-2 TO 26-5 AND FIGS. 26-3 AND 26-4)

- **I.** Airway
- **II.** Breathing
- **III.** Circulation
- **IV.** Drugs
- **V.** EKG
- **VI.** Defibrillation

TABLE 26-2
GUIDELINES FOR VENTILATING PATIENTS

PARAMETER	GUIDELINES
Respiratory rate	6-18/min
Tidal volume	10-20 ml/kg
Inspiratory time	<1.5 sec
Inspiratory/expiratory ratio	1:2 - 1:3
Peak inspiratory pressure	20-25 cm H_2O
Positive-end expiratory pressure	3-5 cm H_2O
Sigh (every 5-10 min)	30 cm H_2O
Assessment of ventilatory adequacy	1. Observe chest wall excursions
	2. Monitor blood gases; preferred method (maintain $Paco_2$ at 40 mm Hg)

TABLE 26-3
TREATMENTS FOR VENTRICULAR FIBRILLATION

Direct-current defibrillators

- 0.5 to 2 Ws/kg internal
- 5 to 10 Ws/kg external
- Small patient (<7 kg)
  5 to 15 Ws internal
  50 to 100 Ws external
- Large patient (>10 kg)
  20 to 80 Ws internal
  100 to 400 Ws external

Alternating-current defibrillators

Small patient
- 30 to 50 V internal
- 50 to 100 V external

Chemical defibrillation

1 mg potassium chloride and 6 mg acetylcholine/kg followed by 1 ml/10 kg of 10% calcium chloride

Unresponsive ventricular fibrillation

- Evaluate ventilation
- Evaluate chest or cardiac compression
- Repeat epinephrine and consider calcium chloride administration (see Table 26-5)
- Administer sodium bicarbonate
- Administer lidocaine
- Repeat electrical defibrillation

Ws, Watt-seconds.

TABLE 26-4

TREATMENT OF CARDIOPULMONARY ARREST

Unwitnessed CPA
↓

Patient evaluation:
1. Ventilations ←
2. Pupillary reflexes
3. Color/refill
4. Heartbeats
5. Arterial pulses
↓

Pulse or heartbeats present? ────────→ No
↓

Yes ←
↓

1. Intubate and ventilate
2. IV fluids
3. Sodium bicarbonate
   (if necessary)
↓

Witnessed CPA
↓

1. External cardiac massage
2. Ventilation (with oxygen)
3. IV fluids

1. Intubate and ventilate
2. External cardiac massage
3. IV fluids
4. Sodium bicarbonate
↓

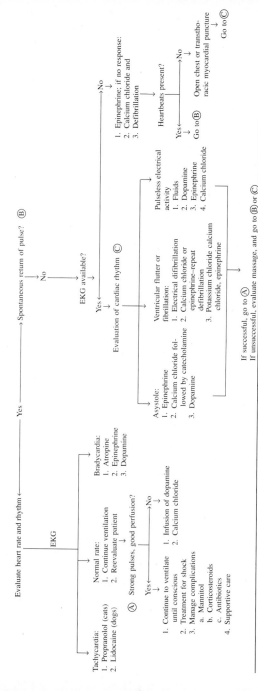

Evaluate heart rate and rhythm

EKG

Tachycardia:
1. Propranolol (cats)
2. Lidocaine (dogs)

Normal rate:
1. Continue ventilation
2. Reevaluate patient

(A) Strong pulses, good perfusion?

Yes →
1. Continue to ventilate until conscious
2. Treatment for shock
3. Manage complications
   a. Mannitol
   b. Corticosteroids
   c. Antibiotics
4. Supportive care

No →
1. Infusion of dopamine
2. Calcium chloride

Bradycardia:
1. Atropine
2. Epinephrine
3. Dopamine

→ Yes → Spontaneous return of pulse? (B)

→ No → EKG available? (C)

Yes → Evaluation of cardiac rhythm (C)

Asystole:
1. Epinephrine
2. Calcium chloride followed by catecholamine
3. Dopamine

Ventricular flutter or fibrillation:
1. Electrical defibrillation
2. Calcium chloride or epinephrine–repeat defibrillation
3. Potassium chloride calcium chloride, epinephrine

Pulseless electrical activity
1. Fluids
2. Dopamine
3. Epinephrine
4. Calcium chloride

If successful, go to (A)
If unsuccessful, evaluate massage, and go to (B) or (C)

No →
1. Epinephrine; if no response:
2. Calcium chloride and
3. Defibrillation

Heartbeats present?

Yes → Go to (B)

No → Open chest or transthoracic myocardial puncture

Go to (C)

CPA, Cardiopulmonary arrest; *IV*, Intravenous.

SHOCK

I. Definition: Shock is an acute disease syndrome characterized by impairment of the cardiovascular system; the key factor in shock is inadequately perfused and oxygenated tissues

II. Etiology (Table 26-6)

    A. Hypovolemic

    B. Cardiogenic

    C. Distributive

    D. Obstructive

III. Pathophysiology

    A. Decreased effective circulating blood volume (Table 26-7)

        1. Endotoxin

            a. Endotoxin-induced extravasation of fluids (third-space loss)

            b. Release of vasoactive substances (histamine, catecholamines, serotonin, bradykinins, prostaglandins, tumor necrosing factor, interleukins, others)

            c. Generalized vasoconstriction (occurs early in septic shock)

            d. Capillary damage with loss of volume

            e. Selective capillary dilatation

            f. Relative hypovolemia

            g. The opening of arteriovenous shunts may result in blood flow bypassing capillary beds regardless of cardiac output

        2. Traumatic, hemorrhagic (see Table 26-7)

            a. Blood loss

                (1) 20% loss: mild signs of shock

                (2) 30% loss: obvious signs of shock

            b. Release of catecholamines

            c. Vasoconstriction

            d. Hypovolemia

        3. Septic, traumatic, hemorrhagic, or cardiogenic shock, if uncorrected, eventually leads to the following

            a. Ischemic anoxia caused by

                (1) Decreased circulatory volume

                (2) Decreased venous return

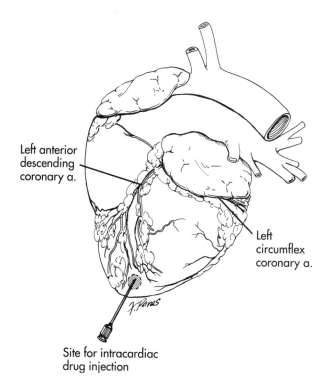

Fig. 26-3
Site for injection of drugs into the left ventricle of the heart.

(4) Reduced cardiac output
(5) Increased total peripheral resistance
(6) Decreased tissue perfusion
(7) Increased catecholamines
(8) Further vasoconstriction

Text continues on p. 430.

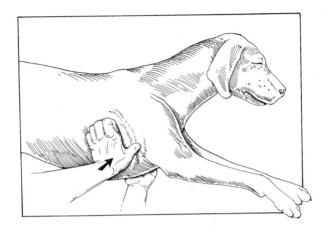

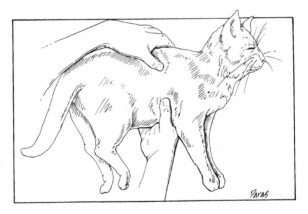

Fig. 26-4
External cardiac massage in the dog and cat.

TABLE 26-5

ESSENTIAL DRUGS USED IN THE MANAGEMENT OF CARDIOPULMONARY ARREST

GENERIC NAME	TRADE NAME	BENEFICIAL EFFECTS (RECOMMENDED USE)	ADVERSE OR SIDE EFFECTS	DOSE AND ROUTE OF ADMINISTRATION
Vasoactive and cardiostimulatory agents				
Epinephrine HCl	Adrenaline	Positive inotrope; initiates heartbeats; increases heart rate and cardiac output; initially increases, then decreases mean arterial blood pressure and coronary blood flow	Intense vasoconstriction of renal and splanchnic vasculature; causes decreased perfusion of these tissues; increases myocardial oxygen consumption and cardiac work	6-10 µg/kg IC 20-30 µg/kg IV 0.1-0.2 ml/20 kg, small animals 1-3 ml/450 kg, large animals
Isoproterenol HCl	Isuprel	Initiates heartbeats; increases heart rate and cardiac output; positive inotrope	Lowers mean arterial pressure, requiring concurrent blood volume expansion; may decrease coronary perfusion; increases myocardial work load and oxygen consumption; arrhythmogenic	1-6 µg/kg IC 2-10 µg/kg IV Use low range for bradyarrhythmias

Continued.

TABLE 26-5—CONT'D.

ESSENTIAL DRUGS USED IN THE MANAGEMENT OF CARDIOPULMONARY ARREST

GENERIC NAME	TRADE NAME	BENEFICIAL EFFECTS (RECOMMENDED USE)	ADVERSE OR SIDE EFFECTS	DOSE AND ROUTE OF ADMINISTRATION
Vasoactive and cardiostimulatory agents—cont'd.				
Dopamine HCl	Inotropin	Positive inotrope; increases heart rate, cardiac output, and mean arterial blood pressure; improves blood flow to coronary, renal, and mesenteric circulation	May produce severe tachycardia if given rapidly; arrhythmogenic; vasoconstriction at higher doses	Give to effect, add 6 mg to 250 ml 5% dextrose; drip slowly at rate of 2-10 μg/kg/min
Dobutamine HCl	Dobutrex	Positive inotrope; has lower chronotropic and vasopressor effect than dopamine	Tachyarrhythmias, vasoconstriction, and arrhythmias at higher dosages	Give to effect, 2-15 μg/kg/min
Epinephrine sulphate	Ephedrine	Vasopressor	Tachycardia, hypertension	5-10 μg/kg
Drugs used specifically to increase contractility				
Calcium chloride		Positive inotrope; used to treat hyperkalemia and electromechanical dissociation	May cause asystole; myocardial calcium overload; "stone" heart	0.05-0.1 ml/kg of the 10% solution IV, IC

Drug	Trade name	Indications/Action	Adverse effects	Dosage
Digoxin	Lanoxin	Positive inotrope; increases vagal tone; used in cases of CPA caused by congestive heart failure	Arrhythmogenic; increases oxygen consumption; causes vasoconstriction when given IV	0.01-0.02 mg/kg IV; given in 4 divided doses; dosed every hour give to effect; monitor EKG
Drugs used to combat acidosis				
Sodium bicarbonate		Buffer acidosis; allows more effective defibrillation	Excessive administration may produce alkalosis, hyperosmolarity, paradoxial cerebrospinal fluid acidosis	1-2 mEq/kg IV, give to effect
Drugs used to treat acute cardiac arrhythmias				
Atropine sulfate		Parasympatholytic effects; may correct supraventricular bradycardia or a slow ventricular rhythm by stimulating supraventricular pacemakers	May cause excessive tachycardia; increases myocardial oxygen consumption; lowers ventricular fibrillatory threshold; may predispose to sympathetic-induced arrhythmias	0.1- 0.2 mg/kg IV
Glycopyrrolate	Robinul-V	Parasympatholytic (anticholinergic); may correct supratricular bradycardia	May cause excessive tachycardia	0.005-0.01 mg/kg IV

Continued.

TABLE 26-5—CONT'D.

ESSENTIAL DRUGS USED IN THE MANAGEMENT OF CARDIOPULMONARY ARREST

GENERIC NAME	TRADE NAME	BENEFICIAL EFFECTS (RECOMMENDED USE)	ADVERSE OR SIDE EFFECTS	DOSE AND ROUTE OF ADMINISTRATION
Drugs used to treat acute cardiac arrhythmias—cont'd.				
Propranolol HCl	Inderal	β-adrenergic blocker; antiarrhythmic; may correct supraventricular and ventricular tachycardia	Decreases contractility, an important adverse effect; may increase airway resistance	1 mg diluted in 1 ml saline; this dilution is given as 0.05-0.1 ml boluses IV give to effect
Esmolol	Brevebloc	$β_1$-adrenergic blocker; treat supraventricular and ventricular tachycardia	Hypertension, bradycardia, heart failure	10-50 μg/kg/min IV
Lidocaine	Xylocaine	Ventricular antiarrhythmic	Dosage must be considerably decreased when used in cats	2-6 mg/kg
Sotalol	Betapase	Ventricular arrhythmias	Hypotension, proarrhythmia	5 mg/kg IV
Acetylcholine KCl cocktail		Chemical defibrillator?	Parasympathomimetic side effects	6 mg/kg ACh + 1 mEq/kg KCl, IC
Drugs used to stimulate ventilation				
Doxapram HCl	Dopram	Direct action on centers in the medulla	Respiratory alkalosis, hyperkalemia	1-4 mg/kg IV 10 μg/kg/min give to effect

Drugs used to combat cerebral edema

Oxygen		Prevents vasodilation	2-4 L/min
Mannitol	20% Osmitrol	Osmotic diuretic; reduces cerebral edema	May cause pulmonary edema with prolonged administration; may suppress ventilatory drive	1-2 g/kg IV
Dexamethasone	Azium	(See section on shock)	May overload the volume of the circulatory system, causing edema	

Drugs used to combat acute pulmonary edema

Furosemide	Lasix	Potent loop diuretic promoting loss of Na^+, Cl^-, and H_2O	May cause dehydration or lead to hypokalemic metabolic alkalosis if used excessively	1-2 mg/kg IV, 2-4 mg/kg IM
Steroids Prednisolone sodium	Solu-Delta-Cortef	Stabilizes lysosomal membranes; induces vasodilation; regulates fluid and electrolyte homeostasis		30 mg/kg IV

Continued.

TABLE 26-5—CONT'D.

ESSENTIAL DRUGS USED IN THE MANAGEMENT OF CARDIOPULMONARY ARREST

GENERIC NAME	TRADE NAME	BENEFICIAL EFFECTS (RECOMMENDED USE)	ADVERSE OR SIDE EFFECTS	DOSE AND ROUTE OF ADMINISTRATION
Drugs used to combat acute pulmonary edema—cont'd.				
Dexamethasone	Azium SP	Increases cardiac output		8 mg/kg IV
Isotonic IV fluids Lactated Ringer's 0.9% saline		Expand the blood volume; hypotension; increase tissue perfusion	May increase edema in cats with congestive heart failure; fluid administration rate generally should not exceed 90 ml/kg/min; administer at high rates initially to improve venous return	20-40 mg/kg/hr until effective
Specific drug antagonists				
Naloxone	Narcan	Narcotic antagonist	None	50 µg/kg
Neostigmine	Protigimine Stiglyn	Cholinesterase inhibitor; used to reverse nondepolarizing neuromuscular blocking agents	Cholinergic effects; a parasympatholytic must be given before drug administration (e.g., atropine, glycopyrrolate)	0.02 mg/kg

Pyridostigmine	Regonol	Cholinesterase inhibitor; used to reverse nondepolarizing neuromuscular blocking agents	Cholinergic effects; a parasympatholytic must be given before drug administration (e.g., atropine, glycopyrrolate)	0.1 mg/kg
Endrophonium	Tensilon	Cholinesterase inhibitor; used to reverse nondepolarizing neuromuscular blocking drugs	Same as neostigmine	0.2-1 m/kg IV
Yohimbine	Yobine	α_2-antagonist; used to reverse α_2-agonists	Excitement, disorientation	0.2-0.4 mg/kg IV
Antipamazole		Same as Yohimbine but more selective for α_2-receptors	Excitement	0.1-0.2 mg/kg IV
Flumazenil	Mazicon	Benzodiazepine antagonist	—	0.1 mg/kg IV

IC, Intracardiac; *IV*, intravenously; *CPA*, cardiopulmonary arrest; *IM*, intramuscularly.

TABLE 26-6
CAUSES OF SHOCK

CATEGORY	CAUSE
Hypovolemic shock	
Exogenous	Blood loss caused by hemorrhage
	Plasma loss caused by thermal or chemical burns and inflammation
	Fluid and electrolyte loss caused by dehydration, vomiting, diarrhea, renal disease, severe exercise, heat stress, or excessive diuresis
Endogenous	Extravasation of fluids, plasma, or blood into a body cavity or tissues (third-space losses) caused by trauma, endotoxins, hypoproteinemia, anaphylaxis, or burns
Cardiac shock	
	Myocardial mechanical problems caused by regurgitant or obstructive defects
	Myopathic defects caused by inheritable traits, chemicals, or toxins
	Cardiac arrhythmias
Distributive shock	
High resistance	Distribution of blood volume and flow to vital organs caused by endotoxins, anesthetic drug overdose, CNS trauma, anaphylaxis
Low resistance	Distribution of blood away from vital organs caused by severe infections, abscesses, or arteriovenous fistulas
Obstructive shock	
	Obstruction to blood flow through the heart (pericardial tamponade, neoplasia, embolism), aorta (embolism, aneurysm), vena cava (gastric bloat, heartworm, neoplasia), lungs (embolism, heartworm, positive-pressure ventilation)

CNS, Central nervous system.

TABLE 26-7

COMPENSATORY AND CORRECTIVE RESPONSES TO A DECREASE IN THE EFFECTIVE CIRCULATING BLOOD VOLUME

Decreased effective circulating blood volume
|
Increased sympathoadrenal response

Compensatory acute changes

Arteriolar constriction
|
Increased vascular resistance
|
Increased blood pressure

Venular constriction
|
Increased venous return

Increased cardiac contractility
|
Increased heart rate

Increased cardiac output

Corrective chronic changes

Increased renin secretion
|
Angiotensin II formation
|
Aldosterone secretion
|
Salt (Na^+) and H_2O resorption

Antidiuretic hormone release
|
Increased H_2O resorption

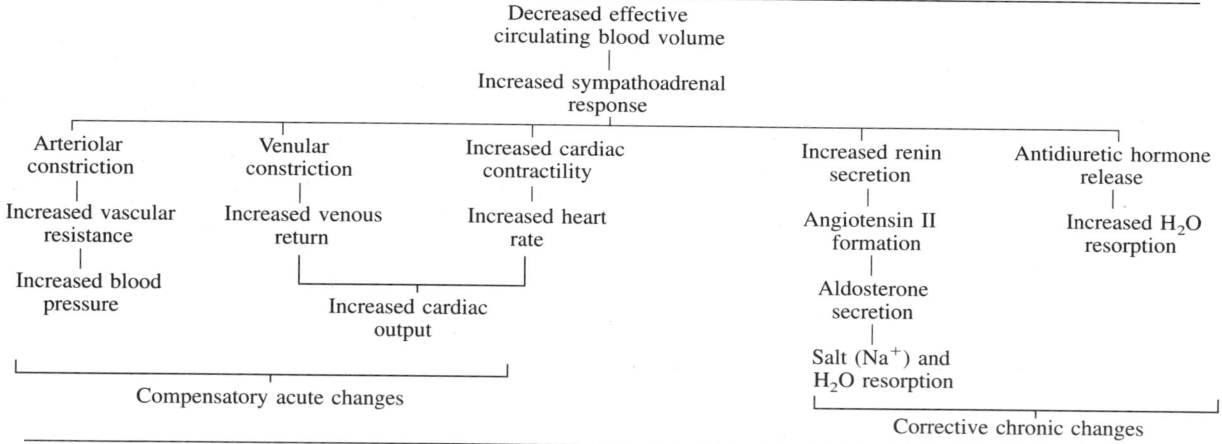

    b. Stagnant anoxia caused by
      (1) Anoxia
      (2) Stagnation
      (3) Acidosis
      (4) Microthrombosis
      (5) Ateriovenous shunting (admixture); bacteria-tissue interaction and/or atelectasis in the lung may contribute to shunting
      (6) Tissue injury
    c. Time; ischemic anoxia to stagnant anoxia may take hours to occur in hemorrhagic shock; it occurs in seconds or minutes in septic shock
    d. The ultimate outcome is cell damage and death
 A. Cellular events
   1. Reduced oxygen and nutrient supply
   2. Anaerobic metabolism
   3. Decreased adenosine triphosphate and energy
   4. Increased membrane permeability
   5. Influx of sodium and water
   6. Efflux of potassium
   7. Cellular edema
   8. Mitochondrial damage (swelling)
   9. Intracellular acidosis
  10. Lysosomal membrane rupture
  11. Extracellular lytic enzymes
  12. Extracellular acidemia
  13. Cell damage and death

CLINICAL AND LABORATORY FEATURES

  I. Shock may be divided into early (reversible) and late (irreversible) stages (Table 26-8)
  II. Laboratory findings: the laboratory data on shock vary greatly and depend, in many instances, on the cause of the shock syndrome and the stage of shock (Fig. 26-5)
   A. Packed cell volume (PCV)
    1. In hemorrhagic shock
      a. Below normal in hypovolemic and progressive phases of oligemic shock; plasma volume increases as interstitial fluid moves into the vascular system

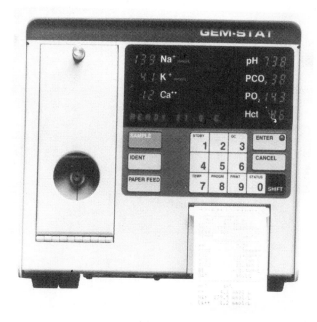

Fig. 26-5
Simple push-button blood chemistry monitors can provide valuable acid-base and electrolyte data.

during the first 30 minutes after hemorrhage (0.25 ml/kg/min); in many species (particularly the horse), the spleen serves as a blood reservoir and buffers the effects of acute blood loss on PCV; because of the ability of splenic contraction to restore blood volume, hemorrhage must be severe before PCV decreases

b. In traumatic burn, endotoxic shock, and colic, PCV increases and hemoconcentration occurs

2. Blood glucose is elevated; epinephrine is released

3. Blood serum protein concentration may be normal or

TABLE 26-8
STAGES OF SHOCK

CHARACTERISTIC	EARLY STAGE	LATE STAGE
Cardiovascular		
Heart rate	Moderately increased	Markedly increased
Heart rhythm	Regular, rapid, normal	Regular or irregular
Pulse pressure	Normal	Reduced (weak, thready pulse)
Capillary refill time	Minimally prolonged	Markedly prolonged (>3 sec)
Mucous membrane color	Pale pink (injected in septic shock)	White (red or blue in septic shock)
CVP	Minimally reduced	Markedly reduced (<1 cm H_2O)
Arterial blood pressure	Normal or decreased (elevated in septic shock)	Decreased (mean pressure <60 mm Hg)
EKG	Normal, tachycardia	Normal, arrhythmic, S-T segment deviation
Respiratory		
Respiratory rate	Increased	Rapid, shallow breathing
Pattern of respiration	Regular	Normal, intermittent dyspnea
Auscultation	Normal, increased tracheal sounds	Increased bronchovesicular sounds, crackles
Tidal volume	Increased	Decreased
Arterial oxygen tension	Normal	Normal or decreased
Arterial carbon dioxide	Decreased	Normal, decreased or increased

Central nervous system

Level of consciousness	Alert, anxious, minimally depressed	Depressed, semiconscious, coma

Laboratory evaluation

Packed cell volume	Normal or increased	Normal or decreased
Total protein	Normal or increased	Decreased
Blood lactate	Normal	Increased
Serum K^+	Normal or decreased	Increased
BUN and creatinine	Normal	Normal or increased
Urine volume and Na^+	Decreased	Markedly decreased
White blood cell count	Increased (left shift)	Decreased (left shift)

CVP, Central venous pressure; *EKG*, electrocardiogram; *BUN*, blood urea nitrogen.

increased early and is generally reduced during later stages of shock

4. Platelet count is usually decreased
5. Blood urea nitrogen and creatinine are elevated, and creatinine clearance is reduced
6. Urinalysis generally shows no specific abnormalities
7. Electrolyte patterns vary considerably, but there is a tendency toward a low serum sodium and low serum chloride
8. Serum potassium may be high, low, or normal
9. Plasma bicarbonate is usually low, and blood lactate is elevated
10. Respiratory alkalosis occurs early in shock and is manifested by a low $Paco_2$ and elevated arterial pH
11. Hypoxia and metabolic acidosis develops as shock progresses with $Paco_2$ values below 70 mm Hg (normal value is 75 to 100 mm Hg)
12. Blood cultures should reveal the causative pathogens, but bacteremia is often intermittent, and the blood cultures are often negative

B. The lung in shock: respiratory failure is the most frequent cause of death in patients with shock, particularly after the hemodynamic alterations have been corrected; this syndrome is characterized by pulmonary congestion, hemorrhage, atelectasis, edema, and the formation of capillary thrombi; pulmonary surfactant decreases, and pulmonary compliance becomes progressively compromised

THERAPY (TABLE 26-9)

I. Support of respiration: in many patients with shock, arterial Po_2 is markedly depressed; oxygen may be administered nasally or by mask; endotracheal intubation and the use of a positive-pressure respirator may be helpful in achieving proper ventilation

II. Volume replacement: with the CVP or pulmonary wedge pressure as a guide, blood volume should be replaced with appropriate fluids; oliguria in the presence of hypotension is not a contraindication in continued vigorous fluid therapy

Text continues on p. 441.

TABLE 26-9
THERAPEUTIC MANAGEMENT OF PROBLEMS ASSOCIATED WITH SHOCK

PROBLEM	TREATMENT	TRADE NAME	DOSAGE	SIDE EFFECTS OR CONTRAINDICATIONS
Hypovolemia—cont'd.				
Fluid loss	Crystalloid	Lactated Ringer's	50-100 ml/kg/hr IV	Hypervolemia, pulmonary edema, hypoproteinemia
Plasma loss	Colloid expander	Gentran 40 (Travenol)	20-40 ml/kg IV	Hypervolemia, pulmonary edema, allergic reactions
Blood loss	Whole blood	—	10-40 ml/kg IV	Hypervolemia, allergic reactions
	Hypertonic saline	7% crystalloid	3-4 mg/kg IV until effective	Adjunct to fluid therapy once hemorrhage has been controlled
Hypotension	Correct hypovolemia first			
	Dopamine	Intropin (Arnar-Stone)	3-10 μg/kg/min IV	
	Dobutamine	Dobutrex (Lilly)	3-10 μg/kg/min IV	
	Phenylephrine	Neo-Synephrine (Winthrop)	10-50 μg/kg IV	

Continued.

TABLE 26-9—CONT'D.
THERAPEUTIC MANAGEMENT OF PROBLEMS ASSOCIATED WITH SHOCK

PROBLEM	TREATMENT	TRADE NAME	DOSAGE	SIDE EFFECTS OR CONTRAINDICATIONS
Hypotension—cont'd				
	Epinephrine	Adrenaline (Parke-Davis)	3-5 µg/kg IV	Hypertension, tachycardia arrhythmias
Cardiac arrhythmias				
Bradycardia	Atropine	—	0.01-0.02 mg/kg IV	Tachycardia
	Glycopyrrolate	Robinul (Robins)	0.005-0.01 mg/kg IV	Tachycardia
Tachycardia	Digoxin	Lanoxin (Burroughs-Wellcome)	0.01-0.02 mg/kg IV slowly	Bradycardia, cardiac arrhythmias
	Propranolol	Inderal (Ayerst)	0.05-0.01 mg/kg IV	Bradycardia, cardiac failure
	Esmolol	Brevibloc	10-50 µg/kg/min	Bradycardia, hypotension
Atrial arrhythmias	Quinidine	Quinidine gluconate (Lilly)	4-8 mg/kg/10 min IV	Hypotension

Ventricular arrhythmias	Lidocaine Procainamide	Xylocaine (Astra) Pronestyl (Squibb)	2-4 mg/kg IV 4-8 mg/kg/5 min IV	CNS excitement Hypotension
Acute heart failure	Dopamine	Intropin (Arnar-Stone)	3-10 µg/kg/min IV	Hypertension, tachycardia, cardiac arrhythmias
	Dobutamine Epinephrine	Dobutrex (Lilly) Adrenaline (Parke-Davis)	3-10 µg/kg/min IV 3-5 µg/kg IV	
Respiratory failure				
Hypoxia	O_2, nasal catheter; oxygen cage		2-4 L/min	Decreased venous return, respiratory alkalosis
Hypercarbia	Doxapram Ventilation	Dopram V (Robins)	1-2 mg/kg $V_T = 14$ ml/kg	CNS excitement Decreased venous return, respiratory alkalosis
Dyspnea	Tracheostomy Chest tubes Ventilation	Heimlich valve	$V_T = 14$ ml/kg	Decreased venous return, respiratory alkalosis

Continued.

TABLE 26-9—CONT'D.

THERAPEUTIC MANAGEMENT OF PROBLEMS ASSOCIATED WITH SHOCK

PROBLEM	TREATMENT	TRADE NAME	DOSAGE	SIDE EFFECTS OR CONTRAINDICATIONS
Sepsis	Surgery			
	Gentamicin	Gentocin (Schering)	4 mg/kg qid IM	Muscle weakness, renal toxicity
	Kanamycin	Kantrim (Bristol)	10 mg/kg qid IM	Muscle weakness, renal toxicity
Metabolic acidosis	Sodium lactate*		Bicarbonate dose = Base deficit × 0.3 × wt (kg) or 0.5 mEq/kg/10 min IV, give to effect	Metabolic alkalosis, hyperosmolarity, CSF acidosis, hyperkalemia, hypocalcemia
	Sodium acetate* Sodium bicarbonate			

Condition	Treatment		Dosage	Complications
Hyperkalemia	Sodium bicarbonate		0.5-1 mg/kg IV	As above
	0.9% NaCl solution		10-40 ml/kg/hr IV	Hypervolemia, hypoproteinemia Tachycardia
	Calcium gluconate		0.5 ml/kg of 10% solution IV V_T = 14 ml/kg	Decreased venous return, respiratory alkalosis
	Hyperventilation			Hyperosmolarity
Hypoglycemia	50% dextrose		1-2 ml/kg IV 0.5-1 g/kg/hr 10% glucose	Hyperosmolarity
Renal ischemia	Fluids	Lactated Ringer's	10-40 ml/kg/hr IV	Hypervolemia, hypoproteinemia, pulmonary edema
	Mannitol (20%)	Osmitrol (Travenol)	0.5-2 mg/kg IV	Hyperosmolality Decreased cardiac output
	Furosemide	Lasix (National)	1-2 mg/kg IM, IV	
Hypothermia	Fluids	Lactated Ringer's	10-40 ml/kg/hr warmed to 37° C	Hypervolemia, hypoproteinemia, pulmonary edema
	H_2O filled heating pad		Warmed slowly to 38° C	

*Questionable efficacy during severe low-flow states.

Continued.

TABLE 26-9—CONT'D.
THERAPEUTIC MANAGEMENT OF PROBLEMS ASSOCIATED WITH SHOCK

PROBLEM	TREATMENT	TRADE NAME	DOSAGE	SIDE EFFECTS OR CONTRAINDICATIONS
Disseminated intravascular coagulation	Correct hypotension	Lactated Ringer's	10-40 mg/kg/hr IV	Hypervolemia, hypoproteinemia, pulmonary edema
	Correct hypoxemia	Nasal catheter Ventilation	2-4 L/min V_T = 14 mg/kg	Decreased venous return, respiratory alkalosis
	Correct acidosis	Sodium bicarbonate	0.5-1 mg/kg IV	
	Heparin		Dog: 500 U/kg tid SC	Bleeding
			Cat: 250-400 U/kg tid SC	
Cellular ischemia	Fluids	Lactated Ringer's	10-40 ml/kg/hr IV	Hypervolemia, hypoproteinemia, pulmonary edema
	Oxygen	Nasal catheter	2-4 L/min	
	Dexamethasone sodium phosphate	Azium SP (Schering)	4-6 mg/kg IV	
	Prednisolone sodium succinate	Solu-Delta-Cortef (Upjohn)	>10 mg/kg	

IV, Intravenously; *CNS,* central nervous system; *IM,* intramuscularly; *CSF,* cerebrospinal fluid; *SQ,* subcutaneously.

III. In addition to fluids, inotropes, antiarrhythmics, antibiotics, and glucocorticosteroids may be indicated; small volumes (3 to 4 ml/kg) of hypertonic saline (7%) in 6% solution have recently been used to help restore and maintain cardiovascular function

    A. Hypertonic (3%, 5%, 7%) saline solutions mixed with 6% dextran 70 solution are being used to treat hemorrhagic traumatic and endotoxic shock with remarkably good response; 3 to 4 ml/kg of 7% produces a beneficial hemodynamic response

IV. Antibiotics: blood cultures and cultures of relevant body fluids or exudates should be taken before the administration of antimicrobial therapy but are often uninformative

V. Surgical intervention: many patients with shock may have an abscess or other local situation for which surgical drainage and excision are required; immediate surgical intervention is of paramount importance; the patient will continue to deteriorate unless the focus is removed or drained

CHAPTER TWENTY-SEVEN

Euthanasia

"Sweet is true love though given in vain, and sweet
is death who puts an end to pain."

ALFRED LORD TENNYSON

OVERVIEW

Euthanasia is a personal and emotional decision often made in the face of incurable disease or uncontrollable pain. Almost all drugs used for chemical restraint and anesthesia have the capability of producing death, provided sufficient drug is administered. Anesthetic drugs offer the advantage of producing total unconsciousness before cardiopulmonary arrest and the elimination of brain electrical activity. This chapter does not presume to identify what technique is the best method of euthanasia but details the various techniques applied to produce euthanasia.

GENERAL CONSIDERATIONS

I. Euthanasia is the act of inducing painless death in animals; death may be defined as permanent abolition of central nervous system (CNS) function
   A. Euthanasia often requires the ability to physically restrain the animal
   B. In many species, capturing and immobilizing the animal for euthanasia may cause a variety of aesthetically unpleasant responses
      1. Vocalization
      2. Avoidance or aggressive behavior
      3. Immobility (the animal may be "frozen with fear")
      4. Urination and defecation

     5. Sweating, salivation

     6. Skeletal muscle tremors, spasms, or shivering

  C. Selection of a method of euthanasia depends on the following factors

     1. Species of animal

     2. Size and weight

     3. Type of physical restraint necessary

     4. Owner preference

     5. Personnel (skill of and risk to)

     6. Number of animals to be euthanatized

     7. Economics

     8. Facilities available

  D. Tranquilizers or other depressant drugs are recommended before administration of euthanatizing drugs in excitable or vicious animals

  E. Pain perception requires a functional cerebral cortex; an unconscious animal does not experience pain; pain-provoking stimuli in an unconscious animal may evoke a reflex motor or sympathetic response

AVAILABLE METHODS

  I. Euthanatizing agents include mechanical, chemical, electrical, and gaseous methods of producing death (Table 27-1)

  II. Euthanatizing agents produce death by three mechanisms

    A. Hypoxia, direct or indirect

    B. Depression of the CNS

    C. Physical damage or concussion of the brain

EVALUATION CRITERIA

  I. Criteria for evaluation of acceptable methods of euthanasia

    A. Production of death without pain

    B. Restraining capabilities of the method used; ability to minimize physical and psychologic stress

    C. Time required to produce loss of consciousness and death

    D. Reliability

    E. Safety to personnel

    F. Emotional effect on observers

    G. Economic considerations

TABLE 27-1
METHODS FOR PRODUCING EUTHANASIA

AGENT	SITE OF ACTION	ADVANTAGES	DISADVANTAGES	GENERAL COMMENTS
Hypoxic agents				
Carbon monoxide (CO)	Carbon monoxide combines with hemoglobin, preventing combination with O_2	Unconsciousness occurs rapidly; inexpensive	Motor activity persists after unconsciousness until death; hazardous to personnel	Acceptable
Muscle relaxants	Paralysis of respiratory muscles by depolarizing or nondepolarizing neuromuscular blockade	Inexpensive	Animal remains conscious until death occurs from hypoxia; no analgesia	Unacceptable
Nitrogen inhalation	Reduced partial pressure of oxygen (Pao_2)	Unconsciousness; inexpensive	Motor activity remains until death	Acceptable
Electrocution (current not through brain)	Spastic paralysis of respiratory muscles and fibrillation of heart	Inexpensive	Slow unconsciousness; pain from muscle spasms; usually followed by exsanguination	Unacceptable

Direct central nervous system depression

Anesthetic gases*	Direct depression of cerebral cortex; death from respiratory and cardiovascular failure	Unconsciousness; analgesia; no motor activity	Potential pollution of environment; expensive; requires closed chamber	Acceptable
Ether				
Chloroform				
Methoxyflurane				
Enflurane				
Halothane				
Barbituric acid derivatives	Direct depression of cerebral cortex; respiratory and cardiovascular failure	Unconsciousness; inexpensive	Transient excitement; requires IV injection of controlled substances	Acceptable
Chloral hydrate and chloral hydrate combinations	Direct depression of cerebral cortex; respiratory and cardiovascular failure	Unconsciousness; inexpensive	Transient anxiety; requires IV injection	Acceptable

Continued.

TABLE 27-1—CONT'D.

METHODS FOR PRODUCING EUTHANASIA

AGENT	SITE OF ACTION	ADVANTAGES	DISADVANTAGES	GENERAL COMMENTS
Physical or mechanical agents				
Electrocution (current through brain)	Direct depression of brain; death from hypoxia	Inexpensive; immediate unconsciousness	Violent muscle contractions	Acceptable
Gunshot or captive bolt	Direct concussion of brain	Inexpensive; immediate unconsciousness	Motor activity may continue after death	Acceptable
Decapitation or cervical dislocation	Elimination of brain blood supply and central nervous system input	Inexpensive; immediate	Aesthetically unpleasant	Acceptable for rodents and some fowl

Modified from J Am Vet Med Assoc Panel on Euthanasia, *J Am Vet Med Assoc* 188:252-268, 1988.

*Although effective, inhalation or gaseous agents are not only expensive, but are hazardous to personnel if adequate precautions are not taken against atmospheric pollution. To avoid pollution, scavenging devices are recommended. Because of the high percentage of concentrations and high gas-flow rates of inhalation anesthetic agents necessary to produce death, their use is not recommended in large animals.

IV, Intravenous.

H. Compatibility with histopathologic evaluation

I. Equipment or drug availability and abuse potential

DRUGS

I. Strychnine, magnesium sulfate, and nicotine are IV drugs that were commonly used for euthanasia in the past; their individual use as the sole euthanatizing agent is absolutely unwarranted; like the neuromuscular blocking drugs (succinylcholine), these drugs have certain properties

A. They do not produce unconsciousness

B. They do not produce analgesia

C. They have no anesthetic effect

D. They lead to specific problems

1. Strychnine produces violent muscle contractions associated with extreme pain

2. Magnesium sulfate causes death from asphyxia

3. Nicotine produces convulsions before death and is extremely hazardous to personnel

II. The most common drug used for euthanasia of dogs, cats, horses, and cattle is pentobarbital sodium, 50 mg/lb IV (100 mg/kg)

Partial Listing of Commonly Used Drugs, Anesthetic and Monitoring Equipment, and Their Manufacturers

ANTICHOLINERGICS

Atropine *(atropine)*
Elkins-Sinn, Inc.
Cherry Hill, N.J.
ROBINUL-V *(glycopyrrolate)*
Fort Dodge Labs, Inc.
Fort Dodge, Iowa

TRANQUILIZERS/SEDATIVES

Dormosedan *(detomidine)*
SmithKline Beecham
Exton, Pa.

Promace *(acepromazine maleate)*
Fort Dodge Labs, Inc.
Fort Dodge, Iowa

Rompun *(xylazine)*
Miles, Inc.
Shawnee Mission, Kan.

Stresnil *(azaperone)*
Pitman-Moore, Inc.
Mundelein, Ill.

OPIOID ANALGESICS

Astromorph *(morphine sulfate)*
Astra Pharmaceuticals, Inc.
Westborough, Mass.

Buprenex *(buprenorphine)*
Reckitt & Coleman Pharmaceuticals, Inc.
Richmond, Va.

Demerol *(meperidine)*
Winthrop Pharmaceuticals
New York, N.Y.

Innovar-Vet *(fentanyl-droperidol)*
Pitman-Moore, Inc.
Mundelein, Ill.

Morphine
Elkins-Sinn, Inc.
Cherry Hill, N.J.

P/M Oxymorphone
Pitman-Moore, Inc.
Mundelein, Ill.

Nubain *(nalbuphine)*
DuPont Pharmaceuticals, Inc.
Manati, Puerto Rico

Sublimaze *(fentanyl)*
McNeil Labs
Fort Washington, Pa.

Sufenta *(sufentanil)*
Janssen Pharmaceutica, Inc.
Piscataway, N.J.

Talwin *(pentazocine)*
Winthrop Labs
New York, N.Y.

Torbugesic *(butorphanol)*
Fort Dodge Labs, Inc.
Fort Dodge, Iowa

LOCAL ANESTHETICS

Carbocaine-V *(mepivacaine)*
   Sterling Drug, Inc.
   McPherson, Kan.

Lidocaine HCL 2%
   Butler
   Dublin, Ohio

INTRAVENOUS ANESTHETICS

Amidate *(etomidate)*
   Abbott Labs
   North Chicago, Ill.

Brevital *(methohexital)*
   Eli Lilly and Co.
   Indianapolis, Ind.

Diprivan *(propofol)*
   Stuart Pharmaceuticals
   Wilmington, Del.

Ketaset *(ketamine)*
   Fort Dodge Labs
   Fort Dodge, Iowa

Pentobarbital *(pentobarbital)*
   Anthony Products
   Arcadia, Calif.

Pentothal *(thiopental)*
   Abbott Labs
   North Chicago, Ill.

Telazol *(tiletamine-zolazepam)*
   Fort Dodge Labs
   Fort Dodge, Iowa

INHALANT ANESTHETICS

Aerrane *(isoflurane)*
   Anaquest, Inc.
   Liberty Corner, N.J.

Halothane *(halothane)*
  Halocarbon Labs
  N. August, S.C.
Metofane *(methoxyflurane)*
Pitman-Moore, Inc.
Mundelein, Ill.

MUSCLE RELAXANTS

Central

Gecolate *(guaifenesin)*
  Summit Hill Labs
  Navesink, N.J.
Valium *(diazepam)*
  Elkins-Sinn
  Cherry Hill, N.J.
Versed *(midazolam)*
  Roche Pharma, Inc.
  Manati, Puerto Rico

Peripheral

Norcuron *(vecuronium)*
  Organon, Inc.
  West Orange, N.J.
Pavulon *(pancuronium)*
  Organon, Inc.
  West Orange, N.J.
Sucostrin *(succinylcholine chloride)*
  E. R. Squibb & Sons
  Princeton, N.J.
Tracrium *(atracurium)*
  Burroughs Wellcome
  Research Triangle Park, N.C.

ANTAGONISTS

α_2

Priscoline *(tolazoline)*
   Ciba Pharmaceuticals Co.
   Summit, N.J.

Yobine *(yohimbine)*
Lloyd Labs
Shenandoah, Iowa

Benzodiazepine

Ro-Mazicon *(flumazenil)*
   Roche Pharmu, Inc.
   Manati, Puerto Rico

Opioid

P/M Naloxone
   Pittman-Moore, Inc.
   Mundelein, Ill.

Peripheral Acting Muscle Relaxants

Prostigmin *(neostigmine)*
   Astra Pharmaceutical Products
   Westborough, Mass.
   Costa Mesa, Calif.

Regonol *(pyridostigmine)*
   Organon, Inc.
   West Orange, N.J.

RESPIRATORY STIMULANTS

Dopram-V *(doxapram)*
   Fort Dodge Labs
   Fort Dodge, Iowa

CARDIAC STIMULANTS

Calcium Chloride
Astra Pharmaceutical Prod.
Westborough, Mass.

Calcium Gluconate
Luitpold Pharmaceuticals
Shirley, N.Y.

Dobutrex *(dobutamine)*
Eli Lilly Industries, Inc.
Indianapolis, Ind.

Epinephrine
Anthony Products
Arcadia, Ca.

Epinephrine
Eli Lilly and Co.
Indianapolis, Ind.

Inotropin *(dopamine)*
DuPont Pharmaceuticals, Inc.
Manati, Puerto Rico

EUTHANASIA SOLUTION

Beuthanasia *(pentobarbital)*
Shering-Plough Animal Health
Kenilworth, N.J.

OTHER PRODUCTS

Azium-SP *(dexamethasone sodium phosphate)*
Shering-Plough Animal Health
Kenilworth, N.J.

Benadryl *(diphenhydramine)*
Parke-Davis
Div. of Warner Lambert Co.
Morris Plaines, N.J.

Dextrose Inj USP
Lyphomed
Div. of Fujisawa Inc.
Dearfield, Ill.

Hypo Tears
IOLAB Corp.
Johnson & Johnson Co.
Claremont, Calif.

Mannitol Inj
Vedco
St. Joseph, Mo.

Sodium Bicarbonate Inj
Vedco
St. Joseph, Mo.

Solu-Delta Cortef *(prednisone sodium succinate)*
The Upjohn Company
Kalamazoo, Mich.

ANESTHETIC AND RELATED EQUIPMENT

Allied Health Care Products, Inc.
St. Louis, Mo.

Bivona, Inc.
Gary, Ind.

Engler Engineering Corp.
Hialeah, Fla.

Henry Schein, Inc.
Pt. Washington, N.Y.

Hudson Oxygen Therapy Sales Co.
Temecula, Calif.

Isotec: Clover Medical
Buffalo, N.Y.

Ispec, Inc.
Georgetown, Ky.

Life Medical Technologies, Inc.
Houston, Tex.

Mallard Medical
Irvine, Calif.

Matrix Medical, Inc.
Orchard Park, N.J.

North American Drager
Telford, Pa.

Ohio Medical Products
　Division of Airco, Inc.
　Madison, Wis.
Spectrum Anesthesia Services
　Louisville, K.Y.
Welch-Allyn
　Skameateles Falls, N.Y.

ANESTHETIC MONITORING AND RELATED EQUIPMENT

Anesthetic Agent Monitor
Biochem Model 8100
　Waukesha, Wis.

Blood Pressure/EKG
Baxter
　Edwards Critical-Care Division
　Santa Ana, Calif.
Cormetrics
　Wallingford, Conn.
Datascope Corp.
　Montvale, N.J.
Gould, Inc.
　Dayton, Ohio
Hewlett Packard
　McMinnville, Ore.

Indirect Blood Pressure Monitors
Critikon, Inc.
　Tampa, Fla.
Doppler Model 811-AL
　Parks Medical Equipment, Inc.
　Aloha, Ore.

Pulse Oximetry

Palco Labs, Inc.
   Santa Cruz, Calif.
SDI, Inc.
   Waukesha, Wis.

Respiratory Monitors

Spencer Instruments
   Irvine, Calif.

Syringe Infusion Pumps

Medfusion, Inc.
   Duluth, Ga.
Travenol Labs, Inc.
   Deerfield, Ill.

Stat Electrolytes

Gem-Stat
   Mallinckodt
   Ann Arbor, Mich.

Blood Gases and pH

PPG Industries, Inc.
   Biomedical Systems Division, Sensors
   La Jolla, Calif.
Radiometer America
   Cleveland, Ohio

Defibrillators

Datascope Corp.
   Montvale, N.J.
Hewlett Packard
   McMinnville, Ore.

Temperature Monitors

Yellow Springs Instruments
   Yellow Springs, Ohio

Water Circulating Heating Pads

Baxter Healthcare Corp.
  Pharmaceal Div.
  Valencia, Calif.

Gaymor
  Orchard Park, N.Y.

Oxygen Cages

Isollette:Air Shields, Inc.
  Hatboro, Pa.

Spectrum Anesth Services, Inc.
  Louisville, Ky.

Physical Principles of Anesthesia

I. Laws

  A. Boyle's law

$$\text{Volume} = \frac{k}{\text{Pressure}}; \quad V \times P = k$$

$$P_1V_1 = P_2V_2$$

  B. Charles' law

$$V = k + T \qquad T = {}^\circ\text{Kelvin (K)}$$

$$\frac{V_1}{V_2} = \frac{T_1}{T_2}$$

  C. Gay-Lussac's law

$$P = k \times T \qquad T = {}^\circ K$$

$$\frac{P_1}{P_2} = \frac{T_1}{T_2}$$

    From above:

$$\frac{P_1V_1}{T_1} = \frac{P_2V_2}{T_2}$$

  D. Gas law

$$\frac{PV}{T} = n\frac{(1 \text{ atm})(22.412)}{273\text{K}}$$

$$PV = nRT \qquad R = 0.08206 \qquad 1 \text{ atm}/{}^\circ K \qquad n = \text{g moles}$$

  E. Henry's law

$$V = \alpha P \qquad \begin{aligned} &V = \text{volume of gas dissolved} \\ &\alpha = \text{solubility coefficient} \\ &P = \text{partial pressure} \end{aligned}$$

The solubility of a gas or vapor in a liquid (α) decreases as the temperature increases

F. Law of partial pressure (Dalton's law): each gas in a mixture exerts the same pressure as it would exert if it alone occupied the same volume at the same temperature; since pressure measurements cannot distinguish different molecules in a mixed sample, the contribution to total pressure made by a given constituent is in proportion to the number of molecules of that constituent

G. Graham's law: the velocity or rate of diffusion is inversely proportional to the square root of the density

II. Terms

A. Vapor pressure
  1. Tendency for a liquid to evaporate
  2. When a liquid and its vapor are in equilibrium, the partial pressure that the vapor exerts

B. Heat of vaporization: the amount of heat required for a liquid to evaporate

C. Volumes of a vapor

$$\frac{\text{Vapor pressure}}{\text{Total pressure}} \times 100 = \text{Vol \%}$$

D. Boiling point of a liquid: that temperature at which its vapor pressure is equal to the prevailing atmospheric pressure; generally stated for 760 mm Hg

E. Critical temperature: when a liquid is confined in a strong container, the temperature at which the contents of the container consists of vapor only

F. Critical pressure: when a liquid is confined in a strong container, the pressure that exists when the container has reached its critical temperature; liquid volumes may be converted to weight by the formula: volume (ml) $\times$ density (g/ml) = grams of liquid

G. Latent heat of vaporization: the amount of heat necessary to evaporate a quantity of liquid to its vapor state without any changes in temperature; expressed in calories/g liquid; this heat is stored in the vapor

III. Specific partition coefficients; the solubility coefficient may be expressed as follows
   A. Bunsen's absorption coefficient: amount of gas (volume) at standard temperature and pressure that dissolves in one volume of liquid when the partial pressure of the gas above the liquid is 1 atm
   B. Ostwald's solubility coefficient: the volume of gas absorbed by a unit volume of liquid when the partial pressure of the gas is 1 atm, the volume of gas being expressed at the temperature of the experiment
   C. The partition coefficient
      1. May be expressed as the ratio of concentration of a substance in the gas phase and in the liquid phase (e.g., milligrams per milliliter)
      2. Partition coefficients are also used to relate the ratios of concentrations in any two phases that are in equilibrium
         a. liquid-liquid (oil-water)
         b. liquid-solid
         c. gas-solid

Drug Schedules

Controlled substances are obtained by prescription and must be used for legitimate medical purposes. Practitioners may not dispense prescriptions from their own offices. The prescriber must have authorization from appropriate legal authorities (usually the attorney general) to prescribe a controlled substance. State and other local regulations must be followed.

CLASSES I AND II

Class I and II drugs must be dispensed by filling out an official order form, which is usually obtained by contacting the Drug Enforcement Agency (DEA). Power of attorney may also be given to one or more people to obtain and use the forms; any theft or loss of these forms must be reported.

If prescriber registration expires, all unused forms must be returned.

All or part of an order may be canceled if both buyer and supplier are informed.

For all controlled substances, the prescription must be dated and signed (as any legal document) on the date of issue. The full name and address of the patient and prescriber name, address, and DEA number must be on the written prescription.

CLASS II

These drugs may be dispensed or administered without a prescription (subject to the above rules).

Oral orders for Class II drugs are permitted in *emergencies,* but only for the amount needed for the emergency period; oral orders must be followed up within 72 hours with a written, signed pre-

SCHEDULED DRUGS	CONTROLLED SUBSTANCES (OR CLASSES)	DESCRIPTIONS	EXAMPLES
Schedule I	C-I	No accepted medical use High potential for abuse	Heroin, dihydromorphine
Schedule II	C-II	Accepted medical uses in United States (may include severe restrictions) High potential for abuse, which may lead to severe psychologic or physical dependence	Morphine, meperidine, oxymorphone, etorphine, pentobarbital
Schedule III	C-III	Accepted medical uses in United States Lesser degree of abuse potential than C-II Abuse may lead to moderate or low physical dependence or high psychologic dependence.	Thiamylal, thiopental, tiletamine-zolazepam
Schedule IV	C-IV	Accepted medical uses in United States Low potential for abuse of C-III Abuse of C-III may lead to limited physical or psychologic dependence	Chloral hydrate, diazepam, pentazocine
Schedule V	C-V	Accepted medical uses in United States Low potential for abuse of C-IV Abuse of C-IV may lead to limited physical or psychologic dependence Some over-the-counter items included in this class (as determined by the Federal Food, Drug and Cosmetic Act may be dispensed without prescription subject to overriding state regulation and provisions on the buyer.	Buprenorphine

All references and laws from Code of Federal Regulations and selected provision and Controlled Substance Act, in *Ohio Drug Laws* Handbook. 1987.

scription, issued to the providing pharmacy for the emergency quantity dispensed. The date of the oral order and "Authorization for emergency dispensing" must be written on the follow-up prescription. Failure to do this will cause action to void all "dispensing without a written prescription" rights.

Oral orders are not permitted in nonemergency situations. Indelible pencil, ink, or typewriter may be used; the prescription should be signed by hand. Prescriptions may be prepared by a secretary or agent, but the prescriber is responsible for all statements.

Class II drugs may not be refilled. A new prescription is required for each filling.

CLASSES III, IV, AND V

Class III, IV, and V drugs may be dispensed by written or oral prescription or may be dispensed or administered from the office without a prescription.

An institutional practitioner may directly administer or dispense (but not prescribe) Class III, IV, or V drugs only if the prescribing physician has done the following:

1. Written and signed the prescription,
2. Given an oral order or had the pharmacist make it into a written order, or
3. Ordered the prescription for immediate administration to the ultimate user.

REFILLS

Class III and Class IV drugs may not be filled or refilled more than 6 months after the original date of issue of the prescription. They may not be refilled more than five times.

Refills must be entered on the back of the original prescription or other appropriate document (medication record).

When retrieving the prescription number, the following information should be available: patient's name, dosage form, date filled or refilled, quantity dispensed, initials of the registered pharmacist for each refill, total number of refills for that prescription to date.

ORAL REFILLS (CLASSES III AND IV)

The total number of refills (quantity) allowed, including the amount of the original, may not exceed five refills or 6 months from the original date.

The quantity of each refill must be less than or equal to the original quantity authorized.

A new and separate prescription must be issued for any more than five refills or after 6 months.

All of the above information may be kept on computer. The physician's name, telephone number, DEA number, and the patient's name and address must also be kept on computer.

Class IV drugs may only be refilled if the prescription is authorized by the prescribing physician.

PARTIALS (CLASSES III, IV, AND V)

Partial prescriptions must be recorded in the same manner as refills.

The total quantity of partials may not exceed the total quantity prescribed.

Class III, IV, and V drugs may not be dispensed more than 6 months past the original date of the prescription.

LABELING

All controlled substances must be labeled with the pharmacy name and address, serial number and date of initial filling, the patient's and physician's names, directions for use, and any cautionary statements.

DISPOSAL

If you are required by the DEA to make reports for all controlled substances, these can be submitted in triplicate on part b of the report form DEA 222 and directed to the Special Agent in Charge of Administististration. If no report is required, list the controlled substances on DEA form 41 and submit three copies to the Special Agent in Charge of Administration.

Guiding Principles for Research Involving Animals and Human Beings

RECOMMENDATIONS FROM THE DECLARATION OF HELSINKI

I. Basic Principles

1. Clinical research must conform to the moral and scientific principles that justify medical research and should be based on laboratory and animal experiments or other scientifically established facts.
2. Clinical research should be conducted only by scientifically qualified persons and under the supervision of a qualified medical man.
3. Clinical research cannot legitimately be carried out unless the importance of the objective is in proportion to the inherent risk to the subject.
4. Every clinical research project should be preceded by careful assessment of inherent risks in comparison to foreseeable benefits to the subject or to others.
5. Special caution should be exercised by the doctor in performing clinical research in which the personality of the subject is liable to be altered by drugs or experimental procedure.

II. Clinical Research Combined with Professional Care

1. In the treatment of the sick person, the doctor must be free to use a new therapeutic measure, if in his judgment it

offers hope of saving life, reestablishing health, or alleviating suffering.

If at all possible, consistent with patient psychology, the doctor should obtain the patient's freely given consent after the patient has been given a full explanation. In case of legal incapacity, consent should also be procured from the legal guardian; in case of physical incapacity the permission of the legal guardian replaces that of the patient.

2. The doctor can combine clinical research with professional care, the objective being the acquisition of new medical knowledge, only to the extent that clinical research is justified by its therapeutic value for the patient.

III. Non-Therapeutic Clinical Research

1. In the purely scientific application of clinical research carried out on a human being, it is the duty of the doctor to remain the protector of the life and health of that person on whom clinical research is being carried out.

2. The nature, the purpose and the risk of clinical research must be explained to the subject by the doctor.

3a. Clinical research on a human being cannot be undertaken without his free consent after he has been informed; if he is legally incompetent, the consent of the legal guardian should be procured.

3b. The subject of clinical research should be in such a mental, physical and legal state as to be able to exercise fully his power of choice.

3c. Consent should, as a rule, be obtained in writing. However, the responsibility for clinical research always remains with the research worker; it never falls on the subject even after consent is obtained.

4a. The investigator must respect the right of each individual to safeguard his personal integrity, especially if the subject is in a dependent relationship to the investigator.

4b. At any time during the course of clinical research the subject or his guardian should be free to withdraw permission for research to be continued.

The investigator or the investigating team should discontinue the research if in his or their judgment, it may, if continued, be harmful to the individual.

GUIDING PRINCIPLES IN THE CARE AND USE OF ANIMALS

Approved by the Council of The American Physiological Society[1]

Animal experiments are to be undertaken only with the purpose of advancing knowledge. Consideration should be given to the appropriateness of experimental procedures, species of animals used, and number of animals required.

Only animals that are lawfully acquired shall be used in the laboratory, and their retention and use shall be in every case in compliance with federal, state and local laws and regulations, and in accordance with the NIH Guide.[2]

Animals used in research and education must receive every consideration for their comfort; they must be properly housed, fed, and their surroundings kept in a sanitary condition.

All experimental procedures must be carried out in accordance with the NIH Guide. Appropriate anesthetics must be used to eliminate sensibility to pain during all surgical procedures. Muscle relaxants or paralytics are not anesthetics and they must not be used alone for surgical restraint, but may be used in conjunction with drugs known to produce adequate analgesia. The postoperative care of animals shall be such as to minimize discomfort and pain, and in any case shall be equivalent to accepted practices in veterinary medicine. All measures to minimize pain and distress that would not compromise experimental results must be employed. If the study requires the death of an animal, the most humane euthanasia method consistent with the study must be used.

The postoperative care of animals shall be such as to minimize discomfort and pain, and in any case shall be equivalent to accepted practices in schools of veterinary medicine.

When animals are used by students for their education or the advancement of science, such work shall be under the direct supervision of an experienced teacher or investigator.

---

[1]Revised 1991.

[2]Guide for the Care and Use of Laboratory Animals, DHEW Publication No. (NIH) 85-23, Revised 1985, Office of Science and Health Reports, DRR/NIH, Bethesda, MD 20892.

Index

B